Trick and T

how 'healthy eating' is making us ill

Trick and Treat

how 'healthy eating' is making us ill

Barry Groves

With a Foreword by
Dr Howel Buckland Jones MB, BS

Hammersmith Press Ltd
London, UK

First published in 2008 by Hammersmith Press Limited
496 Fulham Palace Road, London, SW6 6JD, UK
www.hammersmithpress.co.uk

Printed 2008

British Library Cataloguing in Publication Data: A CIP record of this book is available from the British Library.

ISBN 978-1-905140-22-0

Commissioning editor: Georgina Bentliff
Production by Helen Whitehorn, Pathmedia
Printed and bound by TJ International
Cover design by Veronica Rooke, based on an idea originated by the author

Contents

Acknowledgements

Many people over the years have helped to make this book possible. To name them all would make this already large tome, impractical. But I hereby thank them all.

Three, I think, merit a special mention. They are Dr Joel M. Kauffman, Emeritus Professor of Chemistry and Biochemistry at the University of the Sciences, Philadelphia, PA, who helped enormously by correcting my biochemical mistakes in this book. My thanks, too, to Dr Ignatius F. (Knobbie) Clarke, Emeritus Professor of English at Strathclyde University, and Margaret Clarke for reading it all through to make sure that it was intelligible to a lay readership.

My wife, Monica, also deserves special thanks. She has read the whole manuscript – several times; she also looked after my part of the gardening, while I was slaving over a hot computer.

My thanks also to **Veronica Rooke** who designed the cover, including creating the photograph based on my original idea. Veronica is an artist residing in Australia. She has worked on projects ranging from clothing designs for the tourism industry, newspaper comics, children's picture books, through to socially delicate subjects. She runs the web-based business, '*Fishbitten Designs.*'

Foreword

Don Quixote valiantly and hopelessly charged against imaginary opponents, windmills seen as giants. Barry Groves's text vigorously challenges real powers, entrenched industries, with little prospect of direct success but with every hope that we individuals reading his presentation may reject their intrusion into our lives. His weapons are facts and experience employed with enthusiasm, tackling problems with detail and conviction. His targets are the processed food industry, the pharmaceutical and health industries, and, for good measure, the distortion of medical services and the uncritical acceptance of scientific research.

Wealthy western society has seen two opposing developments: enhanced health and longevity for some, with others precipitated into induced and medicated ill health, many victims of aggressive commerce. Sixty years ago the family shopping basket contained basic commodities and little else; today processed foods and little else. Thousands of items are temptingly on offer displacing traditional diets. Many contain processed cereals and artificial fats; and many list a dozen or more chemical and other artificial ingredients. In consequence thousands of chemicals have been newly added to the nation's diet with incalculable effects.

The official promotion and dominance of refined carbohydrates as principal components in diet have provoked the obesity epidemic, an involuntary physiological compulsion to add excess to excess; and the direct consequences of exposing individuals to thousands of new chemicals involved in processing, previously unknown toxicities, allergies and anaphylactic reactions.

One wonders why many trends in modern society are contrary to good sense and reason: attitudes to medication for example. The pharmaceutical industry has achieved near miraculous success in giving effective treatment for formerly intractable disorders. Not content with this practical benefit, vast quantities of medication are taken for every real and supposed complaint, a commercial bonanza the industry is more than willing to embrace. But good health requires no medication, and ill health the necessary minimum.

Together with the food and pharmaceutical industries, the health industry has grown exponentially, proffering therapies and dietary advice fuelled by fashion and suggestibility, genuine and real benefits becoming diluted by unrealistic expectations.

These three industries which impact strongly on our health are influenced by governmental policy and pressure. It has become the norm for our professional politicians and intrusive government to pronounce and legislate on any and every aspect of our lives far beyond the natural remit of governance. Autocratic government is wilful beyond experience in misuse of power in areas beyond their competence. Transient directives and secondary targets obscure primary objectives. And prescriptions for mass benefit, e.g. statins for males over 50, attempt the impossible.

Research also has a disproportionate influence on policy and attitudes. The blind prestige given to notions of science is in denial of its need for reality and objectivity. Single research studies of complex problems without proper accreditation have minimal significance. Studies require verification, comparison and coordination with related evidence, and in changing circumstances review of their continuing validity. A single study is a piece of a jigsaw puzzle, with others contributing to a fuller picture. Misuse and misinterpretation of science are socially irresponsible.

Part One of this book examines the repercussions of particular developments on community health and welfare. Part Two considers how specific medical disorders may be affected by these changes, not to rewrite medical textbooks but with the prospect that an independent viewpoint may give new insights, most significant perhaps in diabetes, and least in multiple sclerosis. Debate is stimulated disturbing the conventional. Established practices, customs and opinions tend to constancy whereas in changing times resilience is required.

This most detailed text is a valuable contribution to our regaining personal choice and responsibility.

Dr Howel Buckland Jones, MB BS (London), 2008

Introduction

There is no nonsense so arrant that it cannot be made the creed of the vast majority by adequate governmental action.

Bertrand Russell

Early in 2005 a front-page article in *The Daily Telegraph*, headlined 'Vital NHS reforms "in deep trouble"', announced that: 'By 2007-08 the NHS budget in England will have risen to £90.2 billion from £55.8 billion in 2002-03.'[1] The figures were staggering and I wondered: why were we spending so much and apparently getting such a poor service? And where was all the money going?

It wasn't long before two other facts became abundantly clear. Firstly, it came as a surprise to me that there are very few healthy people in our society today; most of us have some minor illness which may or may not eventually lead to serious problems. And secondly, we are being exploited by the biggest and fastest growing industry in the history of mankind.

Compare today's enormous cost with the experience of dentist and explorer, Dr Weston A. Price. He spent 10 years travelling the world in the 1920s and '30s, looking at the diet, and health of indigenous populations who ate their traditional foods, and comparing these with the health of those members of the same populations who had changed to eating our 'civilized' way. When Price visited the Loetschental Valley in Switzerland in 1931, for example, he found those still eating their traditional diet had 'neither physician nor dentist because they have so little need for them.'[2]

The lack of illness that Dr Price found was not confined to one valley in Switzerland; it was universal. From the islands of the South Pacific, through Australia, Asia, Africa, South and North America to Europe, what he found – everywhere – was that those who ate their traditional diets had practically no disease at all, whereas the diseases we are prone to were rife among people of the same cultures who had been influenced by missionaries and traders into adopting our dietary customs. These findings have been confirmed by many other anthropologists, explorers and doctors reporting around the globe from icy waste to tropical jungle. The same is true of animals in the wild: they are almost never sick unless they injure themselves or eat contaminated food. The only chronically sick animals are our 'civilized' pets and food animals: those that have their food controlled by us. That is highly significant. Have you noticed that if you see a fat dog it will invariably have a fat owner?

Set the £90.2 billion figure also against expectation when Sir William Beveridge's team set up the National Health Service (NHS) in the UK in 1948. Although those visionaries realized that any form of universal welfare scheme would be prohibitively expensive initially, they believed the NHS was affordable because, they said: 'there exists in any population a strictly limited amount of illness which, if treated under conditions of equity, will eventually decline.' It was fully expected that if everyone had unfettered access to the best available medical services, disease would be conquered, people would become healthier, and costs would fall as rates of illness declined.

It was a delusion. The NHS is now the largest organization in Europe because no one foresaw so many people becoming sicker at such an alarming rate: the current average expenditure due to illness in the UK runs into thousands of pounds for every man, woman and child through the NHS, hospitals, nursing homes, charities, prisons and other organizations. Ill health is hugely expensive, not just for the taxpayers who fund the NHS, but also for businesses and the people who suffer illness.

Today, we live in a society that has deciphered the human genome; we have learnt many of the mysteries of the complex organisms that are our bodies; we have developed a huge range of drugs and treatments to cure and ameliorate diseases. But despite living in an age when we have a greater breadth and depth of knowledge than ever before in our history, we are also sicker than ever before.

The trouble is that the NHS has lost its way. It is now really a National Illness Service whose members only treat symptoms; they don't promote health by preventing illness.

The situation is even worse in the USA. Total spending on healthcare in the United States grew by 7.9% in 2004 and accounted for 16% of the gross domestic product, according to the National Health Statistics Group of the US Centers for Medicare and Medicaid Services.[3] This amounted to $6,280 (£3,520) per person, or a total for the nearly 300 million population of around $1.9 trillion, says the group's report.[4] 'Medical spending continues to rise faster than wages and faster than economic growth, and workers are paying much more in healthcare premiums than just a few years ago.' With one doctor for every 500 people, the United States is the world's most medicalized country. If you thought that would confer health benefits, you would be wrong. With the highest infant mortality and lowest after-60 life expectancy among industrialized nations, American health is declining.

This is apparent right across the age range. In 2004, Johns Hopkins Bloomberg School of Public Health noted that the health of US children was worse in practically every category relative to children in other industrialized countries. And most elderly Americans have one foot in the grave. The Centers for Disease Control reported that chronic diseases account for seven out of every 10 deaths in the US. At least 80% of seniors have one chronic disease and half have two or more. But statistics are really unnecessary to show Americans are sick, sick, sick. Simply look around and at TV and note the incredible expanding waistlines that have confined most Americans to their sofas.

That yard-stick used to be almost exclusively American. But due to other industrialized countries' governments and the medical establishments' highly successful, but misguided, advertising campaigns exhorting their peoples to eat the same 'healthy diet' that was pioneered in the US, it now affects these other nations in a similar way.

As will become apparent in this book, although ostensibly aimed at reducing conditions such as heart disease, diabetes and cancer, government-sponsored 'health' campaigns are directly responsible for creating and worsening these diseases.

We are making ourselves sick

Few people have 'old age' as a cause of death on their death certificate. Today, we die of cancer, heart attacks, strokes, osteoporosis, diabetes, and so on. And we accept these conditions as normal causes of death. They aren't – and neither are the ill-health, pain and discomfort that make our later years a misery.

It is inevitable that some people will need the ministrations of a physician at some time in their lives: accidents happen. But the high levels of chronic degenerative diseases we see today – obesity, diabetes, heart disease, cancer, senile dementia, and so on, need not – indeed, should not – happen.

These conditions, which were previously rare or even unheard of, really 'took off' in the last century. At the beginning of the 20th century, for example, one person in 27 got cancer and very few doctors had even heard of heart disease, let alone seen a case. Today, the number of people with cancer has increased to nearly one in two and heart disease runs it a close second.

But the 20th century saw not only rapid increases in previously rare diseases, it witnessed the emergence of many new ones. This was despite spending a vast amount of time, money and resources on increasing medical knowledge, diagnostic machines, drugs and treatment protocols. It seems that the more we have learned, the sicker we have become. There is no doubt that something has gone seriously wrong – and we seem to be incapable of learning from our mistakes.

In the case of health, the biggest obstacles to our learning are confusion, doubt, cynicism and preconceived – but unsupported – notions about what is healthy and what is not.

On the other side of the coin are the peoples on this planet who know nothing of our scientific breakthroughs; those who have no lists of nutritional information on the food they eat because the food they eat is entirely natural; those who have never heard of calories but don't get fat; those whose diet is not what our convention would call 'healthy' but don't get heart disease and cancer; those who even seem remarkably resistant to infectious diseases. We call these people 'primitive'; for the last few centuries, we have sent them missionaries and doctors to bring them the 'benefits' of our civilization and to teach them our ways. And we have made them as sick as we are. When Dr Albert Schweitzer set up his mission in Gabon, he could find no cancer amongst the people there – but it was there when he left.

Ill-health is not normal

When I was writing this book, an acquaintance reading it was appalled at what I had written. She told me: 'Who says we are all chronically sick? I certainly am not.' The sad fact is that we accept catching colds and flu as normal; we accept having to put up with aches, pains and discomforts from acne, indigestion, constipation and arthritis, as 'normal' parts of our lives. Women expect to suffer PMT every month, pain when they give birth and distressing menopausal symptoms later in life. They believe these are 'normal' events they have no choice but to live with. We also accept having to wear glasses and hearing aids, have teeth with fillings, false teeth and those ugly braces children and young adults wear today as 'normal'. We even accept as normal such medical procedures as coronary bypasses, hysterectomies, Cæsarean sections, and plastic hip joints.

But none of these things is either normal or natural. While trillions of pounds, dollars, euros and other currencies are wasted as scientists seek ways to treat and cure them, the vast majority need never have happened in the first place.

Although these conditions are caused by a variety of agents in our 'civilized' environment, most can be prevented merely by a change of diet. And many, if you already have them, can be treated so successfully that you will no longer have any symptoms, by the same change of diet and, crucially, without the need for drugs. They range from acne to Alzheimer's, crooked teeth to cancer.

If that claim sounds impossible or unlikely, you only have to consult the medical literature. There you will find ample evidence documented that all of these, and more, can be helped merely by reducing the carbohydrate content of your diet and replacing it with fat.

What has gone wrong?

I believe three major things went wrong in the last century; the evidence supporting that belief is in this book.

The first mistake

The first mistake was made with the best of intentions but then got quite out of hand. About 50 years ago, several international forums agreed that the only way to feed the rapidly increasing world population was to produce and distribute grains and cereals as primary food sources for humans, rather than feed these to animals and then distribute meat and meat products. This approach to avoid food shortages was cheaper and more practical. At about the same time, scientists hypothesized a link between cholesterol and heart disease, pronouncing 'saturated' animal fats to be undesirable foods. These two ideas found common ground and came together in the last quarter of the 20th century to give us:

- The concept of 'healthy eating', which told us to eat less fat, particularly from animals.
- The promotion of polyunsaturated vegetable fats as 'healthy', despite a considerable body of evidence showing that they are biochemically unstable and harmful.
- The replacement of dietary fats with carbohydrates – starches and sugars found in bread, pasta, rice, potatoes, pulses, other vegetables and fruit – as a preferred energy source.
- The rapid growth of a multi-billion dollar industry which provided low-fat, high-carbohydrate 'healthy' convenience foods.
- The even more rapid expansion of a multi-billion dollar dieting industry to combat the rapidly rising tide of obesity that followed as a consequence of the new dogma.
- Pharmaceutical products to control blood cholesterol, appetite, hunger and blood pressure to counter the dramatic declines in health, also as a consequence of the new dietary regimes.
- Two generations of scientists, nutritionists, dieticians and doctors indoctrinated in the 'low-fat' dogma and a consequent decline in the knowledge base.

- The universal acceptance of these developments by governments and health agencies worldwide. ('Healthy eating' doctrine is promoted with huge financial backing.)

This all sparked off an unprecedented obsession about 'health' among western populations. It began in a small way in the 1970s but in the early 1980s there began what has become a crusade of almost religious fervour. Over the subsequent decades the rates at which illnesses occurred rose dramatically. Was this merely coincidence? No, it's a classic example of cause and effect.

All this happened in defiance of scientific knowledge. For example, why should animal fats which we have been eating for the whole of our evolutionary history without any evidence of harm whatsoever suddenly become harmful in the last few decades? There is no evidence that the recent changes have made us healthier – quite the reverse. We are far less healthy now than we were just a few decades ago. This is borne out by the evidence from studies and trials published in the world's medical and scientific journals.

The final standard by which any hypothesis should be judged is how well it accounts for existing findings, and how well it translates into predictions that can be unambiguously tested. It should also be tested against real-life situations. For example, imagine that you are standing on a flat plain at a place where your map says there is a hill. It is your map that is wrong, not the land. The same applies to health: if clinical trials say that lowering cholesterol with drugs will prolong life, but people who *do* lower their cholesterol in this way die younger, it is the trials that are wrong, not the populations who follow their guidelines.

Many eminent scientists have spoken out against this unsupported dogma, to little avail. The crucial point is that no scientist concerned with next year's research grant is allowed to challenge 'healthy' dogma. Neither dare he assert that the recommendations of 'healthy eating' totally ignore our evolutionary background. With discussion and debate stifled, we have developed modern eating habits that couldn't have been better designed to lead to the ill-health we see today if it had been deliberately planned that way.

This dogma is also taught in schools from an early age so that, today, the young have no concept of what real food is or, in many cases, even where it comes from. For example, for many youngsters, milk doesn't come from cows, it comes from supermarkets in cartons; and if eating meat means killing pretty little lambs, then they will be vegetarians. I even find that older people, brought up with a very different dietary regime, have difficulty understanding why their health was better when they ate bread and dripping and fried breakfasts.

This all created an avenue for the second mistake: increasing government tinkering in the name of social justice.

The second mistake

The illusion of protecting the sick, poor and aging originally offered social engineers, parliamentary factions and regulatory agencies a convenient moral pretext for intrusion into, as well as a predatory grip on, the medical industry. Increasingly fierce government intervention followed, founded on the erroneous assumption that more government regulation and control could cure the ills that had been caused by government regulation and control. Third-party financing of medical services brought a radical shift of empowerment from patient and physician to administrative regulators. Universal coverage and unrestricted access also led to a dilution of responsibilities, waste, high administrative costs, a lower quality of care, and ultimately to the general dissatisfaction of all parties involved.

The third mistake

It also allowed the third, and most serious, mistake to happen as we became increasingly medicalized and reliant on health professionals, to the point where we can be – and are – heavily exploited.

In the US, children play a Hallowe'en game called 'trick or treat'. Although it is thought of as a harmless game, it is really extortion with menaces. Our health industry employs a similar strategy, but with a subtle difference: with them it is trick *and* treat – exploiting and fostering unhealthy 'healthy' practices, they first trick us into an unhealthy lifestyle and then they treat the conditions those practices cause. This is not a new phenomenon: a distinguished physician told the Ontario Medical Association:

> 'Far too large a section of the treatment of disease is today controlled by the big manufacturing pharmacists, who have enslaved us in a plausible pseudo-science . . . The blind faith which some men have in medicines illustrates too often the greatest of all human capacities – the capacity for self deception . . .'

Sir William Osler uttered those words in 1909. Nothing has changed for the better since then. Indeed, things have got considerably worse. And that is where this book will set the scene. Our exploitation by the 'health industry' has gone on for far too long. A large proportion of the trillions spent today on health go straight into anonymous pockets to fund lavish lifestyles. Too little is spent on improving health; practically nothing is spent on prevention of disease. Let's face it, how could they make money out of us if we were well?

It must be obvious that the state of the medical establishment is dire. It is also demonstrable that the health and lives of millions of people are being sacrificed in the name of greed. Most of what is spent in western medicine produces only suffering and death. As the late Dr Robert Mendelsohn put it brilliantly in his book, *Confessions of a Medical Heretic*, 'The God of Western Medicine is death. If you want to meet your maker, and soon, then submit to their ministrations.'

The good news is that you don't have to be exploited. If you put your mind to it, not only can you be totally healthy, you can personally help to cut the huge cost of ill-health in this country to a fraction of its current levels. If you are not ill, they can't sell you their expensive drugs. And once that happens, your taxes can be reduced.

It will be easy for you to be sceptical since much of what is contained in this book is not orthodox. I am also fully aware that my message is not 'politically correct'. But I suggest that you defer your conclusions until you have compared this book's findings with the physical and mental status of your own family, your brothers and sisters, their associated families, and of the mass of people you meet in business and on the street. When you look around you, it is important to make the comparison with standards of physical excellence you will find in pictures of 'primitive' groups in the anthropology section of your local library. Look at them, and then at your neighbours.

And since we are the ones who are ill, might it not be a good idea to abandon certain preconceived notions and readjust them to bring them into harmony with Nature's laws? It is Nature, not dogma, which must be obeyed. Many 'primitive' races understand this better than we do. They are not protected by racial immunities; they suffer the same diseases we do when they adopt our ideas of nutrition and health. The supporting evidence for this statement is vast. I have tried to keep it as simple as possible.

While I accept that there is more wrong in modern society than just incorrect diet, this book concentrates on diet as that is something you, yourself, can control.

If you are sick of getting sick, you must understand that disease prevention is entirely down to you. All that is required of you is that you resist the pressures that government and the media, influenced by industry, have spoon-fed you over the years, and look at the facts.

Question government guidelines

In a BBC Radio 4 interview in August 2006, UK health minister, Patricia

Hewitt, said that people should take responsibility for their own health: 'The government's responsibility is making it easier for people to make healthy choices.' I couldn't agree more. But before people can make choices, they must be aware that there *is* a choice. It is essential that the guidelines they are given to help them make those choices are based on a coherent body of reliable evidence, not unsupported dogma. This is not happening.

In his 1909 lecture, Sir William Osler also said: 'We need a stern, iconoclastic spirit which leads . . . to an active scepticism – not the passive scepticism, born of despair, but the active scepticism born of a knowledge.' So be sceptical and question the 'experts'. When they tell you that you must eat such and such, ask for the evidence in support of their advice. If they can't give it, don't swallow it.

If you are one of the millions of people who are overweight, diabetic, have coronary heart disease, cancer, or any one of the many other conditions in this book, you must understand that, to solve these problems, you are going to have to change your lifestyle – for good. There's no going back – if you do the same things you have always done, you will get the same results you have always gotten. It may take a bit of planning, maturity and commitment, but that is all. Do it for yourself and those who love you.

To that end, this book could start you on the road to real health – the way Nature intended; it could call a halt to the corruption in the health professions you will read about, reduce the NHS drugs bill and allow you to keep more of your hard-earned money; it might even, eventually, also allow the NHS to go into retirement, except for accident and emergency cover, as its founders envisaged. But most of all, it could mean that you, your children and their children live long and healthy lives.

The alternative – carrying on as we are – is not a viable option; it can only result in bankruptcy – either of the NHS itself, or of you and me who foot the bill through our taxes. And, of course, your continuing, worsening health.

Part One of this book sets out the extent of the corruption in the 'health industry'; it shows how current 'healthy' dietary guidelines are based more on myth and wishful thinking than any coherent body of scientific evidence. And it gives the evidence for what we should really eat for health.

Part Two lists over 70 common, chronic, degenerative diseases. They range from the serious, such as cancer, heart disease, diabetes and senile dementia, to the less serious but no less distressing like acne and short-sightedness in children. This second part gives evidence that these diseases owe their recent rise in numbers to the diet we are all told to eat.

I am not a medical practitioner and the contents of this book are not based on my ideas. For the most part I simply report the results of research that recognized authorities – scientists, doctors and nutritionists – have carried out. Their findings and their conclusions are a matter of record in the major medical journals. What I have done is to collate them in a way which, I hope, you will find both interesting and informative. Three things I can promise: a rare opportunity to hear the other side of the health argument, a rare opportunity to learn the truth and an opportunity to be healthy again.

Pindar said: 'Not every truth is the better for showing its face undisguised; and often silence is the wisest thing for a man to heed.' I may well be castigated for writing this book, but I cannot be silent.

Part One

The Misappropration of Health

Chapter One

Trick to treat

Medical care is one of the world's largest industries. This chapter sets the scene by detailing widespread corruption, fraud and mismanagement, largely for the benefit of the pharmaceutical industry. Heavily influenced by the drug companies, doctors' training is seriously biased towards prescribing; medical research and publications are rarely independent. There is more interest in wealth than health.

> Western Medicine was founded on deception and, as its behaviour suggests, is motivated by an unquenchable thirst for wealth, not health.
>
> *Shane Ellison*

Every year the amount of money the Chancellor gives to the UK's National Health Service goes up and so do our taxes to provide for it. And every year we hear more and more complaints about falling levels of service, lengthening waiting times for treatment, and worsening levels of hospital-borne diseases. With the billions of pounds we pump into the NHS every year, have you ever wondered why we don't get a better service? The reason seems to be because we *do* pump billions of pounds into the NHS every year.

The *Global Corruption Report 2006*,[1] sponsored by the German government, shows that medical care is one of the most corrupt industries in the world – precisely because of the huge amount of money involved. Bribery of regulators and medical professionals, manipulation of research findings, medicines and supplies going adrift, corruption at the procurement stage, and the over-billing of insurance companies are all daily practices in medicine. The report estimates that the world spends more than three trillion dollars a year on health services. And although much of this goes into the pockets of the corrupt, they are rarely found out. It's almost impossible to put a figure on corrupt practices. Medicine is so inept that a great deal of money is also lost through inefficiencies and honest mistakes, says the report.

One example of this corruption was revealed at a court case in Memphis, Tennessee, where the jury heard that surgeons had received 'donations' of hundreds of thousands of dollars as a small 'thank you' for carrying out some study or other. The *Journal of the American Medical Association* estimated that drug companies spend $13,000 (£7,360) per year on every doctor in order to encourage them to prescribe one drug or another. With a spend of $19 billion a year on marketing to doctors, this is considerably more than they spend on research. But the drugs sold by marketing them in this way make the companies a great deal more so, for them, it is worth it.

The health industry feeds off illness

The ultimate purpose of any business is to generate profits. Medicine is a business just like any other: it derives its income and profits from the sale of treatments for disease, which in most cases means the sale of drugs. If an industry profits from something, then it has a vested interest in that something continuing. So research into the *prevention* of disease is discouraged and ignored in medicine; the focus is on treatment only.

And if the treatment causes damaging side effects, they will give you another treatment for those side effects. And if the disease doesn't go away (and it probably won't as the cause is rarely addressed), then they will gladly refill your prescription. And if nothing seems to be working, don't worry, they are about to announce that they are coming out with a new, better drug next month. (It will probably be only a slight variation on the formula for an existing one, but this will mean they can get a new patent.) Their PR department will spin a story of a revolutionary breakthrough for the newspapers, who will trumpet the good news on the front page. As a consequence, the public will be convinced that this new drug will bring them health, wealth and happiness, and they will all demand it. Arguments about 'postcode lotteries', where some patients are prescribed it whilst others in more prudent areas are not, will mean that very quickly, the National Institute for Health and Clinical Excellence (NICE), will approve it and soon everyone will have to be offered it. The NHS will then need yet more money to fund the treatment, most of which will go to the drug company.

Couldn't happen, you think? Oh, but it does – all the time.

All ill health has the potential not just to make money, but to make it by the barrow load. Almost daily, it seems, we hear of medical breakthroughs that herald an end to one disease or another. It's been the same for decades, and it's a fraud and a delusion. In spite of the 'triumphs' of medical science, medicine is far from decreasing human suffering as much as its practitioners would like us to believe. Paradoxically, in health, epochal discovery has rarely been brought about by medical men. Most of the truly significant discoveries have been made by men who, by standards applicable to their time, could only be considered scientific heretics – men so dedicated and so passionately altruistic that they dared to dream impossible dreams of victory over disease and made those impossible dreams become reality. But the penalty for dreaming such dreams has been severe – derision from their professional contemporaries and the label of fraud, or worse. Medical literature is full of such men.

In the 19th century, Dr Ignaz Semmelweis in Vienna held that germs on doctors' hands caused death in childbirth. He proved it by getting doctors to wash their hands before delivering babies – and the death rate among newborn babies and their mothers plummeted. Doctors refused to see the obvious; Semmelweis went down in utter defeat driven out of his mind into an asylum, and an early death from the very staphylococcus infection that had been killing mothers.

Other heretics included Armand Trousseau, who found that there was an anti-rickets factor in fish liver oil, and Christiaan Eijkman who discovered that eating unpolished rice prevented the dread killer disease, beriberi. And there were, and are, many others. These men were scientists. Scientists aren't like normal men. They ask questions that others are too lazy to research.

The eradication of cholera and typhoid in the 19th century wasn't brought about by medical men, but by improvements in sanitation, clean piped drinking water and better housing. Child deaths from diphtheria, measles, scarlet fever and whooping cough fell dramatically in the early 20th century long before the introduction of antibiotics and widespread immunization. Although other factors helped, most important was the higher resistance of children to disease that followed from better nutrition.

Disease mongering

> 'A LOT OF MONEY CAN BE MADE FROM HEALTHY PEOPLE WHO BE-
> LIEVE THEY ARE SICK. PHARMACEUTICAL COMPANIES SPONSOR
> DISEASES AND PROMOTE THEM TO PRESCRIBERS [DOCTORS] AND CON-
> SUMERS.'

These are not my words; they are from the introduction to an article in the doctors' own *British Medical Journal*.[2] The article goes on to say 'Some forms of "medicalization" may now be better described as "disease mongering" – extending the boundaries of treatable illness to expand markets for new products.'

The article explains how the pharmaceutical industry has four strategies:

1. Find a benign symptom and persuade doctors that it is a discrete disease with a name.
2. Make people anxious about it so that they seek medical treatment.
3. Make out that the 'disease' is widespread so that doctors will see it in every patient.
4. Get at the health professionals who draw up the medication guidelines; shower them with gifts, foreign holidays and consultancy contracts.

And it describes pseudo-treatments for baldness, osteoporosis, erectile dysfunction, and personal or social problems. One example involved the pharmaceutical giant, Roche, who, in a massive publicity campaign, announced that they had a cure for a hitherto undiagnosed psychiatric disorder suffered by one million Australians: Roche called it 'social phobia'. But 'patients' need not worry; Roche had a cure: their antidepressant, *Aurorix*. For what grave medical condition were one million Australians to take *Aurorix* every day? Shyness!

Other examples of 'disease mongering' include:

• Implying that there's something wrong with a normal function which needs treatment, such as a cholesterol level over 5.2 mmol/L (200 mg/dL). The idea that everyone's cholesterol level must be exactly the same regardless of age, sex or circumstance is quite ridiculous.
• Selective use of statistics to exaggerate the benefits of treatment.
• Using a 'surrogate' end point. This is a very common ploy where a believed 'risk marker' is used instead of the real event. For example, high cholesterol is used as a marker instead of what really matters: a heart attack. The two are very different – and not necessarily related.

The use of misinformation to lead people to believe they have a disease that needs to be treated isn't new: doctors in Harley Street, London, used similar methods long before modern pharmaceutical companies got in on the act. The difference now is that where general practitioners were once a bulwark of scepticism against any trading on a gullible public, for the last 30 years they have been used as a cost-effective marketing tool.[3]

Fraudulent drugs advertising

'Our nation is in the throes of an epidemic of controlled prescription drug abuse and addiction . . . While America has been congratulating itself in recent years on curbing increases in alcohol and illicit drug abuse, and in the decline in teen smoking, abuse of prescription drugs has been stealthily, but sharply, rising,' said Joseph A. Califano, Jr., chairman and president of the National Center on Addiction and Substance Abuse (CASA) at Columbia University and a former US Secretary of Health, Education and Welfare.[4] The CASA report provided shocking findings about the abuse of addictive prescription drugs: 'From 1992 to 2003, abuse of controlled prescription drugs grew at a rate twice that of marijuana abuse; five times that of cocaine abuse; sixty times that of heroin abuse.' CASA notes: 'The explosion in the prescription of addictive opioids, depressants and stimulants has, for many children, made their parents' medicine cabinet a greater temptation and threat than the illegal street drug dealer.'

But the CASA report avoids holding the real culprits of the epidemic accountable. This drug epidemic has been orchestrated by physicians and pharmaceutical companies. It is a consequence of the irresponsible prescribing of controlled prescription drugs which have been widely advertised to entice the public – including impressionable children – to take drugs.

The US is not alone. The Institute for Evidence-Based Medicine, an independent research institute in Cologne, Germany, published a study in 2004 of the advertising material and marketing brochures sent out by drug companies to German GPs.[5] The study found that only 6% of the brochures contained statements about drugs that were scientifically supported, while about 94% of the information in them had no scientific basis. They included cholesterol-lowering drugs, blood pressure drugs, and most drugs used for cancer chemotherapy.[6-8] As drug companies spend billions promoting their products, you might expect them at least to get the science right.

In December 2003, Dr Allen Roses, worldwide Vice President at GlaxoSmithKline, Britain's largest drug company, gave an interview to *The Independent* in which he stated that more than 90% of drugs only work in 30% to 50% of people.[9] Not only was someone from the highest echelons of the drug industry, and a high-ranking academic scientist as well (Dr Roses is leading geneticist at Duke University), admitting that a staggeringly high proportion of what is done in the name of medical science is known to be essentially useless, he was also confirming what others had said. Writing in the *British Medical Journal* more than a decade earlier, Dr R. Smith had asked: 'Where is the Wisdom' in medicine? when he pointed out that: 'Over 80% of all healthcare interventions and technologies have no scientific evidence of effectiveness.'[10]

It is actually worse than this because, as well as lacking benefits, the drugs' side effects are known to cause a wide range of harmful side effects: the drugs companies knowingly market drugs that induce heart attacks[11] and diabetes,[12] cause drug dependency,[13] and trigger violent suicidal and homicidal behaviour.[14] Not surprisingly, in 2005, the pharmaceutical industry faced more product liability lawsuits than any other industry.[15]

Despite the obvious failures of 'conventional' drugs, pharmaceutical companies have a strong pecuniary interest in staying in business, ahead of the field. They will only fund research into drugs they can patent and sell; they won't put money into substances which are not patentable; and they will strongly oppose any treatment that does not rely on drugs at all – such as the dietary protocol discussed in this book.

When is a gift not just a gift?

In 2000, an article in the *Journal of the American Medical Association* evaluated the impact of the pharmaceutical industry on doctors' prescribing habits.[16] It found that contact with drug companies began while doctors were at medical school and continued at a frequency of about once a week. The pharmaceutical industry pays for vacations; free air miles are awarded based on the number of prescriptions written; medical equipment is given to practising doctors; and all-expenses-paid trips are organized to 'continuing medical education' seminars – with speakers chosen by the pharmaceutical company.

Most doctors apparently don't realize they are being manipulated in this way. Those interviewed for this article said that they believed the information presented by industry representatives was accurate, and that acceptance of gifts did not affect their prescribing practices. However, after contact with pharmaceutical representatives they tended to favour the prescription of new drugs and reduced their prescribing of generic drugs. In hospitals, changes in prescribing practice were still evident two years after physicians had attended a symposium, which demonstrated the long-term effect of drug promotions on prescribing practices at the institutional level.

The 2000 study reinforced a similar study conducted six years earlier.[17] That showed that doctors who accepted funding to attend a drug company-sponsored symposium changed their prescribing practices, and added the sponsored drugs to their repertoire. Doctors who requested the addition of a new drug to a hospital formulary were five times more likely to have received money from drug companies to attend meetings, give speeches and perform research; 13 times more likely to have met with drug company representatives; and 19 times more likely to have accepted money from those companies, compared with doctors who did not request a particular drug. And requested additions were five times more likely to be for drugs produced by the same companies whose sales representatives met with the physicians, than for drugs from other companies.

These practices aren't confined to richer nations. Multinational drug companies also target doctors in developing countries with bribes of lavish gifts, such as air conditioners, laptops, washing machines, TVs and microwave ovens, as an incentive to prescribe more medical drugs.[18] It is obvious that drug companies' marketing is highly successful in altering physicians' prescribing habits – which is why doctors should stop seeing these representatives, according to a study published in 1999,[19] highlighting doctors' inappropriate and wasteful use of medications after meetings with sales reps.

Doctors' patients are bought
Before any drugs can be used on people, they have to be tested. But where do you find someone silly enough to be a guinea pig? Easy; the drug companies buy them. One common way is to pay university students who are usually broke to take part. But the drug companies also target medical school researchers' patients. In this case the academic researcher is usually offered a per-patient reimbursement by the drug manufacturer that exceeds the per-patient cost to the researcher. And, of course, the researcher can use this money as he wishes. An article in the *Annals of Internal Medicine* stressed that this situation, besides usually being unknown to patients enrolled in the trials, has the potential of creating conflicts of interest. The paper suggested that this could be avoided by re-directing the extra funding to the medical school rather than to the individual investigator. But it points out that, if this were done, the drug company probably wouldn't get the researcher's cooperation.[20]

The drug companies target academia . . .
Official bodies may also contribute to conflicts of interest. There is little point in focusing solely on conflicts of interest related to the pharmaceutical industry while ignoring other important factors that create bias. While scientific and educational meetings routinely require disclosure of conflicts related to industry, they don't ask for disclosures related to clinical income or government grants, both of which are major factors for professional success and involve financial sums much greater than the gifts from industry. If small gifts can create bias, how much worse might these be?

. . . and charities
A similar practice, conducted quietly but growing in popularity, involves drug companies' involvement in charities, according to an exposé published in the *New York Times*.[21] Private-practice doctors across the US set up such charities, which then receive major donations, often in the millions of dollars a year, from drug companies and medical device manufacturers. Concern is rising that drug company payments to such

not-for-profit, tax-exempt organizations bias treatment decisions, lead to suspect research findings, and provide a forum for conflict of interest and misuse of funds. The charities are also closely linked to the doctors' for-profit medical groups, which typically use the products and devices made by the drug companies funding them.

Drug companies boycott conference following speech

But the drug companies won't play if their ploys are disclosed. In November 2006, a young medical researcher almost stopped an entire conference in New Mexico after her talk about drug company influence on medical education.[22] The speaker, Professor Adriane Fugh-Berman of Georgetown University, told her audience: 'Drug representatives are paid to be nice to us, as long as we cooperate, sustaining our market share of targeted drugs and limiting our continuing medical education lectures to messages that increase drug sales.' At that, one drug company representative said her company would immediately withdraw its sponsorship and no longer support the annual conference; the next day there was a near total exhibitor boycott as only one exhibitor showed up. A physician friend of Professor Fugh-Berman remarked: 'Maybe he missed your talk.'

Fraud in medical journals

The drug companies use even more deceitful methods which compound their duplicity. Trials of new drugs, conducted as they are firstly on animals and then on humans, usually over many years, are hugely expensive. It's understandable that drug companies want to recoup their costs, but what happens when a particular drug doesn't live up to the drug company's hopes and expectations? Do they abandon all that work? It seems that the answer is often, No. According to a well-referenced exposé by Shane Ellison, an internationally-recognized authority on therapeutic nutrition with first-hand experience in drug design, companies use deceit to bypass the usual controls, and medical ghostwriting and 'checkbook science' are the most prominent manifestations of this deceit.[23]

Medical ghostwriting is the practice of hiring scientists with PhDs to write drug reports that hype benefits while hiding side effects. The ghostwriters then bow out and qualified physicians are recruited to add their names as the authors. According to Ellison, the reward for ghostwriters can be up to $20,000 per report; the scientists are rewarded with the prestige of having been published.

This practice is much more common than you might think. The *New England Journal of Medicine* relaxed its conflict-of-interest rules in 2002.[24] The following year Professor David Healy, of the University of

Wales, suggested that half of the journal's drug review articles were written by ghostwriters.[25] Dr Richard Smith, editor of the *British Journal of Medicine* acknowledged that medical ghostwriting was a 'very big problem'. He told *The Observer*: 'We are being hoodwinked by the drug companies. The articles come in with doctors' names on them and we often find some of them have little or no idea about what they have written.' He continued: 'When we find out, we reject the paper, but it is very difficult. In a sense, we have brought it on ourselves by insisting that any involvement by a drug company should be made explicit. They have just found ways to get round this and go undercover.' The deputy editor of the *Journal of the American Medical Association* concurred: 'This is all about bypassing science. Medicine is becoming a sort of Cloud Cuckoo Land, where doctors don't know what papers they can trust in the journals, and the public doesn't want to believe.'[26]

'Checkbook science'

According to Dr Diana Zuckerman of the National Center for Policy Research for Women and Families, Washington, DC, the greatest danger to public health might be 'checkbook science', which she defines as 'research intended not to expand knowledge or to benefit humanity but to sell products.'[27]

Drs Joe Collier and Ike Iheanacho, of the Medicines Policy Unit in London, say that cheque-book science explains why deadly drugs are approved. Drug companies have enormous financial power. They choose the investigators from medical academies and government institutions and in many instances involve them in the collation, interpretation and reporting of data. Akin to medical ghostwriting, this practice allows drug companies to hide the dangers associated with drugs while highlighting benefits.[28]

'Sometimes,' say Collier and Iheanacho, 'their commercially determined goals represent genuine advances in healthcare provision, but most often they are implicated in excessive and costly production of information that . . . can risk undermining the best interests of patients and society.'

As with medical ghostwriting, cheque-book science is extremely common. Universities and similar teaching organizations should be independent and unbiased. But, despite increasing awareness of the potential impact of financial conflicts of interest on biomedical research, many academic professors have personal financial ties to drug makers.[29] Justin E. Bekelman and colleagues at Yale University School of Medicine say that: 'Approximately one fourth of investigators have industry affiliations, and roughly two thirds of academic institutions hold equity in start-ups that sponsor research performed at the same institutions.'

US government institutions are guilty, too. The National Institutes of Health (NIH) were once considered: 'an island of objective and pristine research, untainted by the influences of commercialization.' Their supposed objectivity influences medicine and health not just in the US but in other countries, including the UK. However, according to an in-depth article published in the *LA Times*, top scientists at NIH also collect pay cheques and stock options from the drug industry.[30] To substantiate this claim, the *LA Times* published a list of scientists and their gratuities from drug companies; the sums involved were up to more than $600,000. NIH officials apparently allow almost all of their own top-paid employees to keep 'consulting' fees confidential. When it comes to disclosing financial conflicts of interest, NIH is reckoned to be the most secretive agency in the US government.

While it is understandable that the drug companies aren't in business for their health, they don't seem to be in it for the sake of anyone else's health either.

The Bayh-Dole Act

You might wonder how on earth this has been allowed to happen. The answer lies in a 1980 amendment to US patent law, called the Bayh-Dole Act. It was the brainchild of President Reagan's science advisor, George Keyworth II. Keyworth had been watching the United States get beaten in world markets by the Japanese. The Act was intended to stimulate advanced technological invention and speed its transfer from university laboratories into private industry, where it could be put to work for the US economy; to allow universities to commercialize products and inventions without losing their federal research funding. It looked like a great idea and several private drug companies contributed billions of dollars of much needed research money to the universities at a time when research costs were increasing dramatically.

This helped to launch the biotech industry and speed several lifesaving products to market. It also allowed the pharmaceutical industries to buy the expertise of the best academic clinicians at the medical schools for a fraction of the costs of in-house teams; it ensured lower costs and access to a bigger market for their drugs. The academics not only received the research grant money; they could augment their incomes with $1,000-a-day consulting contracts with pharmaceutical companies, patent royalties, licensing fees, and stock options.

But there was a serious downside: Bayh-Dole has fostered increasingly close relationships between the academics upon whom not just the US but the world depends for unbiased medical information, and private drug companies which are anything but unbiased.

It is assumed that professional medical journals, which are regarded by the medical profession as their bibles, offer the hard science behind any given drug. This assumption is false. Thanks to widespread medical fraud, medical journals can't be trusted.

Publication bias

There is one further phenomenon to be considered: publication bias. Not all studies produce the result that researchers were hoping for. This is particularly true of drug trials. Drug companies will not normally publish such results, and the medical journals don't like to publish them either. For this reason, only data that appear to convey a benefit will be published; data which are negative will not. This leaves readers with the impression that the evidence for a procedure or drug is all positive, when, in many cases, it may be marginal at best.

Political censorship is even worse than this. Editors of once great journals, such as *Nature*, jump through hoops in order to prevent the publication of critiques of establishment dogma.

The 31 May 2003 issue of the *British Medical Journal* ran no fewer than six articles saying that too many of the published drug studies are no more than industry-sponsored 'infomercials', citing the selective reporting bias whereby only pro-industry studies are published. It suggested that it was: 'Time to untangle doctors from drug companies.' Time, yes, but there is little sign yet that this state of affairs will cease. As a result of this bias the word 'cure' has all but vanished from the medical literature.

Pharmaceutical company bias

The effectiveness of a drug is usually established by a trial of the drug versus a placebo. These trials are expensive and usually funded by manufacturers. But when researchers from the University of California investigated 192 published trials for cholesterol-lowering statin drugs, they found that the results were 20 times more likely to be favourable, and the researchers 35 times more likely to give their conclusions a favourable spin, when the drug company was paying than when the funding was from an independent source.[31] In fact the greater effectiveness of a drug over placebo seems to disappear when tested independently. A systematic search of the Cochrane Database of Systematic Reviews, considered by many to be the most objective medical science reporting of all, showed that all of the industry-funded meta-analyses of drugs recommended the experimental drug without reservations, while none of the Cochrane reviews did so, even though the estimated treatment effects were the same in both cases.[32] Peter Gøtzsche at the Nordic Cochrane Center in Copenhagen, a co-author of the meta-analyses report, said that he would now ignore any meta-analyses funded by drug companies.[33] But drug trials are worthwhile investments for drug companies for, once a drug has received a favourable review in a so-called 'scientific' trial, it is well on the road to millions of dollars of sales.

This probably wouldn't be the case, however, if the drug companies published their data showing that their drugs were useless or harmful. Not surprisingly, they don't. Whenever a study doesn't come up with the 'right answer', they keep quiet about it. To combat this, the Labour Party's 2005 election manifesto promised to: 'require registration of all clinical trials and publication of their findings for all trials of medicinal products with a marketing authorization in the UK.' However, under EU legislation, it seems that forcing drug companies to publish negative trial results is illegal![34] So we can't even trust those whose duty it is to protect us.

Misleading abstracts

There is one last point that must be made in this context. There are some 30,000 medical journals published throughout the world. No busy doctor can be expected to read more than a handful at most. The papers they contain are often long and complex, so many doctors will simply read the 'abstract' (summary) and, perhaps, the conclusions. It is important, therefore, that the abstract be a true reflection of the paper. It is worrying that a review of the accuracy of abstracts in six of the most prestigious and most read journals found that up to 68% of their abstracts were inaccurate. The authors of the review conclude: 'Data in the abstract that are inconsistent with or absent from the article's body are common, even in large-circulation general medical journals.'[35]

The result

We now have a situation where caring and conscientious General Practitioners and hospital doctors have no way of knowing which drugs or other treatments have any benefit and which may cause harm to their patients. Having to rely on the papers published in medical journals is, for them, fraught with danger. They are caught in a trap not of their making, but which has conferred on them an unenviable reputation as harmers of our health, as we will see later.

And how are their patients to make informed treatment choices if they cannot rely on the efficacy and safety of the treatments that are recommended to them by their physicians?

Health or wealth?

Drugs companies aren't philanthropic organizations and they must make a profit to survive. This means that a treatment which doesn't make money is of no interest to them. Dr Bernard Dixon, writing in the medical journal, *Lancet*, in 2003, asked whether the recent outbreak of SARS in Asia might be treated by the well-tried, century-old technique of 'passive immunity' – that is injecting antibodies derived from infected patients and multiplied in some neutral organism. This method can be greatly improved by modern biotechnology. 'Would it not work?' he asked. A drug company executive told him: 'Of course it would. But we've looked at it and there's no money in it.'[36]

Are new drugs any better than the old ones?

Drug companies make most of their profits from the sale of new drugs; when patents run out, so does their income. New drugs are always launched with a promise that they are far better than the drugs that they replace. And human nature being what it is, we tend to believe this.

In reality, the new drugs are often no better; indeed, they are often only a little different from the ones they replace. It's true that they are usually far more powerful, but that often means they come with an even greater risk of causing a serious adverse reaction.

When a new drug comes on the market, everyone expects the prescribing doctor to report any adverse reactions in his patients. But a new Portuguese study has discovered this doesn't happen as often as it should in Portugal, with less than 10% of the numbers expected according to the World Health Organization.[37] The US, Canada, Italy, Sweden and the UK also have very low reporting rates, say the researchers. Nonetheless, health authorities often recommend newer – and more expensive – drugs even though medical trials consistently discover that they are no more effective, or safer, than the older generations of drugs.

To combat this (we are told) we have institutions such as NICE in the UK and the FDA (Food and Drugs Administration) in the US. But just what is their role? Is it to protect us, the public, or to help the drug companies generate greater profits?

Psychiatrist, Dr David Healy (by now a Professor), from the North Wales Department of Psychological Medicine, writing in the *British Medical Journal*, wanted to know why a drug company had written to him, admitting that its antidepressant, *paroxetine*, might increase the risk of suicide six-fold, while the official data from the regulators painted a far rosier picture.[38] 'Many people expect drug companies to be slow to concede that a drug causes hazards, but we do not expect our regulators to be even slower,' he said.

The reluctance of the drug regulators to issue warnings about drugs happens on both sides of the Atlantic. Dr Healy pointed out that 'every antidepressant licensed since 1987' was associated with a higher risk of suicide compared with placebo, and yet America's drug regulator, the FDA, continued to obscure this vital fact. The FDA was aware that drug manufacturers had tried to muddy the waters by wrongly blaming some suicides and suicide attempts on the placebo rather than the drug itself, and yet had done nothing about it.

Dr Jerry Avorn, writing in the *New England Journal of Medicine*, points out that: 'Since 1992, the United States has relied heavily on the pharmaceutical industry to pay the salaries of Food and Drug Administration scientists who review new drug applications.' More than 40% of the budget of the FDA division that reviews new drug applications is contributed by those drug companies. Avorn tells how colleagues at the FDA are worried that the organization is accountable to the industry it regulates. 'One FDA scientist who was often criticized for being too concerned about drug-risk data was told by his supervisor to remember that the agency's client was the pharmaceutical industry. "That's odd," he replied. "I thought our clients were the people of the United States."'[39] Pressures on the FDA by drug companies to rush the drug-approval process have led to the FDA's regulatory review times being among the shortest in the world.

Consumer, beware

In view of the wide range of harmful side effects, you might expect that compensation should be forthcoming in the event of harm. You would be wrong. So many people in the US have brought lawsuits against drug companies for the harm caused by their drugs that something had to be done. And it probably isn't what you might expect. In February 2008, the US Supreme Court's decision gave the biotech drug and device industry immunity from liability for marketing defective products that kill.[40] American consumers now no longer have any recourse if they are harmed by defective drugs, vaccines or medical devices that carry the FDA seal of approval. That seal of approval is a licence to market even poorly tested, defective drugs, vaccines and medical devices that kill. And these drugs can be used in other countries as well as the US.

So, beware: if you blindly accept and use any prescription drug and it harms you, it's your own fault!

The American model

The main driving force behind American medicine is wealth rather than health. There is plenty of insurance money so doctors have no compunction about cashing in on it. This, of course, increases medical insurance premiums, which means even more money . . . and so on.

According to a new survey which was conducted for the Commonwealth Fund, a non-partisan foundation that supports research into health and social issues, 40% of adults polled reported having serious problems paying for health insurance or for their own or a family member's healthcare in the past two years. A similar number reported having serious problems getting appointments to see a doctor when they were ill; and that the time needed to handle paperwork or deal with disputes related to medical bills and health insurance was a serious problem. Three-quarters of US adults now: 'believe the US healthcare system needs to be fundamentally changed or rebuilt completely.'

High healthcare costs have long been a problem in the US. With an average household income of $44,000, half of those earning up to $50,000 report difficulties paying for healthcare. There are also concerns that costs are 'moving up the income ladder'; worries about whether they would be able to afford high-quality care when needed were found in groups with incomes as high as $75,000. Not surprisingly, 'the findings indicate that more than half of all households experience stress when paying for medical care.'[41]

The health industry milks the system for all it can get. The British NHS could find itself in similar trouble unless the hold the drug companies have on it is not broken soon.

Approve our drug or else . . .

If anyone still believes the pharmaceutical industry's main concern is to help mankind they might be interested in the way drug company executives lobby UK government ministers. In an exposé, *The Guardian* reported on notes made at meetings between drug company lobbyists and government ministers, which have just been made public under Freedom of Information legislation.[42]

The article reveals bully-boy tactics and threats from the drug company executives to get their new expensive drugs 'fast-tracked' by NICE for acceptance within the NHS. Over the eight months from October 2005 to May 2006, senior executives from ten drug companies met ministers to press for favourable decisions on their products. The executives were highly critical of NICE. Although NICE is an independent expert body the government invariably accepts NICE's final recommendations. At one meeting, the health minister, Jane Kennedy, was confronted by eight managing directors, vice-presidents and senior executives from six drug companies who lobbied hard for a NICE ruling to be overturned by the government; two companies lobbied ministers for wider access by

patients to their drugs, both of which were later turned down by NICE on
the grounds that they were not effective enough and too expensive; and
Pfizer executives suggested they could withdraw their investment in the
UK unless NICE reconsidered its refusal of one of Pfizer's drugs.

This giant US company, with annual revenues of $52.5 billion (£26 bil-
lion), suggested that it might 'take its business elsewhere' unless the
government helped create a more 'robust' environment for pharmaceuticals in the UK. Richard Marsh, director of external affairs at Bristol-Myers
Squibb, who also attended one of the government meetings, said drug
companies wanted to invest in countries with a 'favourable environment'.

With a total investment in research and development of more than £3.4
billion in 2004, the pharmaceutical industry is a major contributor to the
UK economy. So, in effect, the government is being told it must either
approve drugs, without all the time-consuming safety and efficacy
checks, or lose substantial inward investment. It's a powerful lobby
which has no regard for the patient or the tax-payer.

And it's not just the drug companies that are lobbying for this. It seems
that there is also intensive lobbying by the White House to grant American pharmaceutical giants unrestricted access to the UK market. If it is
successful, it means every new, approved drug would become immediately available on the NHS as part of a free-market initiative. US deputy
health secretary, Alex Azar, has also intimated that the American system
of advertising drugs directly to the patient would also be introduced.[43]

. . . and pay a higher price for it
In another story, *The Guardian* reported that GlaxoSmithKline had won
a partial court victory in an attempt to block wholesalers from buying its
drugs cheaply in Spain and selling them in the UK and other European
countries where prices are higher.[44] Drug companies set different prices
for their medicines in each country according to what they think the
market will stand. It is called 'parallel trading'. Prices in the UK are relatively high, so wholesalers will buy up cheaper stocks in Spain, Portugal
or Greece and sell them to UK high street pharmacies at discount prices.
This saves the NHS £200m a year. Major pharmaceutical companies,
however, argue that it damages innovation by reducing the profits available to invest in research and development (R&D) of new medicines.

Fat cats and your local GP
When we talk of fat cats in industry, few people think of their family
doctor. In 2006 a study of tax returns forced a rethink.[45] As the NHS's
cash crisis deepened and hospitals shed thousands of jobs, it emerged
that GPs' average annual earnings rose by 63% in 2006; some are

earning up to £250,000 a year – the equivalent of ten nurses' salaries. Whether such huge incomes deliver value for money is subject of much debate. Then Prime Minister, Tony Blair, robustly defended this, saying: 'It's right we make our GPs the best paid in Europe.' He neglected to add that NHS Trusts were concurrently closing wards and sacking staff to balance their books as they ran short of money.

This turn of events may be because of yet another ploy used by the drug companies: according to the *New York Times*, they use governments to endorse and recommend their products. The way they do this is by rewarding physicians with outrageous bonuses and appointments. But not just any physicians; these are the doctors who are on official government panels that set the policy on which drugs will be recommended. It is vital that you understand that this is the way the system operates if you are to resist it.

It was entirely government incompetence combined with mercenary advice from a malevolent drugs industry that led to this sorry state of affairs. The UK's New Labour government seemed more interested in 'targets' than in people's health. It used targets to measure how healthy we were. When the government introduced this method of measuring healthcare, the way GPs were paid changed so that around two-thirds of their income was linked to whether they delivered 'quality services' in certain areas. Targets varied from record keeping to providing a range of clinical services such as cholesterol tests, cancer screens and flu jabs. For the GPs, the more targets they met, the more points they earned, and the more points they earned, the more pounds they found in their pockets. That might not seem like such a bad idea: it would give doctors an incentive to work harder and we would all be healthier as a result, wouldn't we? It hasn't worked that way.

The Quality and Outcomes Framework (QOF) provides 1,050 points for targets across all of the clinical domains, with 550 related to heart disease alone. Each point is worth £124. If doctors manage to get all their patients on all the schemes, that's an extra £126,000 on top of their already not inconsiderable salaries of around £106,000. It's a very powerful incentive for doctors to comply with government targets whether they believe it is doing any good or not. And there's another dimension: with QOF points being written into the national contract and dicta coming from NICE, it is clear that clinical judgement is no longer required; indeed, it will have to be suspended where NICE 'advises' clinicians on best practice. The average physician will depart from 'approved practice' at his peril – the penalties for not toeing the party line being abandonment by his medical defence organization and having no professional support from his colleagues.

We now have healthcare by committee decision, arbitrary order and censure; and the professional wilderness awaits clinicians who dare to use their medical experience and knowledge to question or challenge this orthodoxy.

The UK government defends its policy, of course, saying that it is helping to ensure preventative measures such as health checks take place. And that will make us all healthier and save money in the long term. It's cloud cuckoo land, as we will see in the next chapter.

Patients' groups, underwhelmed by these tactics, complain that GPs are so busy 'ticking the boxes' so that they can earn money for reaching targets that there is little time left for patients' real health problems. Niall Dickson, chief executive of the independent medical think-tank, the King's Fund, says the GPs' contract has not only *not* increased GPs' productivity, it may actually have reduced it.

In the UK, this 'payment by results' scheme has resulted in many GP practices reaching the specified targets. Overall, practices attained 93.2% of the total available points for diabetes.[46] But it's a total waste of money because, as physicians pick up their bonuses, the numbers of cases of degenerative diseases such as diabetes are increasing at an alarming rate.

Whatever happened to the concept of 'First do no harm'?

Another of the reasons for the increase in NHS costs is a constant demand for more and more doctors, nurses and hospitals. Try to close a hospital or even a ward and all hell breaks loose in the local press. But it might be better for our health if, instead of demanding more doctors, we did reduce their numbers. Not only would that cut costs; there is very strong evidence that fewer doctors might actually result in us being healthier.

Doctors strike – and death rates fall

Doctors don't often go on strike, but it has happened sufficiently often for a disturbing trend to be noticed. During the rare times that they have gone on strike – in several countries – the death rate has always gone down.

In 2000, Israeli doctors employed in public hospitals pursued a course of industrial action. This included the cancellation of outpatient clinics and the postponement of all routine surgery. And this limited strike action had some unusual consequences. Throughout Israel, while the doctors were on strike, death rates fell. The coastal city of Netanya has only one hospital whose staff members had a 'no strike' clause in their contracts. As a result, doctors in Netanya continued to work normally – and death rates remained stubbornly the same, failing to reflect the reduction that was shown in almost all of the rest of the country.[47] And it wasn't the first time; doctors in Israel went on strike in 1973, and reduced their total daily patient contacts from 65,000 to just 7,000. The strike lasted a month and during that time the death rate, according to the Jerusalem Burial Society, dropped by half.

It doesn't just happen in Israel. The 1960s saw physicians in Canada go on strike and the mortality rate dropped. In 1976, in Bogota, Colombia, doctors refused to treat all but emergency cases for a period of 52 days, and in that time the death rate fell by 35%.[48] In the same year the death rate dropped 18% during a 'slow-down' by doctors in Los Angeles. After the strike, deaths rates jumped to 3% *above* normal for more than five weeks as the Los Angeles doctors caught up on their paperwork.[49]

And it is a standing joke among cardiologists that death rates fall during their conferences because fewer of them are attempting to cure moribund patients by doing dangerous surgery. Their treatment can be worse than the disease. It may come as no surprise, therefore, that a major report by Australian medical researchers posed the question 'WILL MORE DOCTORS INCREASE OR DECREASE DEATH RATES?' The report, written by scientists at the Centre for Health Program Evaluation, hypothesized that an increase in death rates in that country was caused by an increase in the number of doctors. Although the report was concerned only with the situation in Australia, there is strong evidence to suggest that this question also needs to be addressed in many other developed countries including Britain and the US.

You may think that the question and hypothesis are outrageous. After all, *Primum non nocere*, 'First, do no harm', is a central tenet guiding medical practice, and most doctors treat this tenet very seriously. Yet the reality is that, with the state of healthcare as it is, our continual calls for more doctors, and expansion of the NHS and our dependence on it, may actually be increasing rather than decreasing illness in our lives. With the world's highest concentration of doctors – one for every 500 people – you might expect that the US would be the healthiest country. Far from it; data from a health survey of the top thirteen wealthiest industrialized countries were published in the summer of 2000. The US came twelfth.[50]

One reason why medical care may increase death rates is the large number of adverse events associated with it. The Australian report mentions a 1995 study of 14,000 hospital admissions. Of those admitted almost 17% suffered an adverse event. One in seven adverse events resulted in a permanent disability and one in 20 of the individuals affected died.[51]

Even that may be an under-assessment. Research on under-reporting of serious adverse drug reactions in the United States and Canada suggests that formal reporting rates may be as low as 1.5% of the real total. US estimates place adverse drug reactions as the fifth most common cause of death after heart disease, cancer, stroke and pulmonary disease.[52] These figures are not always easy to acquire. It is well known that doctors and hospital consultants are notoriously bad at reporting drug side effects. Although there is a new national reporting system in the UK designed to flag potentially dangerous drugs and remedies, pharmacists said they tend not to report a side effect if patients have been harmed; they are more likely to report only those incidents where a protocol has been broken.[53] They fear that they will be blamed for any side effect, and so feel it is not worth running the risk. Why might they act in this way? It seems that they are ashamed to admit to their patients that they were wrong.[54]

In modern society there is an increasing tendency, typified by the human rights movement, to shame governments, professions and individuals into complying with a particular organization's ideas for social change. Shame is hard to deal with. It engenders embarrassment and guilt; it makes professionals feel flawed. It is, perhaps, no surprise that they fall back on silence. Shame is probably the major reason why most doctors don't report adverse drug effects or change their views on the usefulness and harm of drugs.

A second possibility, which the Australian researchers call 'the dependency hypothesis', is the idea that the more doctors are available, the more dependent on them people become to maintain their health. This leads patients to adopt an exaggerated confidence in the effectiveness of medical care and its ability to offset the harmful effects of their own self-neglect. But that is not a healthy attitude because getting involved with the medical profession can be decidedly dangerous. In 1999, doctors in the US were recognized as the third leading cause of death.[50] Four years later another review had elevated them into first place.[55] The number of Americans killed by FDA-approved pharmaceuticals is equivalent to dropping a nuclear bomb on a major US city every year.

We in Britain are not immune to this trend. On 13 August 2005, an astonishing article appeared on the front page of *The Times*. Based on an independent report published in the *British Medical Journal*, it confirmed that medical accidents and errors were directly blamed for the deaths of 40,000 Britons per year. This made them officially Britain's fourth-biggest killer. But the report went on to state that less than a third of an estimated 900,000 medical mistakes are properly reported each year. The figure also excluded errors committed in primary care such as in GPs' surgeries.

Later in the year came a Parliamentary Public Accounts Committee Report, *A Safer Place for Patients: Learning to Improve Patient Safety*. It stated that some 22% of medical mistakes that lead to a serious reaction or even death go unreported in the UK. This is because, while you may read 'the patient died from complications of surgery', the truth is often 'the surgeon killed the patient'. Only one in four hospitals owns up to the patient (or relatives) when something goes wrong; the rest blame it on the disease itself; while just one in 25 drug reactions is ever reported. This massive under-reporting of mistakes is an acknowledged problem. It is usually because of fears of litigation.

Government officials were shocked to hear that nobody knows how many of the reported blunders end in the death of the patient. But based on the known, reported accidents, one in 10 people admitted to a hospital in Britain every year will suffer an incident that will harm them, said Tory MP Edward Leigh, chairman of the Commons Public Accounts Committee. These included 974,000 medical 'accidents'.[56] This is a conservative estimate; government officials accept the figure is more likely to be 1,190,000. We should then add 300,000 hospital-acquired infections, and 250,000 serious adverse reactions to a prescription drug, a figure which is again a very conservative estimate as it is based only on reported reactions – a truer figure may be closer to 1,200,000 every year, according to officials. This means that some 2,690,000 people, or 4.5% of the entire population, could be harmed by medical mishaps every year. 'The numbers of blunders could have been halved if staff had learned from earlier errors,' the report said. Edward Leigh added: 'No public health system should tolerate a failure to learn from previous experience on this scale.'

The lapses cost the NHS (actually, you and me, the taxpayers, of course) an estimated £2 billion in extra bed days and £540 million in litigation and compensation.

All of this may be why the late Dr Robert Mendelsohn, a physician himself, wrote: 'Doctors in general should be treated with about the same degree of trust as used car salesmen.'[57]

However, we do need doctors; no matter how healthy we are, there will always be accidents and emergencies. Doctors are intelligent, good and caring people. Nonetheless, intensely busy and inundated with information and the need to meet government targets, they just cannot keep up. So, hard-working doctors at the sharp end should not be blamed if they get it wrong occasionally. They are being manipulated as much as their patients are.

But when a society's healthcare system is one of the major killers in that society then that system is a failed system in need of immediate attention.

Doctors are the most trusted people in Britain
In view of all that has been written above, you might be surprised to

learn that according to a Mori Poll taken in 2006, an overwhelming 91% of the population voted doctors the most trustworthy professionals in the UK for the 22nd year running.[58] But that might be because the British Medical Association, the UK doctors' trade union, funded the poll.

Do doctors get the wrong training?

If you go to your doctor today, it's extremely unlikely that he will tell you that whatever you have wrong with you is curable. When you use the word 'cure' around him, he will interpret the word to mean 'treat'. His medical school training will have taught him that everything is 'treatable' but practically nothing is 'curable'. For example, take adult onset (type-2) diabetes, which has reached epidemic proportions throughout the industrialized world over the last decade or so. Conventional treatment means taking an increasing number of drugs for the rest of your life as the illness progresses and your health declines. Yet this form of diabetes has been curable for some 70 years. It is also probably the easiest disease both to cure and to prevent, without resorting to drugs, as we will see in Chapter 20.

Your doctor will also never tell you that not so long ago, obesity, high blood pressure, high cholesterol, high blood glucose and insulin levels, strokes, heart failure, poor wound healing, peripheral nerve damage and many other non-contagious disorders were once well understood to be no more than symptoms of diabetes.

There may be two reasons why doctors think in this way. Firstly, there is the drug companies' influence on medical education.[59] Doctors are taught to think drugs, drugs, drugs. Despite this, David Webb, Professor of Therapeutics and Pharmacology at the University of Edinburgh, said: 'Patients are becoming ill and some are dying as a result of poor prescribing . . . A substantial proportion of that is undoubtedly avoidable.' This is because doctors are no longer being taught the basics about drugs and how they work – they are led by drug salesmen, who make great claims for their drugs while underplaying the dangers. It's an alarming situation that is worrying medical students, who have privately expressed their concerns about their lack of prescribing knowledge.

This level of doctors' drug knowledge is especially worrying at a time when drug company hype and influence have reached fever pitch, and when drugs have become more complex and dangerous.

The second training fault seems to lie in the simple fact that, as Dr G. T. Wrench pointed out in the Introduction to his 1938 book, *The Wheel of Health*, during all their years at medical school physicians are taught entirely about disease, not about health:[60]

'After debating the question – Why disease? Why not health? – again and again with my fellow students, I slowly, before I qualified, came to a further question – Why was it that as students we were always presented with sick or convalescent people for our teaching and never with the ultrahealthy? Why were we only taught disease? Why was it presumed that we knew all about health in its fullness? The teaching was wholly onesided. Moreover, the basis of our teaching upon disease was pathology, namely, the appearance of that which is dead from disease . . . By the time, however, we reached real health . . . the studies were dropped. Their human representatives, the patients, were now well, and neither we nor our educators were any longer concerned with them. We made no studies of the healthy – only the sick.'

The experience that Dr Wrench had in medical school has changed little over the subsequent decades. Doctors today still get little or no training in nutrition even though a person's nutrition is probably the most important single factor influencing his or her health.

Hippocrates' admonition to 'Let food be thy medicine, and let thy medicine be food' is as meaningful today as it was two millennia ago.

Drug companies control patients' groups
So, if you can't trust your doctor as an impartial source, who can you turn to? One answer might seem to be an independent patient support group that supplies helpful information and advice on specific diseases. Sorry, that probably won't help either: these groups are also targeted by the drug companies. They call it 'astroturfing'.

The Ekbom Support Group which helps advise people with restless leg syndrome was discovered to have been 'astroturfed' by Glaxo-SmithKline (GSK), the manufacturer of *Adartrel*, a drug for restless leg syndrome. GSK helped Ekbom set up its website and Ekbom was found to be actively promoting *Adartrel*. This underhand trick might never have come to light if the website hadn't started to promote the drug some eight months before it had been approved.

The *British Medical Journal* investigated 28 other support groups. They found that 27 were being funded by drug companies, and were presenting information that was, at best, 'partial'. The journal found they all seemed to be pushing specific drugs to treat conditions, while downplaying risks. The latest is a new pan-European pressure group, Cancer United (CU), which was launched in Brussels on 19 October 2006. It described itself as a pioneering coalition of doctors, nurses and patients, pushing for equal access to cancer care throughout Europe. Many MPs, MEPs and leading figures in European cancer charities, including the head of the European Cancer Patients Coalition, joined CU's board. Then it became clear that things weren't all they seemed to be. It turns out that

CU is merely a front for the drug giant, Roche, which makes *Herceptin*, the new breast cancer 'wonder drug', and *Avastin*. Not only is Roche funding the coalition; a senior Roche executive is sitting on CU's board, and Roche's PR agency, Weber Shandwick, which has been heavily promoting it to clinicians and journalists, is CU's secretariat.[61] Roche's action is further evidence of the pressing need for transparency and accountability in the pharmaceutical industry. A Consumers International study earlier in 2006 found that the top 20 drug companies in Europe all flout their own industry guidelines on corporate social responsibility.

The religion of health

Medical politics has slowly assumed the trappings of a religion whose dogmas we are expected to follow without question. Doctors and nutritionists have become health priests whose verdicts we must accept blindly. School teachers, elected and appointed public health officials, TV and radio pundits, even TV chefs and chat show hosts, have become lay-preachers so that they, too, can help to spread the gospel. People cannot be blamed for acquiescing as many have received this indoctrination since childhood, just as happens in other religions. And anyone who objects or tries to preach a different gospel is ridiculed, ostracized and vilified. This is particularly true of people within the medical profession.

The late Dr Robert Mendelsohn wrote: 'There's no room for compromise because churches never compromise on canon law . . . in medical politics there is a rigid authoritarian power structure which can be moved only through winner-take-all power plays. Historically, doctors who have dared to change things significantly have been ostracized and have had to sacrifice their careers in order to hold to their ideas. Few doctors are willing to do either.'

Many religions are evangelical; 'Health' is no different. It sets out with evangelical zeal to convert unbelievers. In the next chapter, we will see the lengths to which the medical establishment will go to increase its 'congregation'.

Of course, not all doctors are taken in. An Australian doctor, Herbert Nehrlich, summarized the financial aspect in limerick form:

> Any doctor today must have stealth,
> as he deals with his patients' ill health.
> Let me tell you, my friend,
> what goes on in the end
> is a state-sanctioned transfer of wealth.

Chapter Two

What's behind the screens?

> Screening for disease is promoted as a preventive measure. It is not: if a disease is found it hasn't been prevented. With considerable evidence of adverse effects, medical screening seems merely a pretext to increase the 'patient base' and identify a market for increased drug sales, with precious little evidence of benefit to the 'patients'.

> In absolute terms less than 1% of women who are invited for screening will benefit from it, whereas a greater percentage will have to face the problems of false alarms, unnecessary surgery, unnecessary labelling as having cancer.
>
> *Professor M. Baum*

Not so long ago every other child had its adenoids or tonsils removed; a hysterectomy was performed on any woman who had menstrual problems; appendectomies were performed on symptom-free patients 'just to be on the safe side'; and circumcision of the sons of middle-class parents for reasons of 'hygiene' were commonplace. These examples of ritualized brutality happened in the middle of the 20th century; they were the medical fads of their time. If you believe that medicine has come a long way since then, you would be wrong. Fads may change but fixations that owe more to passion and political correctness than to evidence or logic are still common and still visited on a trusting populace. They also provide the medical world with something to do and a ready source of income.

The latter half of the 20th century saw the emergence of a belief that any disease could be eradicated if enough were spent on research and if the diseases could be found before the patient knew he/she had them. And if you want to sell drugs, then identifying people who might 'benefit' from them is a major priority. So the medical profession began to spend a great deal more time and money looking for diseases which had no symptoms.

The government, no doubt influenced and advised by vested interests, reinforced the message with a sense of moral mission which forces submission to 'check-ups' at every routine visit to the doctor's surgery.[1] Try to say 'no thanks' and you will be branded as ungrateful or downright irresponsible. In the US blackmail is used: a child who hasn't had this or that vaccination isn't allowed in school. And it has become a punishable crime to believe there might be evidence which refutes your doctor's unasked-for advice. Don't take your statin, and you could be struck off as a patient.

Prevention is better than cure, we are told. Screening is a 'good thing'. Finding and treating diseases increases life-expectancy, reduces expenses in the National Health Service and promotes health. That's the belief. Actually there is no evidence that the progress of any disease targeted today is much influenced by the treatments we have for them; finding them earlier merely increases the burden of worry. And if the government is so naïve as to believe that health costs will be reduced, they might reflect that the elderly cost significantly more both in their medical and social requirements and in their pensions. You don't save money by promoting longevity. Only the health industry makes money out of screening programmes.

The incentive for patients

In 1986, British General Practitioners were required to offer three-yearly health assessments to adult patients under 75 years of age, and were encouraged to offer health promotion services to all their patients. In the middle of 1991, the government announced a green paper, *The Health of the Nation*. It marked a significant change of emphasis for the NHS. The government said that tens of thousands of premature deaths could be avoided if people could be persuaded to change their lifestyles. According to the strategy proposed by the paper, the main causes of diseases believed to be preventable would each be 'targeted' in a concerted attempt to reduce their incidence over the next two decades.

The major targets included cutting premature deaths from coronary heart disease by 7,500 per year by the end of the 20th century; reducing cancer deaths, 85% of which it believed were preventable; and reducing stroke deaths by 30% by the end of that century. Other areas where the paper suggested that health could be improved included obesity, diabetes, asthma, mental illness, child health, and food-borne diseases.

The fallacy that prevention is always better than cure

This shift of interest towards 'preventive' medicine appeared to be a good thing. There were good historical examples of where taking preventive measures had resulted in large reductions in disease. But to say that prevention is better than cure in *all* cases involves a fallacy.

Preventive medicine in Britain today is confined almost exclusively to screening the population for diseases. This is not *prevention* of the disease; if a disease is found, it *hasn't* been prevented. Nevertheless, for such procedures to be of benefit a number of criteria are well established.[2] Firstly, the disease must be both common and serious, as screening for an uncommon disease will throw up many false results which will inevitably incur the cost of further testing, and cause unnecessary anxiety which itself is harmful. Secondly, there must be an effective treatment for the disease available, as there is no point in detecting a disease for which there is no effective remedy.

After screening comes the second phase of 'preventive' measures. This usually involves changing one's lifestyle in some way, at a price which may be high. We know that a smoker is more likely to get lung cancer than a non-smoker. The preventive measure here is to stop smoking and, in this case, the lost pleasure of smoking is balanced by having more money to spend on other treats. In other cases, however, there may be no compensating benefit. For example, we can avoid being hit by a bus by staying at home. But would you want to?

We understand how infectious diseases are caused and can combat most of them. However, many modern diseases are caused by the way we live or the stresses placed on us. Increasing those pressures has been shown to increase the incidences of such diseases – and screening for disease increases those stresses.

Screening for cancer

Not so long ago, the diagnosis of cancer was thought to be a death sentence; today we tend to believe that any cancer can be cured if it is caught early enough. It may appear at first sight that cancer is an ideal disease at which to aim a pre-emptive strike, before it spreads. But on closer examination that turns out to be a misconception. While there have been advances over the past few decades in the treatment of some of the rarer cancers such as childhood leukaemia, melanoma and testicular cancer, there have been no similar advances in treatments of the more common cancers despite the vast resources that have been thrown at them. By telling us of death rates we have been persuaded that mass screening programmes are justifiable. In fact, only if it can be shown that death rates are *falling* can one say that screening for cancers is really worthwhile. As yet there is little sign of any significant reduction in the number of deaths from the common cancers. In *The Cancer Business*, Dr Patrick Rattigan wrote in 1990: 'In Britain, at the present time, around one third of general hospital patients are suffering from cancer. Two out of five of the population have, or will develop, the disease. If we accept the figures for cancer incidence of 30% in 1980, 40% now and 50% in the year 2010, at the present rate of increase the figure will reach 100% around 2080.'[3] So far Rattigan's figures are proving to be remarkably accurate.

Breast cancer screening

In 1971, the year that President Nixon declared 'War on Cancer', 11,182 women in England and Wales died of breast cancer; in 2005 the number was 11,040.[4] As you can see, not a lot has changed over those 34 years, despite countless trillions spent trying to find a cure or useful treatment for the condition.

It's even worse in the US where breast cancers have increased at an alarming rate over recent years. In the 1940s, a woman's lifetime risk of breast cancer was one in 22. By 2004, it had tripled to one in seven. More American women have died of breast cancer in the last 20 years than the total number of Americans killed in World War I, World War II, the Korean War and the Vietnam War together.[5]

You might expect that discovery of breast cancer earlier would enhance the chances of a successful treatment. But by the time a breast cancer is large enough to be detectable by hand, it has usually been growing, on average, for some eight years. Mammography may detect it at about six years. Mammography will only make an appreciable difference to the outcome, therefore, if the tumour metastasizes (spreads) during the two years in between – and there is no reason to believe that it will.[6]

To complicate things, whether a breast tumour will kill seems to depend more on what type of cancer it is than its age. In many cases removal of a breast is irrelevant to the eventual outcome. Mortality statistics show that, as yet, there has been no really significant reduction in the numbers of women dying of the disease – even with breast removal.[7] Nevertheless, early detection of a lump and removal of a breast seems to be the most frequent course of events, involving disfigurement and much consequent psychological distress. Some American doctors actually advise women with no sign of the disease to have both breasts removed merely as a precaution. It is inevitable that far more women will suffer this mutilation than would ever have contracted a breast tumour.

'Relative' or 'absolute' risk

So just how much benefit can you truly expect from regular mammography? How effective is it in terms of saving lives? Before I answer those questions we need to understand the difference between *relative* risk and *absolute* risk.

Table 2.1: Benefits of mammography – breast cancer deaths

Trial	HIP New York	Two Counties Sweden	UK	Malmö Sweden
Reduction in *relative* risk of death	35%	29%	14%	5%
Reduction in *absolute* risk of death	0.02%	0.008%	0.006%	0.001%

If one person in every 100,000 of a population suffers an ailment, then the *absolute* risk is 1 per 100,000, or 0.001%. If the number of people suffering the disease doubles, there has been an apparently spectacular increase of 100% in the *relative* risk, but the *absolute* risk, at 0.002%, or 1 in 50,000, is still extremely small. When the pharmaceutical industry and the media want headlines, it is the more eye-catching *relative* risks that are quoted; the unspectacular absolute risks are rarely mentioned. Yet the *absolute* risks are the ones that matter: they are the ones that predict the likelihood of any one person suffering a complaint.

The effectiveness of mammography

In the trials tabled above, although *relative* benefits from mammography in four trials may look worthwhile, the reduction in *absolute* risk is very small; two of the results were so small that they did not achieve statistical significance.

You might argue that even a small chance of saving a life is worth doing and you might be right – if the screening process enhanced the likelihood of a cure, but there is absolutely no evidence that it does. Professor Samuel Epstein, of the University of Illinois, and colleagues pointed out the lack of benefit from breast cancer screening in 2001, saying:

> 'Even assuming that high quality screening of a population of women between the ages of 50 and 69 would reduce breast cancer mortality by up to 25% . . . the chances of any individual woman benefiting are remote. For women in this age group, about 4% are likely to develop breast cancer annually, about one in four of whom, or 1% overall, will die from this disease. Thus, the 0.75 relative risk applies to this 1%, so 99.75% of the women screened are unlikely to benefit.'[8]

On 20 September 1995, *Independent Television News* broadcast the news that breast cancer screening was a success. To demonstrate the benefits of mammography in detecting malignancies, the item stated that doctors had saved 7,000 women's lives. Let's look at that figure. Breast cancer screening is conducted routinely on women between the ages of 50 and

69. So that is the age group where benefits, if any, will be seen. In 1994, the most recent figures available at the time of that *News* report, the number of women in that age group who had died of breast cancer was 4,621.

By 2005, (the latest figures published at the time of writing this book), the reduction from 1994 was only 790. So where, I wondered, did that 7,000 figure come from? I was told that the reduction they claimed was a reduction from what they *thought figures would have been if nothing had been done.* They make it up as they go along!

Breast cancer screening has been recommended in Sweden since 1985. As a study published in 1999 found no decrease in breast-cancer mortality in that country, Drs P. C. Gøtzsche and O. Olsen at the Rigshospitalet, Copenhagen, did a meta-analysis themselves.[9] They concluded that: 'Screening for breast cancer with mammography is unjustified,' and continued:

> 'If the Swedish trials are judged to be unbiased, the data show that for every 1000 women screened biennially throughout 12 years, one breast-cancer death is avoided, whereas the total number of deaths is increased by six.'

Naturally, publication of this study caused a flood of letters disagreeing with its findings. The Swedes, however, were supported by the Canadian National Breast Screening Study-2 (CNBSS-2). That had been following more than 39,000 women assigned either to annual physical examination or to examination plus mammography since the mid-1980s. This found that, although mammography did lead to the discovery of smaller, earlier stage tumours, it still did not improve breast cancer survival rates over examination alone.[10]

Adverse effects

Modern mammography is so sensitive that it can detect very small abnormalities, the vast majority of which turn out to be quite harmless. For this reason, the value of mammography in detecting tumours is estimated to be less than 10%, meaning that more than nine out of every 10 of all positive results are false positives. Such over-diagnosis then leads to unnecessary breast removal and the trauma that accompanies such an operation. It also means that a great many unnecessary biopsies are performed. X-rays, exploratory surgery and biopsies themselves can all promote tumour formation.[11]

Mammography can start a cancer

When you have a mammogram, your breasts are X-rayed. It is no secret whatsoever that X-radiation causes cancer. We have known that for a century. 'Oh but, when a breast is X-rayed the dose is very small,' women are told. But according to the textbook, *Clinical Oncology for Medical Students and Physicians*: 'Tumor induction information for extremely low doses [of radiation] . . . has been difficult to obtain . . . [It] is the subject of great debate.'[12] In other words, we don't know! While one X-ray may not do much harm, radiation damage is cumulative, so what are the consequences of having annual mammograms for several years?

Mammography can spread cancer

When a breast is X-rayed, it is squashed between two plates, with enough force to cause pain. According to *Clinical Oncology*: 'Massage of a tumor is followed by massively increased numbers of circulating tumor cells in the bloodstream in animals. A few clinical studies suggest the same phenomena [in humans]'. Mammography is far more brutal than massage.

Mammography often turns up something that doesn't look as it should. When this happens, women are asked to return for a second examination – and another chance to do more damage.

Biopsies spread cancer

Breast cancer among women aged between 50 and 64 years has been increasing by 1.8% every year since 1990, an inexorable rise that cannot be fully accounted for by improved scanning programmes identifying more cases. When mammography finds things that cannot be resolved with a second mammogram, oncologists delve inside the breast to see what is there. This procedure, where tissue is removed for examination, is called a *biopsy* – more usually a 'needle biopsy' because a hollow needle is inserted through the breast tissue to the spot where the abnormality is thought to be and a piece is snipped off.

But biopsies themselves can promote tumour formation in two ways: firstly, by the inflammation and trauma in the surrounding cells, as inflammation increases the risk of starting a tumour;[11] and secondly, according to *Clinical Oncology*: 'a needle track may harbor nests of cells which may form the basis for a later recurrent spread.'

Researchers in a new study fear that biopsy may be playing a part in the spread of early-stage breast cancer, especially among women aged over 50 years.[13] It is the 50- to 64-year-olds who are more likely to have a biopsy; all other age groups have shown a decline in breast cancer rates over the same period.

In the vast majority of cases the borderline abnormalities revealed by mammography might be better left undisturbed.

Case history
My mother was an example of what can happen. She went into hospital
in August 1994 because she was suffering from a hiatus hernia. It was an
uncomfortable condition but hardly life-threatening. While she was
there, doctors gave her a full examination and found a lump in her
breast. My mother said she had known about this lump, which had given
her no symptoms, for over 20 years. However, the doctors did a biopsy
and pronounced the lump a malignant cancer. The following April, at
the age of 85, my mother died from a metastasis in her liver. Was it just
coincidence that her breast tumour spread at that time?

A study by researchers from the Nordic Cochrane Centre in Denmark
found that mammograms may harm 10 times as many women as they
help.[14]

Trials of mammography still go on. A study led by Joann Elmore, Professor of Medicine at the University of Washington School of Medicine,
Seattle, put women with and without breast cancer into two groups.[15] The
authors opined that if screening prevented women from dying from breast
cancer then the cancer-free group would contain a higher proportion of
women who had been screened. However, screening rates in the two
groups were the same. Checking cancer deaths over a 15-year period in
women aged 40 to 65, they say: 'We observed no appreciable association
between breast cancer mortality and screening history [regardless of age or
risk level].'

As breast cancer screening has potential adverse effects, Dr M. Baum,
Professor of Surgery at the Royal Marsden NHS Trust, London, believes
that women should be told the truth so that they can make an informed
choice as to whether they want to participate or not. Dr Baum is uncomfortable with the suggestion that General Practitioners should coerce
women into the programme without this information, but he could see
why the medical profession might not want to let women know – they
might stay away.[16] Dr Baum wrote:

> 'In absolute terms less than 1% of women who are invited for screening
> will benefit from it, whereas a greater percentage will have to face the
> problems of false alarms, unnecessary surgery, unnecessary labelling as
> having cancer . . . true informed consent for an invitation to screening
> might reduce rather than increase acceptance.'

If women really understood this issue, perhaps the practice could be
stopped. But they don't. An Irish study published in the *European Journal
of Cancer* found that although women and men were aware of breast cancer, they lacked accurate knowledge about it.[17] The researchers say: 'The
ignorance highlighted by this study makes it unlikely that the general

public or at-risk females could currently make sensible or informed decisions on a range of breast cancer issues . . . These problems might be redressed somewhat if impartial healthcare agencies provided accurate information.' But if they did that, would women subject themselves to the barbarity of mammography? And mammography may not even be the best way to detect breast cancer. Canadian researchers say that mammography screening is inadequate for detecting breast cancer in women who are at high risk of developing the disease.[18] They recommend MRI scans, which are less harmful, but more effective. The problem with MRI is that it is more expensive.

Cervical cancer screening

Cervical cancer is much rarer than breast cancer. This inevitably means more false positives and false negatives. The 10% of the female population found to have 'pre-cancerous cells' is some 100 times greater than the number of women who will go on to develop the disease. In other words, only one out of 100 positive results is likely to be cancer. Realistically, cervical cancer screening is so inefficient as a predictor of cancer that it is not worth doing.

Women given a positive result have shown considerable adverse psychological consequences.[19] In a study published in the *British Journal of Obstetrics and Gynaecology*, nearly 65% had anxieties about cervical cancer, 68% suffered tension, over 70% had mood swings, 50% found their sexual interest was impaired and over 40% had difficulty sleeping. Even where a negative (clear) result was given and women should have been reassured that they had no cancer, many had similar anxieties: over 43% worried about cervical cancer, 75% suffered tension, 68% had mood swings, 31% had impaired sexual interest; and more than a quarter had difficulty sleeping.

Two hundred and twenty-four women were screened for cervical cancer in a trial at Temple University, Pennsylvania, in 1990. Of them, 106 had normal test results which required no follow-up, but 118 were recalled for a further examination. Of the 65% who turned up, not one was found to have a cancer.[20] Imagine, however, how they must have felt when they got the letter calling them back for re-examination; and imagine how worried the 35% who did not go back must have continued to be.[21]

Between 1988 and 1993, 225,974 women were screened for cervical cancer in the Bristol Screening Programme. Abnormal cells were found in 15,551 of them; nearly 6,000 were referred for colposcopy (insertion of a fibre optic into the vagina for an optical examination). Dr A. E. Raffle and colleagues in Bristol pointed out that these numbers are excessively high compared with the actual numbers of cases of cervical cancer.[22] The number of women who would be expected to develop cervical cancer in a five-year period before screening began 40 years ago was in the order of 150 to 200. So, even if screening had controlled the numbers of deaths which otherwise would have occurred, that figure would not have exceeded 220. Thus over 15,000 women were wrongly told they were at risk and 5,800 investigated and treated – and left with lifelong worries about a cancer which they would never have suffered.

Despite a high take-up of invitations for screening, there has been no detectable reduction in deaths from cervical cancer as a result of screening. Over the country most of the women who die of cervical cancer *have* been screened.

Recently, the guidelines came under considerable criticism because of the lack of scientific evidence on which they were based.[23] One of the guidelines' authors was particularly outspoken on the subject.[24]

Cervical cancer is a violent and fast-acting cancer. Testing for it every three years inevitably means that most cancers will be missed. Professor James McCormick of Dublin University Medical School concluded that this screening: 'is an expensive contribution to ill health because the harm exceeds the possible benefits by a substantial margin.'

Many general practitioners would agree with that. But if they do not comply with guidelines set for them by government, that they get 80% of their female patients screened, they are liable to suffer financial penalties. And so they continue with this useless process.

Prostate cancer screening

In the early 1990s, it was fashionable in the US to screen men for prostate cancer although no trials into possible benefits had been done. It was politically correct to give men the same benefits as women. The same began to be applied to British men. And so another expensive screening programme was begun. Again there are serious doubts about its usefulness. Prostate cancer is a quiescent cancer which is very common in elderly men. But, since the operation is more radical than simply the removal of the prostate and often leaves the patient incontinent and impotent, it is unjustified in men who feel all right as they are.

The way that prostate cancer is tested for is either with a blood test to measure *Prostate-Specific Antigen* (PSA) or a digital rectal examination. Because men don't like the doctor to stick his finger up their backside – and doctors don't like doing it either – a PSA test is the normal method used.

But PSA is not only raised by cancer; it is also raised in *benign prostatic hyperplasia* and in *prostatitis*, neither of which is cancerous.

Being overweight or obese can also affect PSA levels: PSA goes down as weight increases; and riding a bicycle can raise PSA; and men can have advanced prostate cancer, yet also have a PSA reading of zero. It is now probably too late to undo the damage done to a generation of men who have undergone a PSA test and been treated because of the readings. Urologist, Professor Peter Whelan said of testing for PSA that it: 'promotes stress and anxiety'.[25] Which is assuredly true.

And after all this hoo-ha, a major study in 2005 suggested that, even if a man were found to have prostate cancer, the best thing for him to do was nothing.[26] In which case there isn't much point in testing for it. The fact is that many men will develop prostate cancer if they live long enough. But by far the majority die with it, rather than of it.

Early detection does not prolong life

Even if a cancer is discovered earlier, that doesn't necessarily mean the patient will live any longer. The cancer industry tends to measure its effectiveness in terms of 'five-year survival rates'. In other words, if you live for five years from first diagnosis of cancer, you are a 'success'. Let's look at a hypothetical case from two points of view:

Scenario One:

Mary discovers a lump in her breast when she is 50 years old. It is biopsied and confirmed as cancer. After treatment, the cancer metastasizes and Mary dies of it at age 54. As Mary didn't survive for the critical five years, the treatment is listed as a failure.

Scenario Two:

A routine mammogram finds that Mary has a breast tumour when she is 48 years old. It is biopsied and confirmed as cancer. After treatment, the cancer metastasizes and Mary dies of it at age 54. Mary did survive for the critical five years and she is logged as a success.

And this is exactly what does happen. Finding a cancer earlier merely gives a longer time between diagnosis and death. This means that Mary is scored as a victory for the cancer industry, even though she lived not one day longer.

Incidentally, if you die as a result of the cancer treatment you receive, you are also classified as a success – because you didn't die of cancer!

Summary

The problem is that the cancer industry is a multi-billion dollar industry, rife with conflicts of interest. Most contributions to cancer research go toward paying salaries and upkeep of buildings, not into cancer research – and certainly not to cancer prevention. Few in the cancer industry seem to be actively trying to prevent cancer. If they succeeded, they would all be jobless.

In the 20 years from 1970 to 1990, the cancer industry was worth an estimated one trillion dollars ($1,000,000,000,000) in the US alone.[27] That included contributions from a generous – but misled – public, treatment centres, and sales of chemotherapy drugs. Today the figure exceeds six times that amount. Yet we are no closer to finding a cure than we were 50 years ago. Despite President Nixon's famous 'War on Cancer' in 1971, we are still being prescribed the same three failing treatments for cancer: surgery, radiation treatment and chemotherapy, or slash, burn and poison, as they are more commonly called.

The central harm of screening for cancer is that it can detect pseudo-disease: an abnormality that meets the definition of cancer but either does not progress, or grows so slowly that an individual dies from another cause before the cancer ever causes symptoms. As screening tests become increasingly sensitive, the detection of pseudo-disease is bound to become an increasingly common problem. The follow-up procedures and psychological aspects engendered by such screening probably cause far more harm than any of the cancers screening is supposed to prevent.

Coronary heart disease screening

Because heart attacks are our 'biggest killer', it is fondly hoped that screening can be of the greatest benefit in this condition. But even today, we do not know what causes coronary heart disease and, without knowing its cause, cannot know how to cure or prevent it. As there is no point whatsoever in detecting a disease for which there is no known effective treatment, screening for it is a total waste of time and resources.

But some will say that we do know the cause of coronary heart disease: it is high cholesterol, or too much fat in our diets, or smoking, or not taking enough exercise, or one or more of 246 'risk factors' for heart disease that were identified in 1981.[28] That number is now several hundred more – which tells us that we really have little idea what causes coronary heart disease.

So, the first problem lies in deciding what to test for. As a predictor of coronary risk, total blood cholesterol turns out to be irrelevant,[29] and merely testing for that is regarded by many experts as misguided. Far more reliable, they claim, is measurement of HDL (the 'good' cholesterol). However, in tests of the accuracy of checking for HDL at various laboratories,[30] values differed by as much as 40% in 95% of the samples tested. A test of 16 instruments manufactured by nine companies in 44 laboratories found that, although the inaccuracies of the machines were lower at 3.6% to 4.4%, biases attributed to the methods used ranged from -6.8% to +25%.[31] A third study to evaluate the ability of cholesterol screening to detect individuals with blood cholesterol abnormalities concluded that 41% of those with abnormal levels would not be detected using present guidelines.[32]

To compound the machines' errors, an individual's blood cholesterol is constantly changing. There is a gradual increase in the general level throughout life quite naturally and this seems to be protective. It also changes from day to day and even from minute to minute quite naturally. Raised blood cholesterol is part of the 'fight-or-flight' reflex. If you run to the surgery your cholesterol will be higher than if you walk; if it is tested sitting down, it will be higher than if you are lying; if you are anxious about the result, that can elevate the level. Imagine that you are asleep in bed at 2.00 AM, and you are woken suddenly by what you are certain is a burglar. You will know how quickly your heart starts to race – well, that is how quickly your blood cholesterol level will rise – and for the same reason. The difference can be as much as 23%.[33] To put it in perspective, let us assume that you are around 30 years old and your cholesterol level is a perfectly respectable 6.0 mmol/l (230 mg/dL). You hurry to the surgery and are anxious about the result. This could raise it by 25% to 7.5 (288 mg/dL). If it is sent to a laboratory giving high readings it could be raised by a further 1.3 (50 mg/dL). Your perfectly normal 6.0 is now a high 8.8 (338 mg/dL)!

So many variables affect cholesterol levels that a one-off test is a waste of time and an unnecessary worry for the patient. Yet one-off readings are used as a basis for the prescription of a class of drugs that are the biggest money-spinners of all time – the cholesterol-lowering drugs called statins.

Statins

Have you ever wondered why the figure 5.2 mmol/L (200 mg/dl) became the 'healthy' level of cholesterol? According to a professor at the University of Maryland (who prefers to remain anonymous), it was an entirely political decision made on the floor of the National Institutes of Health Mazur Auditorium in December 1984. She told me: 'The decision would allow the National Heart, Lung and Blood Institute (NHLBI) to have yet another even more extensive long-term "trial" to work on. The NHLBI could not get more money from Congress for more large trials such as the MRFIT (Multiple Risk Factor Intervention Trial) or LRC (Lipid Research Council) and they were developing the National Cholesterol Education Program. With the cutoff number at the lower end of the normal range (200 mg/dL), they could include all of the healthy normal citizens in the range that would need treatment with diet, and since the diet would never work to permanently lower those normal levels to below 200 mg/dL, they could recommend that all these people should go onto cholesterol-lowering medications. The three men who were heading the NHLBI [I won't include the names] were standing together in the Mazur Auditorium just before the Cholesterol Consensus Conference began. They were discussing the cutoff level of serum cholesterol to put into the consensus report. One said to the other two, "but we can't have the cutoff at 240; it has to be at 200 or we won't have enough people to test." Several of us from the University of Maryland, Department of Chemistry Lipids Research Group were standing directly behind them and within clear earshot. We looked at each other and of course were not surprised when the final numbers came out.'

In 2001 the *Journal of the American Medical Association* published a 'Financial Disclosure' of the doctors who had set that 'healthy' cholesterol level.[34] It told readers that most were connected financially with the manufacturers of cholesterol-lowering drugs, and it named them.

The heart disease screening situation is similar to that of cancer screening: the expenditure of lots of money and resources with little perceivable benefit other than the sale of drugs!

Statins are the drugs of choice for high blood cholesterol (*hypercholesterolaemia*). There is no definition for hypercholesterolaemia, but if American doctors accept the NCEP guidelines, as they will be obliged to do when the guidelines form part of their 'standard of care' programme, nearly all Americans will soon be on a statin. And the rest of the developed world will not be far behind, because we all seem to follow the US example. We in Britain are actually ahead of the US as statins are already available here without prescription.

The statins whose patents haven't run out sell at over £1 per pill and they are taken at the dose rate of one pill, per person, per day – for life. As screening for 'high cholesterol' with a cut-off at 5.0 (recently down from 5.2, and they are currently talking of lowering it again to 4.0) will find that most people 'need' to take them, drug companies can look forward to an extremely lucrative period, at least until their patents run out. Currently the worldwide market for statins is worth upwards of £30 billion a year.

Between 1996 and 2002, prescriptions of cholesterol-lowering drugs, mainly statins, increased in Britain nearly six-fold from 3.1 million to 17.6 million items, costing the NHS a total of £571 million in 2002 compared with £93 million just six years earlier. You would expect that such a huge increase in expenditure would be supported by a similarly huge reduction in hospital admissions for heart problems. It wasn't. During the period, the

number of hospital admissions for heart attack or other heart problem fell by a meagre 4%.[35]
But that is only half the problem. Statin drugs have a wide variety of adverse side effects. Serious adverse events (SAEs) comprise one component of safety and are potentially the most important outcome measure in randomized trials. Regulatory bodies require SAEs, which include any untoward medical occurrence that results in death, is life-threatening, requires hospitalization or prolongation of hospitalization, or results in persistent or significant disability, to be collected in all clinical trials. In studies of statins these are rarely reported.[36]

Statins are now among the best-selling prescription drugs in the world and are widely viewed as very safe. Yet adverse effects reported with statins include gastrointestinal and neurological effects, psychiatric problems, immune effects such as lupus-like syndrome, potentially fatal muscle wasting, erectile dysfunction and breast enlargement in men, rashes and other skin problems, and disturbed sleep.

The only light on the horizon for some sanity is in the recently published Incremental Decrease in End Points Through Aggressive Lipid Lowering (IDEAL) study which compared the two most common statins: *simvastatin*, marketed as Zocor, and *atorvastatin*, marketed as Lipitor.[37] It was the first and only study so far to give a true report of adverse effects: nearly all of the participants suffered an adverse effect, half of which were listed as severe.

Despite these data, the British government is still bowing to commercial pressure and aggressively bribing doctors to prescribe statins, even to those who cannot possibly benefit from any cholesterol lowering.

Statins are not suitable for the elderly . . .

Irritability or short temper is a problem that occurs with statin therapy and resolves with its discontinuation.[38] This might seem a trivial problem, but for elderly patients who depend on others for assistance, irritability and its impact on their relationship with caregivers may have special implications.

Table 2.2: Adverse effects: the IDEAL Study (Data from the IDEAL's Table 4)

	Zocor	Lipitor
Numbers of participants	4449	4439
	No. (%)	No. (%)
Any adverse event	4202 (94.4)	4204 (94.7)
Any serious adverse event	2108 (47.4)	2064 (46.5)
Any adverse event resulting in		
permanent discontinuation of study drug	186 (4.2)	426 (9.6)

Heart failure may also occur in patients taking statin therapy. In some people, the heart-damaging effects of statins may impair heart pumping function.[39] However, in patients with reduced pumping function due to coronary artery blockages, statins may help heart pumping by improving blood flow to the heart.[40] It depends on the person whether benefit or harm dominates with statin therapy.

Statins inhibit the body's production of cholesterol. But they also inhibit the production of Coenzyme Q10 (CoQ10), which is enormously important for the heart, one of the biggest users of CoQ10.

One side effect of particular note for the elderly population, is that the PROSPER trial found a significant *increase in cancers* with statins.[41] Because statins have been reported to cause cancer in animals, the significant increase in cancer in this trial cannot be dismissed as necessarily a fluke. While a similar increase has not been seen in studies of statins in younger people, older people have poorer stores of the cancer-protecting antioxidant nutrients that low-density lipoprotein cholesterol helps to transport to body tissues. Even if the fractional change in risk were similar, the elderly have a higher risk of cancer.

While middle-aged men at high risk for heart disease did appear to get a small mortality benefit from statins,[42] no trend toward overall survival benefit is seen in elderly patients at high risk for cardiovascular disease.[41] Despite this, the elderly are seen by many GPs as at high risk for a heart attack and put on statins.

. . . or for women

I have seen many advertisements for statins in women's magazines, but women need to know that lowering cholesterol has not been shown to be of benefit to women of any age, whether or not they have had a heart attack.

Read the fine print

Lastly, if you need any more convincing that statins are not worth the huge amount of tax money that is spent on them, it's worth reading the fine print on the medication. In the US, where it's wise for manufacturers to be more open about their products, the blurb for the biggest selling statin, Pfizer's Lipitor, states:

> 'Important information: Lipitor (atorvastatin calcium) is a prescription drug used with diet to lower cholesterol . . . *Lipitor has not been shown to prevent heart disease or heart attacks.*' (emphasis added)

And it's the same with other statins. Since preventing heart attacks is the only reason for suffering this harmful drug, why on earth should anyone take it? The other statins also carry a similar disclaimer – although you might need a magnifying glass to read it.

Statins summary

The trials into statins actually disproved the cholesterol hypothesis as what protective effects were demonstrated were the same whether cholesterol was lowered a lot or not at all. It has become quite clear that the meagre benefits of statins are not related to lowering of cholesterol but to an anti-inflammatory property.[43] The current goal of lowering LDL to an arbitrary value, which is often difficult to achieve, inevitably ensures increasingly higher doses for longer periods of time.[44] This means more money for drug companies – and more adverse side effects, many of which are ignored or suppressed.[45,46]

The evidence of fallacy

The proponents of screening for heart disease risks want us to modify our lifestyles to avoid or minimize those 'risk factors'. But there is already a considerable body of evidence from expensive long-term trials that such a programme does not work. The five major studies, totalling a massive 828,000 man-years of study, came up with the following results: deaths due to coronary heart disease in the intervention groups totalled 1,015, and in the control groups, 1,049; the number of deaths from all causes was 2,909 in the intervention groups against 2,947 in the controls. That, at less than one death fewer in 2,500 men per year, is well within the limits of chance. In three trials where blood cholesterol had been the target, 115,176 man-years of observation showed a reduction of eight deaths from heart disease in the intervention group compared with the controls, but 35 more deaths in total, tending to confirm yet again that lowering blood cholesterol may do more harm than good.

Real confirmation came in an analysis of 35 randomized clinical trials. The paper's authors conclude that: 'population screening . . . whether in the high street or the general practitioner's surgery is not currently indicated. Such screening may, indeed, result in large numbers of people being treated for whom there are no benefits, or even net adverse effects.' They conclude that: 'Population cholesterol screening could waste resources and even result in net harm in substantial groups of patients.'[47]

Doctors are bribed to prescribe statins

The medical evidence does not support the notion that lowering cholesterol is a 'good thing'. Many other peer-reviewed studies, which we will look at in Chapter 22, are quite clear: lower cholesterol is associated with an earlier death. Despite this, General Practitioners are now signing new contracts of employment that include the Quality and Outcomes Frame-works (QOF), a system which awards points to GPs' practices for meeting government targets. Of the 1,050 QOF points available across the board, heart disease has some 550 points attached to it. The extra cash which can be earned by prescribing statins is around £64,000 per practice per annum. With incentives like this, GPs are going to be treat-ing patients primarily because of the extra cash it will bring them and treatment based on clinical judgement will become a thing of the past.

The question is: why on earth is the government so keen to pay GPs so much extra to do the job that they are already well paid to carry out? I can only think that the government wants to get everyone on statins be-cause the increasing numbers of elderly people are too expensive in terms of pensions, hospital beds, care homes, and so on.

It's a waste of resources

But that consideration aside, surely it is blatantly obvious today that the skills needed for *prevention* of lifestyle diseases are utterly removed from those of *treatment*. By relying on early detection of disease and treatment of symptoms found, no medical intervention will ever make a person healthy, however skilled, knowledgeable or well organized the practitioner is. Nevertheless, the fallacy that early diagnosis and various screening programmes will make us healthier still remains the priority today for most enthusiasts for prevention.

Dr P. Thomas, in a letter to the *British Medical Journal* in 1992, point-ing out that only one intervention trial had ever shown any evidence of benefit, told how 'well-man' screening makes men feel worse and causes depression.[48]

Conclusion

What we hear from those who would have us change our lifestyles is that, if we change, thousands of lives will be saved. This involves the fallacy of cheating death. We are not an immortal species, but have a biological life-span which is probably about 85 years. Some of us are programmed genetically to die earlier and others destined to get a telegram from the Queen. But not one of us will live for ever even if all diseases were totally eradicated.

As life expectancy is approaching biological lifespan in the western world, further increases in life expectancy are likely to be minimal. In these circumstances, even the gains which might be achieved by such un-realistic goals as the total elimination of cancer and heart disease must be relatively small. It has been calculated that if there were no cancer deaths before the age of 65, which is a pipe dream, mean life expectancy would be increased by only seven months. The best that all the screening and the mass interventions based on it can be said to have achieved is to transfer the cause of death from one category to another, an achievement which has no importance unless, perhaps, it is accompanied by the prolongation of useful and happy life.

Although screening to detect disease early sounds like a good idea, it hasn't proved to be so in practice. Figures show no evidence that screening for any disease is of much benefit to the consumer. Dr Halfdan Mahler, then-Director General of the World Health Organization, recognized this when he remarked in 1984 that the: 'major and most expensive part of medical technology as applied today appears to be far more for the satis-faction of the health professions than for the benefit of the consumers of health care.'

Dr Mahler's remark was confirmed in 2008. According to a *Guardian* article, NHS staff don't believe that their patients are the top priority; it is marketing and financial targets that matter most.[49]

The headlong dash by the 'health industry' to make ever bigger profits has led to a disaster of epic proportions. Professor Ian Roberts at the London School of Hygiene and Tropical Medicine recently described it as 'industry slaughter'.

Not only does screening appear to serve very little useful purpose, it is extremely costly. Costly but worthless interventions seem to be a recur-ring theme within the cash-strapped NHS. This whole screening programme, to which more conditions are likely to be added, does abso-lutely nothing to prevent any of the diseases targeted. It's aimed only at finding an existing 'disease' so that it can be treated.

There is a much better – and far less costly – way: don't treat disease, prevent it.

Chapter Three

How we got
to where we are

Since we were introduced to 'healthy eating' our health has deteriorated dramatically. How on earth did this sorry state of affairs come about? We look at how the battle against cholesterol and development of the 'diet/heart' hypothesis radically changed dietary recommendations for the worse.
The roles of cholesterol are explained.

> I beseech you, in the bowels of Christ, think it possible you may be mistaken.
>
> *Oliver Cromwell*

The reduction of blood cholesterol levels is a business worth billions to pharmaceutical companies, physicians and the producers of margarine, even though it is totally irrelevant, hazardous and quite frequently life-threatening. How on earth did we become so dependent on medicine, allow the 'health industry' to get such a hold over us, and to make us so ill? For the answer, we have to look at a piece of recent history. In the 19th century, we were free of most of the chronic diseases we are now suffering, so it is worth looking at what happened in the 20th century.

The British should eat more fat

Throughout our history a healthy diet was based mainly on foods of animal origin and high in fat. In Britain, the wealthy, who ate meat and dairy produce regularly, had average life spans which were comparable with or better than those of today. It was the poor who could not afford such foods who suffered high levels of infant mortality, poor growth and shorter, less healthy lives.

In the 1920s, Sir John Boyd Orr conducted a number of studies which compared growth rates of children in fee-paying schools with those in the state-run schools.[1] He found that those from wealthier backgrounds were significantly taller than their poorer peers. After examining their relative diets and changing the constituents, Boyd Orr proved conclusively that children of the socially deprived, who lived on a largely carbohydrate diet of bread and potatoes, benefited from a diet supplemented with full-cream milk.

Boyd Orr's studies found confirmation in observations by many other scientists. General Sir Robert McCarrison, a colonial medical officer, studied the peoples of India. He noticed that the southern Indians, who ate very little in the way of dairy produce, were of 'stunted growth' and prone to disease. He compared them with their neighbours to the north, the Sikhs. The Sikhs drank a great deal of milk and were fit and healthy.[2] Similar research in Africa contrasted the tall, slender and healthy Maasai, who lived almost exclusively on blood and milk from their cattle, with their unhealthy vegetarian neighbours, the Kikuyu.[3] That added to the weight of evidence. Boyd Orr concluded that the food intake of half the British population was seriously deficient in a number of what he called 'protective constituents' which were necessary for good health. Chief amongst these were foods of animal origin.

In the late 1930s he proposed that the British people should drink more milk, and eat more dairy produce and meat. The British government of the time recommended that milk consumption should be doubled and introduced free school milk. The British Medical Association advised that the population should consume 80% more milk, 55% more eggs, 40% more butter and 30% more meat. And later, with the advent of television advertising, the government sponsored its own 'go to work on an egg' campaign.

Except for the period of food rationing during the 1940s and early 1950s, Boyd Orr's recommended diet was the standard British fare. We ate breakfasts of eggs and fatty bacon fried in lard; dripping, the fat from the Sunday joint, was saved to have on bread and toast; we drank full-cream milk and ate butter. Only the poor ate margarine; and only they had high levels of disease. The recommendations to eat a relatively high-fat, high-animal protein diet led to a spectacular reduction in a wide range of diseases. Rickets, called the 'English Disease' because it was so widespread in England, together with a number of other deficiency diseases largely disappeared. Child deaths from diphtheria, measles, scarlet fever and whooping cough also fell dramatically – long before the introduction of antibiotics and widespread immunization. Although other factors helped, most important was the higher resistance of children to disease that followed from better nutrition.

However, a dramatic change was to come. Coronary heart disease was so rare before 1920 that most doctors had never seen a case, even if they had heard of it. During the next three decades all that changed as the death toll from coronary heart disease, originally called *angina*, rose dramatically. By the 1940s it had become a major cause of premature death. The rapid increase in the number of cases immediately set doctors searching for a cause.

Coronary heart disease

In 1915 a German pathologist published two reports of examinations of the coronary arteries of 140 soldiers who were killed during the First World War.[4, 5] The soldiers' average age was 27.7 years and yet, 65 of them had fatty build-ups, called *atheroma*, in their coronary arteries.

In 1951 pathologists were sent to Korea to learn about war wounds, again by dissecting the bodies of dead soldiers.[6] As they worked, they too noticed signs of coronary heart disease. So the pathologists launched a concerted study of the dead soldiers' hearts, performing a detailed dissection of the next 300.

When the small coronary arteries were dissected, the pathologists had expected to find their interiors to be slick and smooth. Instead, in 30% they found deposits sticking to the walls. Although these posed no immediate threat, they did show that degeneration of the arteries was well advanced long before the age at which heart attacks start to become frequent. In a further 41% they found fully formed lesions; in 3% of the soldiers these lesions were sufficiently large that they blocked at least one coronary artery. Thus, three-quarters of all the men examined showed evidence of serious coronary heart disease – and they were barely out of their teens.

Since the publication of those findings, other studies have been conducted which concentrate on younger bodies to evaluate the natural history of coronary artery plaques. One study, from New Orleans, found that everyone over the age of three who was tested had at least some fatty streaks in their aortas, and fibrous plaques had started to develop by the time they were in their teens.[7] By 1960 the New Orleans studies were extended.[8] The later studies revealed that fatty streaks were rare in the coronary arteries before the age of 10 but were more frequent in those in their teens, particularly in white males and, after the age of 20, were present in over 90% of all subjects regardless of colour or gender. By the age of 40, most also had fibrous plaques and advanced lesions in their coronary arteries.

These results stimulated the development of an international programme to compare them with findings in another 14 countries.[9] Data from studies of over 23,000 subjects showed wide geographical and racial differences: those from western industrialized nations generally had about three times as many lesions as those from less developed cultures.

The widespread and variable nature of the results from all these studies presented doctors with a problem. As there are no symptoms associated with the partial blockage of the coronary arteries, how could they tell, without a direct examination of those arteries, who was in danger? They had to find what was different in those with the disease and those free of it.

Cholesterol is blamed

The underlying condition in heart disease is the narrowing or hardening of the arteries that transport blood to various organs in the body. This transportation ensures that oxygen and nutrients are delivered to all areas of the body. The process by which arteries become narrow or hardened due to a build-up of material in their walls is referred to as *atherosclerosis*. This greatly inhibits circulation, and as the heart muscle is supplied in this way, a heart attack occurs when there is insufficient oxygen reaching the heart muscle.

In 1913 a Russian physiologist named Anitschkow conducted an experiment on rabbits that was to change the history of atherosclerosis for most of the following century.[10] The experiment consisted of feeding huge doses of cholesterol to rabbits, an animal which would never normally eat any food that contains cholesterol and whose liver is not equipped to excrete the excess. Not surprisingly, the rabbits' cholesterol shot up to very high levels and the concentrations proved toxic; some atherosclerosis of the blood vessels was discovered at autopsy. Anitschkow was no fool; he realized that this experiment had no practical significance for humans. Similar experiments on dogs, rats and humans showed that the rises in blood cholesterol and atherosclerosis didn't happen in them. This is because cholesterol is a natural part of their diets and their livers are equipped to cope with any excess.

In 1950, a team led by Dr John Gofman hypothesized that blood cholesterol was to blame.[11] Quickly, trials were conducted on rabbits based on Anitschkow's study and rabbits fed a high-cholesterol diet again developed blockages in their arteries. Several scientists pointed out that the results were more likely to be an allergic reaction to their unnatural diet. One, Ancel Keys, pointed out the error of the approach when he wrote in 1956: 'For many years there was argument as to whether cholesterol in the diet promotes atherosclerosis in man. One cause of the disagreement resided in the persistent error in attributing to man the same responses seen in rabbits and chicks fed large amounts of cholesterol . . . *It is now clear that dietary cholesterol per se, which is contained in almost all foods of animal origin, has little or no effect on the serum cholesterol concentration in man'.[12] (emphasis added).*

Is cholesterol really to blame?

If cholesterol does cause atherosclerosis, then the more cholesterol there is in the arteries, the more plaque there should be within the arterial walls. And as cholesterol decreases, so should the plaque. Gofman's group obviously weren't thinking clearly or, instead of playing around with rabbits, they would have done what two other scientists had done 14 years earlier.

In 1936, Drs Kurt Landé and Warren Sperry of New York University's Department of Forensic Medicine measured blood cholesterol levels in a large number of accident victims' blood and, by dissecting their arteries, measured their degree of atherosclerosis.[13] Landé and Sperry fully expected to find that the two were related. To their surprise, what they found, as you can see in Figure 3.1, was that they were not.

Landé and Sperry were very cautious, thorough and methodical; their study was well conducted. If those who later promoted the idea that blood

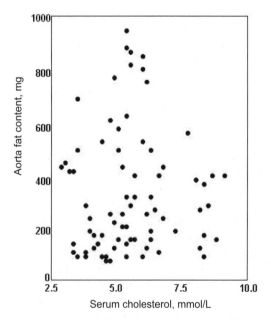

Figure 3.1: Blood cholesterol and atherosclerosis

cholesterol was to blame for coronary heart disease (CHD) had read this paper before they began their research, they might well have dropped the idea right there.

Landé and Sperry's results were confirmed by further studies in the 1960s. In 1961, levels of cholesterol and the degree of atherosclerosis seen at autopsy within the arteries of 20 recently deceased patients as well as 200 more cases selected from medical libraries were measured.[14] In all cases the measurements were taken shortly after death.

Again there was no correlation between these patients' blood cholesterol levels and the amount or severity of atherosclerotic plaque within the arteries. Cholesterol levels, whether high or low, had no impact on the growth of atherosclerotic plaque.

In 1962, another team led by Dr Z. Marek searched for a correlation between cholesterol levels and atherosclerosis in a further 106 cases and came up with similar results.[15]

Today we no longer need to wait for people to die; we can use electron beam computed tomography (EBCT) to look at and measure atherosclerosis and check cholesterol levels while people are still alive. Two scientists in New York did exactly that in 2003.[16] They were particularly concerned with atherosclerosis and LDL (the 'bad' cholesterol) levels. They chose 182 men as their subjects and then lowered their cholesterol levels with drugs. Then, over time, they measured atherosclerosis. What they found was that lowering cholesterol made not the slightest difference. They were forced to conclude that, with respect to LDL lowering, '"lower is better" is not supported by changes in calcified plaque progression.'

There have been many trials of cholesterol-lowering with a wide variety of drugs. As yet, there is no evidence, even with the latest statins, that any of them prolong life.

And there is actually no reason to suppose that it would, as LDL cannot be the cause of coronary artery disease, as we will see later.

Dietary fat

In 1953 Ancel Keys suggested that a fatty diet might play a part as a cause of CHD.[17] Using data from just six countries, Keys compared the death rates from CHD and the amounts of fats eaten in those countries to demonstrate, he said, that heart disease mortality was related to fat intake. As Figure 3.2 shows, there is an almost perfect fit (countries in bold).

And so the 'lipid hypothesis' (*lipid* is a word that encompasses fats, waxes and sterols) was born. However, at that time, data from another 16 countries were available. If they are added the picture is a lot less clear.

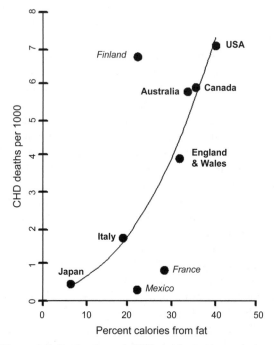

Figure 3.2: Fat intake and CHD deaths in six countries

For example, Finland near the top has seven times as many deaths as France, but Finns eat less fat; and Mexico has the lowest number of deaths, yet Mexicans have three times the fat consumption of Japan. These are three of the countries Keys didn't use.

Despite its faults, some of which didn't become apparent until later, Keys had what looked like a plausible hypothesis to explain the high levels of heart disease in some countries.

Now, anyone can have a hypothesis. What you have to do then is prove it. In medicine, the usual way is to select two groups of people, as identical for sex, age, and lifestyle as possible. One group, called the *intervention group*, tries the new diet, drug or whatever, while the other, called the *control group*, carries on as normal. After a suitable time, the two groups are compared and differences noted.

Keys' 'fatty diet-causes-heart disease' hypothesis was persuasive, but was it true? To test it, many large-scale, long-term, human intervention studies were set up in many parts of the world. These involved hundreds of thousands of subjects and hundreds of doctors and scientists and cost billions of dollars in an attempt to prove that a fatty diet caused heart disease. What they found was the opposite of what they expected.

The Anti-Coronary Club Project, launched in 1957 compared two groups of New York businessmen 49 to 59 years old. One group followed a 'Prudent Diet' which replaced butter with corn oil and margarine, eggs with cold cereal and skim milk, and beef with chicken and fish. A control group ate eggs for breakfast and meat three times per day.[18]

The report noted that the cholesterol levels of those on the Prudent Diet were significantly lower than the control group eating eggs and meat – but there were eight deaths from heart disease among the Prudent Dieters and no deaths from heart disease in the control group.

The longest running and most respected study is the Framingham Heart Study. It was set up in the town of Framingham, Massachusetts, in 1948 and is still going on today. It was this study that gave rise to other 'risk factors' with which we all are so familiar today: lack of exercise, smoking and so on. The Framingham researchers thought that they knew exactly why some people had more cholesterol in their blood than others – they ate more in their diet. To prove the link, they measured cholesterol intake and compared it with blood cholesterol.

As Table 3.1 shows, although subjects consumed cholesterol over a wide range, there was little or no difference in the levels of cholesterol in their blood and, thus, no relationship between the amount of cholesterol eaten and levels of blood cholesterol was found.

Next, the scientists studied intakes of saturated fats but again found no relation; there was still no relation when they studied total calorie intake. The researchers then considered the possibility that something was masking the effects of diet, but no other factor made the slightest difference. After 22 years of intense expert study and analysis, the researchers concluded: 'There is, in short, no suggestion of any relation between diet and the subsequent development of CHD in the study group.'[19] That was in 1970, and no finding since has changed that view.

The other studies also showed little convincing correlation between either the amount of fat eaten and heart disease or the type of fat eaten and heart disease, but there were a handful of exceptions. These supportive trials are cited far more often than the much larger number of unsupportive ones.[20]

Table 3.1: Cholesterol intake – the Framingham Heart Study

	Cholesterol intake mg/day	Blood cholesterol in those below median intake, mmol/L	Blood cholesterol in those above median intake, mmol/L
Men	704 ± 220.9	6.16	6.16
Women	492 ± 170.0	6.37	6.26

One that did seem to support the 'healthy' recommendations was a Finnish trial involving 1,222 men published in 1985.[21] Men in the intervention group were seen regularly and advised about diet, physical activity and smoking. Those with high blood pressure or high cholesterol levels were treated with drugs. The men in this group did as they were advised and, as a result, the 'predicted risks' for CHD were halved during the trial. It was hailed as a great success because: 'The program markedly improved the risk factor status.' In other words, they succeeded in changing their subjects' diets, and so on. In December 1991, the results of a 15-year follow-up to that trial were published.[22] During this period the intervention group had continued to be instructed on diet, smoking and exercise and treated for high blood pressure and cholesterol when present. Were they healthier? Did they live longer? The results are shown in Table 3.2 below.

These figures show that not only did those who continued to follow the carefully controlled, cholesterol-lowering diet had more deaths in total, they were also more than twice as likely to die of heart disease as those who didn't – some success!

Dr Michael Oliver, Professor of Cardiology at Edinburgh University's Cardiovascular Research Unit, commenting on these results in the *British Medical Journal*, wrote that:

> 'This runs counter to the recommendations of many national and international advisory bodies which must now take the recent findings from Finland into consideration. Not to do so may be ethically unacceptable. . . We must now face the fact that the evidence from large, well conducted trials gives little support to hopes that altering the lifestyle of the community at large, when started in middle age, will reduce cardiac deaths or total mortality.' [23]

If heart disease really did result from eating saturated fats – as we are told – it would be reasonable to expect to find more heart disease in the 19th century when the fats we ate were all from animal sources; and we could have expected a decrease in heart disease with the introduction of vegetable-based margarines and consequential reduction in intakes of butter and other animal fats in the early 20th century. Yet the reverse is true.

Results of some early studies of fats and coronary thrombosis suggested

Table 3.2: Deaths during 15-year follow-up

	Intervention Group	Control Group
Total deaths	67	46
Heart disease deaths	34	14

that individual saturated fatty acids were likely to cause blood platelets to clump together and form clots (thromboses). But these studies were conducted *in vitro* (in glass dishes), a method now known to give entirely the wrong results. For example, an *in vitro* study from 1962 reported that the saturated fatty acid, stearic acid, found widely in animal fats, considerably shortened the time needed for a clot to form whereas unsaturated fatty acids had almost no such effect.[24] In the model used, other saturated fatty acids commonly found in animal fats also increased clot formation. But contradictory results from other studies meant that results taken together were inconclusive. In 1996 a study looked at this whole vexed question by testing individual saturated fatty acids *in vivo* – in real, live people.[25] It showed the exact opposite of what had been observed in the laboratory studies: the saturated fats suspected of increasing the risk of a blood clot actually reduced the risk of clotting.

Another worry about saturated fats, that they might contribute to heart disease by adversely affecting blood cholesterol sub-fractions (HDL and LDL), has also been shown to be unwarranted. A study, presented at the Canadian Institute of Food Science and Technology's conference in June 2001 by Margaret French, of Canada's Department of Agricultural, Food and Nutritional Science, found that 112 grams (4 ounces) of beef eaten twice daily raised neither total nor LDL cholesterol any more than diets that were primarily of chicken, beans and pulses.[26] French also noted that saturated fats had benefits such as lowering stress hormone levels and improving blood flow.

CHD and saturated fat in Tokelau vs Pukapuka

Studies of human populations in a natural setting rarely allow us to compare like with like so that a single difference in diet can be studied. But two populations of Polynesians living on the Pacific atolls, Pukapuka and Tokelau, do provide such an opportunity. In 1981 the relative effects of their diets on cholesterol levels was studied.[27] Coconut is the chief source of energy for both groups; being over 90% saturated, coconut oil is the world's most saturated natural fat. The sole difference between the two populations is that Tokelauans obtain 63% of energy from coconut, compared with 34% among the Pukapukans. You won't be surprised to know that with almost twice the saturated fat intake, blood cholesterol levels are higher in Tokelauans. However, cardiovascular disease is equally uncommon in both populations.

Margarine causes more illness

With animal fats denigrated and the backing of the medical world, the vegetable oil and food processing industries who were the main beneficiaries of any research that found fault with traditional foods, began promoting cheap-to-produce vegetable margarines and cooking oils. These could now be sold at prices which rivalled the price of butter and animal fats. In 1983 a multi-year British study, the WHO European Collaborative Trial in the Multifactorial Prevention of Coronary Heart Disease (CHD), involving 18,210 men aged between 40 and 59, showed clearly that eating these was ill-advised.[28] Men who switched to 'healthy' margarines and vegetable oils had twice the death rate of those on an 'unhealthy' saturated fat diet, even though the men on the saturated fat diet also continued to smoke. Despite this, the authors perversely reported that: 'There was no clear effect on hard CHD end-points (coronary deaths and myocardial infarction) or on all-causes mortality.'

They continued: 'However, there was a 36% reduction in the rate at which intervention subjects reported ill with other CHD (principally angina) during the study, and at the end fewer intervention men gave positive responses to a self-administered questionnaire on angina and chest pain.' So was there some benefit? Apparently not. The authors say: 'These apparent benefits were not substantiated by electrocardiographic evidence, suggesting that participation in a heart disease prevention campaign may bias reporting of symptoms.' Ultimately, they ignored their own findings and presented a politically correct conclusion, saying: 'The implication for public health policy in the UK is that a preventive programme such as we evaluated in this trial is probably effective . . .'

Scientists at the Wynn Institute for Metabolic Research, London, compared the fatty-acid composition of artery blockages. What they found was a high proportion of both omega-3 and omega-6 polyunsaturated fatty acids; what they did *not* find was saturated fatty acids. They suggested that 'current trends favouring increased intake of polyunsaturated fatty acids should be reconsidered.'[29]

Ten years later two further studies published simultaneously in the *American Journal of Clinical Nutrition* reinforced the findings that saturated fats actually protected against heart disease. The first found that a so-called 'healthy' carbohydrate-based diet increased the rate at which older women's arteries degenerated and that increasing intakes of saturated fat actually slowed down the progress of their atherosclerosis.[30] The second study found what its authors called a 'paradox' when they showed 'that a high-fat, high-saturated fat diet is associated with diminished coronary artery disease progression in women with the metabolic syndrome, a condition that is epidemic in the United States.'[31]

Dietary paradoxes

'Paradox' is a word that is increasingly used in the context of diet and heart disease. This is because there are so many populations who eat pro-digious amounts of so-called 'unhealthy' foods but have low levels of heart disease.

The *French Paradox*, first described in 1987,[32] is perhaps the best known. It concerns the observation that the French have high consumptions of meat and fat, yet have low rates of heart disease. This is thought to be down to their intakes of red wine and olive oil,[33] but this hypothesis doesn't explain the other paradoxes.

For example, there is an *Alpine Paradox* in Switzerland where a great deal of high-fat cheese is eaten, red wine is conspicuous by its absence and olives don't grow;[34] and a *Greek Paradox*, where meat consumption is also higher than average.[35]

The *Spanish Paradox* is a good example of how researchers simply could not understand that these 'paradoxes' are not paradoxes at all; they actually provide evidence that high animal fat diets are the truly healthy way to eat. You will see what I mean when you read their findings and then their conclusions. This study noted that between 1964 and 1991 in Spain bread consumption fell by 55%, rice consumption fell by 35%, and potato consumption fell by 53%. Over the same period, there were also some spectacular increases: beef consumption rose by 96%, pork consumption went up by a huge 382%, 312% more poultry was eaten, and full-cream milk consumption rose by 73%.

The study noted that, during this period, heart disease deaths fell by 25% in men and by 34% in women; high blood pressure rates improved; and there were fewer stroke deaths.[36] Under the circumstances, you might expect that the authors would suggest that the dietary changes might have been responsible for the changes in patterns of heart disease. But paradoxically, they didn't. To say such a thing, when 'everyone knows' that fats and meat are bad for you, isn't politically correct. In their conclusions they state: 'Nevertheless, our results, in the context of current knowledge about the relation between diet and health, suggest several dietary recommendations that might be applied to the prevention of CVD [cardiovascular disease] in Spain: Promote moderate consumption of all meat (beef and pork in particular), increase consumption of foods rich in complex carbohydrates (bread, rice and so on) and encourage use of skim milk and low-fat cheese.'

In other words, they suggest that the Spanish should stop eating their protective and truly healthy diet, and change to our version of 'healthy'!

The *Italian Paradox* is not a dietary one, but is still another paradox as it runs counter to politically correct health advice. This concerns the observation that the Italians have very little cardiovascular disease – yet they are a nation of heavy smokers.[37,38]

Social deprivation is another 'risk factor' for heart disease. The *Albanian Paradox* concerns the fact that, although Albanians have the highest level of social deprivation in Europe, they have a coronary mortality rate which is similar to that of Italy, and only half the United Kingdom rate.[39]

In fact all across the Mediterranean region, heart disease rates are low regardless of the supposed 'risk factors' in various regions.

The *Northern Ireland Paradox* concerns a population with a great deal of coronary heart disease, but which doesn't have high rates of the expected 'risk factors'. Belfast has a coronary artery disease death rate that is more than four times higher than in Toulouse, France, despite almost identical coronary 'risk factors'.[40,41]

On the other side of the coin are those countries which do eat so-called 'healthy' foods but have higher heart disease deaths. One such is Sweden where a *reduction* in saturated fat consumption was followed by an *increase* in heart disease.[42]

The *Israeli Paradox* is similar – cardiovascular disease is high despite a high consumption of 'healthy' polyunsaturated vegetable oils.[43] Having one of the highest dietary polyunsaturated to saturated fat ratios in the world – Israel has a consumption of omega-6 polyunsaturated fatty acids 8% higher than the USA, and 10 to 12% higher than most European countries – Israeli Jews could be regarded as a population-based dietary experiment of the effect of the widely recommended polyunsaturated vegetable oil diet. However, despite such 'healthy' national habits, Israel has, paradoxically, a high prevalence of cardiovascular diseases, hypertension, type-2 diabetes and obesity. There is also an increased cancer incidence and total mortality rate, especially in women, compared with western countries.

And then there is the *Indian Paradox*, an observation that a high prevalence of coronary artery disease in urban Indians is associated with *low* saturated fat intake.

In 1967 Dr S. L. Malhotra, Chief Medical Officer for the Western Railway system, reported that in Madras, in the south of India, the population was vegetarian, living mainly on rice.[44] The principal fat in their diet was polyunsaturated peanut oil.

Malhotra compared the Madrasis with a population who lived in the north near Udaipur. Their religion allowed them to eat meat and their fat intake was almost entirely from animal sources and highly saturated. They cooked in ghee (clarified butter) and had what was probably the highest butterfat consumption in the world.

Present-day wisdom would predict that the vegetarians would have the lower rate of heart disease, but Malhotra found the opposite: the vegetarian Madrasis had 15 times the death rate from heart attacks compared with the northern Indians even though those in the north ate nine times as much fat – and that fat was animal fat. Twenty years later, a paper in the *Lancet* noted an increase in heart-attack deaths amongst the northern Indians.[45] By this time the northerners' diet had been made 'healthier' by replacing the traditional ghee in their diets with margarine and refined vegetable oils. This finding was confirmed by a third study conducted 10 years later when researchers found that a low saturated fat diet did not prevent heart disease in the citizens of the city of Moradabad in northern India.[46]

And lastly, another paradoxical pattern is seen in Japan. After the Second World War, and influenced by US eating patterns, the Japanese increased their consumption of meat and animal fats, and cardiovascular deaths fell.

These examples are hard to reconcile with the current paradigm of the causes of heart disease until you realize that they are not really paradoxes at all. What they really demonstrate is that our 'healthy' paradigm is wrong.

What about people who have already had a heart attack?

People who have had a heart attack are obviously at higher risk. They are invariably told by their doctors to cut out butter and use polyunsaturated margarines instead. But, as long ago as 1965 patients who had already had one heart attack were assigned to one of three study groups. These were given polyunsaturated corn oil, monounsaturated olive oil or saturated animal fats respectively. Blood cholesterol levels were lowered by an average of 30% in the polyunsaturated group, while there was no change in the other two groups. At first sight, therefore, it seemed that men in the polyunsaturated group had the best chance of survival. However, at the end of the trial only 52% of the polyunsaturated group were still alive and free of a second heart attack. Those in the monounsaturated group fared little better: 57% survived and had had no further attack. The saturated animal fats group fared the best with 75% surviving and without a further attack.[47] So yet again, saturated fat turns out to be the healthiest.

Cholesterol and women

Women seem to worry more about their cholesterol levels than men. Yet, for women, the evidence is that a high cholesterol level is healthier than a low one. In 1992 a report of 19 major studies published over the previous 20 years suggested that public policy for reducing blood cholesterol should be reviewed. The report's author, Dr Stephen Hulley, published figures showing the relative risk of death from all causes associated with

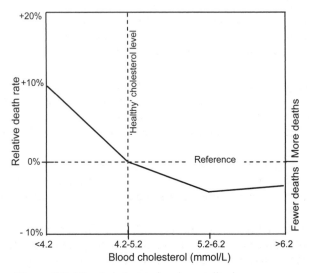

Figure 3.3: Blood cholesterol and mortality in women

levels of blood cholesterol in men and women. As can be seen in Figure 3.3, it is clear that risk for women increases as cholesterol levels fall.[48]

This confirmed a study published three years earlier by Dr Bernard Forette and a team of researchers in Paris. They found that elderly women with very high cholesterol levels lived the longest, and showed that the death rate was more than five times higher for women who had low levels of cholesterol in their blood.[49] In their report, the French doctors warned against lowering cholesterol in elderly women.

But they could just as well have warned against cholesterol lowering in women at any age as no study has ever found that lowering cholesterol in women is beneficial. In 2002 a report from the Framingham study showed that 80% of their women subjects who went on to have CHD had exactly the same total cholesterol concentrations as those who did not.[50]

Women will also be pleased to know that in a paper entitled *A Practical Diet For Weight Reduction*, Dr Broda Barnes of Colorado State University, noted that: 'No heart attacks have occurred during the use of diets rich in saturated fats for over 25 years.'[51] That was written over 40 years ago – and it is still true today.

What is cholesterol?

Having discussed cholesterol and heart disease, you might like to know just what cholesterol is and what it does.

The first thing is that cholesterol is not a fat: chemically it is an alcohol.

Cholesterol is one of a number of *sterols* widely distributed in plants and animals (although cholesterol is found only in animals). The richest sources of cholesterol are brain, fish roe, eggs, liver, hard cheese and butter.

Because of the propaganda, you can be forgiven for thinking that cholesterol is a harmful, alien substance which should be avoided at all costs, but nothing could be further from the truth. Cholesterol is an essential ingredient for many body processes:

- Body cells are being broken down and replaced all the time. Obvious examples are finger nails, hair and skin cells, but almost all body cells are replaced many times over during a person's life. Cholesterol is a major building block for this process.
- If you radically restrict your cholesterol intake to the point that there is not enough cholesterol to repair and build tissue, cell growth is disrupted.
- Cholesterol is vital for keeping cell membranes throughout the body intact and permeable so that nutrients can pass into the cells, and waste products can leave them.
- It is also found in the brain and nerve cells, where it is essential for nerve transmission and for brain function.
- It is used to maintain normal hormone production including the sex hormones in both men and women.
- It is essential for the proper functioning of the immune system.
- It is used, in conjunction with sun on the skin, to make Vitamin D_3.
- It is used to make bile acids, essential for proper digestion of fats and in ridding the body of waste products.
- Cholesterol is so important that practically every body cell can make it.

'Good' and 'bad' cholesterol

At this point, let me scotch another myth: there is no such thing as 'good' and 'bad' cholesterol. That is perhaps one of the most pervasive medical myths out there, created and perpetuated by pharmaceutical advertising. Cholesterol is one chemical compound and *all* cholesterol is exactly the same. Talking of LDL and HDL as if they were two different types of cholesterol is misleading.

Cholesterol is not water soluble so it cannot travel freely in the bloodstream to where it is needed. It is transported in little packets together with other materials, notably fats and proteins. These little packets are called *lipoproteins*, a contraction of the words 'lipid' and 'protein'. LDL stands for *Low-Density Lipoprotein* and HDL is *High-Density Lipoprotein*. LDL and HDL are not cholesterols, they are merely the *carriers* of cholesterol. LDL carries cholesterol from the liver out around the body to where it is needed for cell repair and all the other jobs that cholesterol does; and, as the body abhors waste and is a great recycler, HDL carries 'second-hand' cholesterol from cells being replaced back to the liver for re-use. Neither HDL nor LDL is 'bad'; both are essential.

Studies shatter the HDL = 'good', LDL = 'bad' myth

As I was writing this, three studies really scotched the myths about LDL and HDL. The first, published in the *Journal of the American College of Cardiology*, was to determine the relationship between established cardiovascular risk factors such as cholesterol, LDL, triglycerides, C-reactive protein, and others, and the extent of coronary atherosclerosis.[52] The most significant finding as far as this chapter is concerned was that LDL was *not* a predictor of greater disease. This was confirmed by a joint Canadian and American group who also found that levels of LDL did not predict CHD.[53] To rub this in, the third research team showed that it was raised levels of *HDL* which predicted recurrent coronary events in some heart attack patients.[54] Studying the interaction between LDL, HDL and inflammation in the THROMBO (Postinfarction Thrombogenic Factors and Recurrent Coronary Events) study, researchers showed that in a subgroup of patients, only elevated HDL was a significant and independent predictor of risk. What these studies say, therefore, is that LDL is not 'bad' after all and HDL isn't necessarily 'good'. Which, of course, is the exact opposite of what we are told.

Confirmation of the falsity of the LDL = 'bad' myth became apparent in 2007 with a study which showed that of 270,655 hospitalizations from 541 hospitals, fully half the patients hospitalized with coronary artery disease had very low LDL levels of less than 2.6 mmol/L (100 mg/dL);[55] and more than one in six had LDL levels below 1.8 mmol/L (69 mg/dL).

High cholesterol protects the heart

Another study published in 2006 said that the idea that high cholesterol levels cause heart failure and heart disease may be one of the greatest myths of modern medicine. In fact, high cholesterol levels may protect some people from a fatal heart attack, and the widespread use of cholesterol-lowering drugs such as statins may have little or no benefit.[56] These conclusions were supported by a separate study which criticized the new recommended low levels of LDL. Researchers from the University of Michigan concluded that the new low levels for cholesterol had no scientific validity; the drive to reduce LDL to the lowest levels ever recommended for patients at highest risk may be a wild goose chase.[57] Dr Andrew Clark of Hull University and one of the research team members said: 'In contrast to what you might imagine, having a high level of cholesterol might be good for you.'

Eat as much cholesterol as you like

Your body can absorb only about 300 milligrams of cholesterol per day from the foods you eat and, as your body needs many times that amount, it then makes up the difference. Although the major proportion is manufactured in the liver, almost all body cells can make cholesterol. For this reason, if you cut down on the amount you eat, your body simply makes more. And you can eat foods containing as much as five times the usual 300 mg without it having any significant effect on the amount of cholesterol in your blood. So it doesn't matter how much cholesterol you eat.

Summary

Although the media and food companies still warn against cholesterol in diet, it has been repeatedly demonstrated over the last 35 years that the amount of cholesterol you eat has little or no effect on the level of cholesterol in your blood, and that cholesterol – whether total, HDL or LDL – is *not* a good indicator of possible heart attack risk. It has also been shown that the only fats which are harmful are the ones found in polyunsaturated margarines and cooking oils, and manufactured products which contain them: cakes, biscuits, commercially fried foods, and many more. 'Such discrepancies', says Dr Uffe Ravnskov, an internationally renowned expert on cholesterol and heart disease, 'indicate that the association between high cholesterol and CHD is not due to simple cause and effect. The most likely interpretation is that high cholesterol is not dangerous in itself but that it is a marker for something else.'

What has become quite clear is that blood cholesterol is a relatively poor predictor of who will have a heart attack. It is also clear now that the hypothesis that a fried breakfast is a 'heart attack on a plate' is based more on myth than on any coherent body of supportive evidence.

No mechanism means no hypothesis

People have been led to believe that atherosclerosis is a build-up of fat or cholesterol inside the arteries, with LDL being the major culprit. But that is not the way it works. The plaque that is atherosclerosis actually forms not in the bloodstream in the arteries but within the artery walls. The walls of the tubes that are arteries have three distinct layers. The innermost layer is the *endothelium*, a smooth and slick lining that is only a single cell thick but is completely impervious to blood. Around that is a much thicker layer of smooth muscle cells; and around that is the third layer which holds it all together and stops the artery bursting.

The cholesterol hypothesis tells us that LDL passes through the endothelium, into the smooth muscle cell area. It is then oxidized and, since our bodies recognize that oxidized LDL is harmful, cells called macrophages which are designed to mop up harmful bacteria, particles, and so on, engulf the oxidized LDL. As macrophages don't know when to stop, they keep on eating away until they turn into foam cells. This is the basis of an atherosclerotic plaque. As this is going on, smooth muscle cells migrate into the area, expanding the plaque so that it reduces the area of the artery, restricting blood flow. The plaque eventually ruptures, putting pieces of debris into the artery which can cause a blockage further downstream.

But there are some questions that need to be answered before this hypothesis can be accepted. For example, plaques only form in certain arteries, never in veins or capillaries, and not in the pulmonary arteries which carry blood to the lungs to be oxygenated – despite the fact that these are bathed in the same 'bad' LDL, and all blood vessels are essentially the same.

And think about it: if blockages of this kind were the cause of coronary artery disease, you would expect the smaller arteries to become blocked before the larger ones, yet the opposite is the case.

Then there is the big question of how LDL gets through the endothelium in a healthy person, because the endothelium is a barrier to LDL. Despite 50 years of research no-one has yet been able to show by what mechanism this process is supposed to happen. There are other problems as well, but if you don't have a mechanism, you cannot have a hypothesis; without this, the whole LDL hypothesis falls flat on its face.

And then we come to the so-called 'good' HDL. Just like the Seventh Cavalry, HDL comes along, sees all this going on in the artery wall, screeches to a halt, sucks the LDL from the plaques and returns it to the liver. And just as nobody has found a mechanism by which LDL is supposed to do its dastardly work, neither is there an explanation of how HDL is supposed to operate in this way. The whole idea is based on unfounded speculation.

This is the shaky basis for an enormous health industry which is proving to be such an unmitigated disaster as, since 'healthy eating' was introduced two decades ago, the numbers of cases of the diseases covered in this book have rocketed. As will be demonstrated, this is not a coincidence; it is cause and effect.

To be fair, not all of this clinical evidence had been published when the American Heart Association and British COMA committees launched 'healthy eating' on us in 1982 and 1984 respectively. But a lot of it was, and there was a great deal more that was not only available but potentially far more valuable, which appears not to have been considered at all. But why is it not considered now? If I can find this information, why can't those in the establishment?

So why are we still trying to lower cholesterol?

The reason seems to be because some doctors jumped the gun. The Framingham Heart Study's first pronouncement wasn't until 1970, but people were dying of heart disease, and the arguments for fat being a cause seemed to make sense. In 1968, Dr J. B. Hickie in Melbourne, Australia, suggested that the situation was too urgent to wait for convincing evidence from organized trials.[58] He estimated that by changing to a low-fat diet and taking more exercise, mortality from heart disease would drop by 40% in men over 40 years of age. Many other doctors had similar faith. By the time the large human intervention studies started to be published in the 1970s and 1980s, doctors had been telling people to cut down on fats for so long that most couldn't reverse their advice without the risk of losing face and credibility. But some did speak out. In 1983 Professor Michael Oliver reminded doctors:

> 'Oliver Cromwell wrote in 1650 . . . "I beseech you, in the bowels of Christ, think it possible you may be mistaken." This admonition might now be appropriately addressed to some of the epidemiologists and the many overenthusiastic health educators concerned with the prevention of coronary heart disease, for the evidence against substantial benefit to the community from multiple risk factor intervention is increasing.'[59]

You won't be surprised to learn that Professor Oliver went unheeded. The juggernaut had already started to roll the previous year when the American Heart Association published its dietary guidelines recommending a reduction of fat intake and a change to polyunsaturated oils.[60] Britain followed immediately in 1983 when the National Advisory Committee on Nutrition Education (NACNE) published a discussion paper which suggested cutting fat intake;[61] and the following year the Committee on Medical Aspects of Food Policy (COMA) published official guidelines for dietary policy.[62] All three were remarkably similar. By now the 'fatty diet causes heart disease' dogma was official. Nothing would be allowed to stop it. And over the last quarter of a century, our health has gone inexorably downhill.

It's getting silly

Figure 3.4 shows that at least one Texas laboratory now includes 0 mg/dl

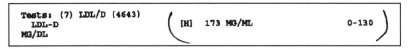

Figure 3.4: Detail from patient's blood test result showing LDL. (The 0-130 on the right indicates the 'normal' range.)

in the normal reference range for LDL cholesterol.

You might consider that, in view of the very important part cholesterol plays in our bodies, having none at all is extremely hazardous. In fact, of course, the only living things that have cholesterol levels that low are plants!

It really is getting very silly indeed.

Conclusion

Since 1982 in the US and 1984 in UK, when we were introduced to the concept of 'healthy eating', many studies have demonstrated that far from being a killer, the so-called, unhealthy diet we are told to avoid by the nutritionists may actually protect us against heart disease!

Now we need to know why.

Chapter Four

Learning from history

If we are to right the health of western societies, we could do worse than look at the way populations we call primitive manage to stay entirely healthy, despite (or because) they have none of our advanced scientific knowledge. The story of pemmican tells how nutritionists, even a century ago, consistently undermined traditional healthy dietary practices.

> If we do not learn from the past, we remain in the infancy of knowledge.
>
> *Cicero*

After the advent of 'healthy eating' nutritionists and dieticians started to dictate dogmatic recommendations based, they said, on the findings of dietary studies. But the studies they used were conducted in clinical settings and were biased by what was perceived as a healthy diet. So, instead of looking at the real world – the real experts on diet are those who live long, healthy lives on their particular diets – they based all their advice on studies conducted in unnatural conditions. And that has led to *unhealthy* advice. It is no secret at all that cases of obesity, diabetes and associated conditions have increased spectacularly since 1984. This, as I hope to show, is not a coincidence, but a prime example of cause and effect.

In this book I have included examples of nutritional nonsense which should be obvious even to those with no background in nutrition or dietetics. I have also included contradictions that regularly issue forth from such bodies as the British Dietetic Association, or American Diabetic Association. It is they who advise doctors and government. When you read these, you will begin to realize why our health has declined so alarmingly since we were introduced to 'healthy eating', and why it is so difficult to find dietary advice today that may actually do some good.

But first, let's look at the real world, the healthy world.

Back to the future

In his 1939 book, *Nutrition and Physical Degeneration*,[1] Dr Weston A. Price presented descriptions and photographs of primitive peoples and their environments in their primitive state and, for comparative study, descriptions and photographs of members of the same tribes who had been in contact with Europeans. He recorded the effects of that contact as expressed in physical and character changes. To make this a worthwhile contribution to our knowledge, it was necessary for Price to study a wide variety of primitive groups and physical environments. This work entailed 10 years of travelling around the world.

In order to help our society, Dr Price thought it important to find out not so much why we succumbed to so many diseases, but why primitive people did not. His purpose was to glean information that would be, in his words, 'useful in preventing race decay and deformities, in establishing a higher resistance to infective diseases, and in reducing the number of prenatal deficiency injuries. These latter include such expressions as mental deficiencies caused by brain defects in the formative period, which result in mental disturbances ranging from moderate backwardness to character abnormalities.'

What Price found was that all societies, eating traditional foods, were healthy; and all those who had succumbed to 'civilized' ways of eating were not.

Many other doctors, medical missionaries, explorers and anthropologists have found the same thing: people eating their traditional diets had (and still have) none of the degenerative diseases we are prone to today.

There may be other reasons than this for this lack of chronic illness in 'primitive' societies, but it is certainly possible that our health professionals are at least in part responsible for our present sorry condition.

Pemmican and the nutritionist

Let me give just one example of how nutritionists have always seemed to be wrong with the story of pemmican.

Pemmican was a food made by the indigenous North Americans long before Europeans invaded their country; it was also copied and used by European hunters, trappers, explorers and anthropologists for hundreds of years. On a diet of pemmican alone, they performed amazing feats of endurance and exploration.

Pemmican is a simple food which traditionally has just two ingredients: lean meat and fat; anything else was considered accidental and extraneous. The first step in the making of pemmican is to dry the lean meat of buffalo, caribou and moose or, later, beef. To ensure it dries quickly, all the fat is removed and the lean meat is sliced thinly.

The next step is to pound the dried meat into shreds. After this, special rawhide bags, about the size of a pillow case, are made to hold the finished product. With the bag prepared, it is filled lightly and fluffily with shredded lean meat.

Fat, often suet from around the kidneys, which is the hardest fat, is then rendered down and poured into the bag so that it percolates everywhere, a film of it covering every shred of lean meat. The finished mix is 50% lean meat and 50% fat by weight. And traditionally that is it.

Disputes over pemmican

Throughout anthropological texts you will find nothing but praise for pemmican. What is interesting to read is what those who actually ate pemmican say of it, compared with the comments of nutritionists who generally had no such experience. In his 1873 book, *Ocean to Ocean*, Dr George Monro Grant wrote:

> 'Pemmican is good and palatable uncooked and cooked . . . It has numerous other recommendations for a campaign diet. It keeps sound without being canned or salted for twenty or thirty years, is wholesome and strengthening, portable, and needs no medicine to correct a tri-daily use of it . . . All joined in its praises as the right food for a journey, and wondered why the Government had never used it in war time . . .'[2]

Both while in the army and later, Brigadier Hiram Martin Chittenden made a special study of pemmican. His book, *The American Fur Trade of the Far West*, published in 1902, is generally recognized as the greatest work in this field. Chittenden says of pemmican:

> 'The Indians had another process of curing buffalo meat, equal, if not superior, to the most approved canning processes, and wholly free from the use of chemicals . . . This was the much used pemmican . . . it would last indefinitely and was always ready for use without cooking. It formed a very palatable as well as nutritious food.'

Admiral Robert Edwin Peary was one of the greatest Arctic explorers. In his book, *Secrets of Polar Travel,* Peary wrote that:

> 'Too much cannot be said of the importance of pemmican to a polar expedition. It is an absolute *sine qua non.* Without it a sledge-party cannot compact its supplies within a limit of weight to make a serious polar journey successful . . . With pemmican, the most serious sledge-journey can be undertaken and carried to a successful issue in the absence of all other foods.
>
> 'Of all foods that I am acquainted with, pemmican is the only one that, under appropriate conditions, a man can eat twice a day for three hundred and sixty-five days in a year and have the last mouthful taste as good as the first.'[3]

The Admiral added that in 20 years of use he and his men never tired of pemmican, 'Yet nutritionists of the United States Navy are responsible for instructions that pemmican shall not be used in that service.'

The famous anthropologist and explorer, Dr Vilhjalmur Stefansson, wrote a great deal about pemmican in his book, *The Fat of the Land*. He also discussed at length the differences of opinion between those who had actually used pemmican and nutritionists who had not.[4]

According to Stefansson, pemmican's 'most impressive record as the exclusive diet, or nearly so, of large numbers of men for long periods, is from transportation crews of the fur trade working twelve to eighteen hours a day and straight through the noon period with its scorching or steaming heat.'

The history of pemmican shows that it was a complete food: a man could live healthily and work hard in any climate for years at a time. It was the only food which ever met such demanding calls upon it. But despite all this evidence, there were those who opposed pemmican saying that it was not a complete or a wholesome food, that it was not capable of maintaining full health and strength indefinitely. They also said that it was 'so unpalatable that this quality by itself would prevent its use'.

There were similar disputes about how long it would keep without going bad. There was no disagreement among Native Americans, European trappers and hunters, explorers or historians of the North American frontier: for all of them, pemmican was 'among the most preservable of foods. Cases are on undisputed record where packages of pemmican, wrapped only in rawhide, were in good condition after twenty and more years, without any preservative, and without protection from the weather other than that given by the leather covering.' On the other side of the debate, nutritionists during World War II stated that: 'the control of enzyme action in pemmican is as yet an unsolved problem and that the food will spoil rapidly unless canned.'

There was such animosity to pemmican that a war was fought over it in North America. Stefansson relates:

> 'The Pemmican War of 1814-1821, although mainly in Canada, spilled over into the United States, and reference to it can be found in works such as the *Dictionary of American History*. The disputes between those who wanted to use pemmican in the Second World War and those who were determined it should not be used became so emotional, violent and broadly spread, at home and abroad, that it was suggested we had a war within a war, the Second Pemmican War within the Second World War.'

Nutritionists 'improve' pemmican

This 'war within a war' came about because of nutritionists' misguided ideas on what constituted a healthy diet. Ideas differed very little in the 19th century from what is preached today. Note that many who actually lived on pemmican said how palatable it was and that they could eat it every day without ever becoming tired of it, while others said that it was so unpalatable that they couldn't eat it. These discrepancies become understandable when we learn that nutritionists had changed the recipe for pemmican to make it 'healthy'.

Admiral Peary wrote: 'On a still later expedition I was persuaded to purchase some so-called pemmican of a foreign make. This, after I had sailed and it was too late to remedy the error, I found to be largely composed of pea-flour.' The reason for the pea flour was the theory current at the time that 'fat burns only in the flame of the carbohydrates'. It was an entirely false belief that fat couldn't be utilized by the body unless it was eaten with carbohydrates. The pea flour had been added to the pemmican to provide enough carbohydrate to do the 'burning'.

For permanent good health there must be a certain minimum amount of protein. Pemmican furnished this through its shredded or powdered lean meat. The fat element, which is largely used as the energy source, could, however, be replaced by a carbohydrate – starch or sugar – as both provide a source of energy. However, because of the lower energy density of carbohydrates, every gram of fat removed needed to be replaced by about two grams of starch or sugar. If dried fruit, such as berries or raisins, was added, as it frequently was, the case was even worse: it takes far more than two grams of raisins to make up in nourishment for one gram of fat. Nevertheless, that was exactly what was done – and that not only changed pemmican; it degraded it with disastrous results.

Pemmican's chief claim to excellence was that it got the maximum energy from the minimum weight and bulk. The nutritionist-formulated 'pemmican' that contained raisins, shredded coconut, pea meal, sugar, and the like, was no longer light or compact in proportion to energy value, and it ceased to have the real pemmican's great advantage over other food. So, by progressively adding more and more fruit, sugar or flour to make the food more 'healthy', bulk and weight were increased with no increase in nutritional value. This meant that either a great deal more needed to be carried, or shorter campaigns and expeditions must be undertaken.

The change of recipe had other, serious consequences as well. True pemmican, made exclusively of dried lean meat and rendered fat, was as good, fresh and palatable after 20 or 30 years as the day it was made. Pemmican which had dried berries in it went bad rapidly unless canned. 'Pemmican' made for use in World War II, contained not only a great deal of sugar, vegetable oil and peanuts but even had chocolate to take the place of the lean beef.

It was this 'healthy' pemmican that was unpalatable and detested by the troops.

Case history

In 1912, Captain Robert Falcon Scott and his South Polar expedition team all died on their way back from the Pole, only 11 miles from their home base. The blame for this is put on the fact that they were trapped in a storm and ran out of food. The real cause, I believe, was that they didn't have traditional pemmican with them, but a heavier, lower energy, 'healthy' sort of candy bar. With proper pemmican, which weighed a great deal less and which would have provided them with far more nourishment, they could have carried sufficient for a much longer time. I am convinced that Scott's party was effectively killed by their nutritionists.

A high-fat diet is also ideal for the tropics

Another claim by nutritionists was that, while high-fat food might have some merit in Arctic conditions, it was no use at all in a temperate or hot climate. However, the Plains Indians used pemmican chiefly as a summer food. Journeys were usually made in summer and as pemmican was light and kept well, it was the food of choice for travelling 'where midsummer temperatures go above 120°F [49°C] in the shade occasionally and above 100°F [38°C] frequently'.

Earl Parker Hanson wrote extensively about the diet he found among tropical peoples in both Africa and South America.[5] His experiences with pemmican were based on a personal conviction that meat 'including the proper amount of fat' was 'every bit as necessary for health and energy in the tropics as in the North' and he tells of how 'the pygmies of the tropical Ituri forest will run miles to gorge themselves on the fat of a recently killed hippopotamus.'

Hanson had long wondered about the glaring discrepancies in the nutritionists' arguments to the contrary. 'On the one hand', he tells us, 'they say that fat is the most efficient energy food known; on the other they talk in doleful tones about the "debilitating" effects of the tropical climate. Why you should be careful to avoid energy-giving foods in a climate that supposedly saps your energy has always been beyond me.'

Hanson's first experience with fat shortage came on his 1931-1933 Orinoco-Amazon expedition. It started when his canoe Indians almost went on strike because he hadn't included sufficient lard or other fat in his supplies. That was a situation that almost every newcomer to the Orinoco ran into, and the Indians made sure, before starting a journey, that their hirer had plenty of fats with him. Hanson says:

'I bought enough fat to please my Indians, and then proceeded to eat on the journey from a separate pot, because I "couldn't stand their greasy food." It wasn't many weeks, however, before I avidly grabbed at every turtle egg I could get hold of – for its rich oil as I now realize – and at every Brazil nut, avocado pear, and every other source of vegetable fat, when I couldn't get animal fats.'

If he were going on another journey to the Amazon basin, Hanson says he would either take pemmican with him from the United States or spend some time in Brazil making pemmican before starting an expedition.

Hanson wasn't without his critics in the US. When he claimed that any healthy white man could stay in perfect health on any diet that keeps native populations and 'primitive' peoples in health, one ethnologist told him that he was quite wrong. She said she had tried such a diet for some weeks in Mexico, with almost disastrous results. Hanson asked her if she hadn't had trouble adjusting her taste to the 'greasy' food of the Mexicans. She replied that 'of course' she and her companions had eaten 'exactly what the Mexicans ate', but had taken pains to prepare the food in a more appetizing way by leaving out the grease! The 'disastrous results' she then described were typical symptoms of fat-shortage: constant hunger, discomfort, lack of energy, distended stomach, and so on.

Hanson's experiences had a profound effect on him. On returning to the US and a mixed diet, he changed his food habits: where previously he had cut the fat off his meat and left it, he now ate all the fat he could get hold of. Despite this he said that: 'In fact, there are times now when I have a real craving for fat, and a longing to return to the pemmican regimen . . . As soon as wartime restrictions are lifted on meats, and such animal products as cheeses, my diet is undoubtedly going to consist very largely of such foods. And if I return to the Amazon basin, I will never again differentiate between my meals and those of my Indians on the ground that the latter are too fat.'

An amusing but frustrating occasion occurred when Hanson decided to experiment with three types of pemmican: in terms of calories, Type A was 80% fat and 20% lean; Type B was 70% fat and 30% lean; and Type C was 60% fat and 40% lean. The dieticians warned him when he started that he would endanger his health, because they 'knew' from years of research that a fat intake of more than about 35% of calories was dangerous.

Hanson wasn't deterred. 'At first I preferred the lean "Type C" pemmican, because I wasn't used to eating much fat,' he wrote. It wasn't long, however, before he began to realize that it was unsuitable. He tried the other two and found that the fat Type A pemmican was completely satisfying. When he had only the lean Type C pemmican for several days, Hanson emphasized that he had 'a craving for fat' and even then still felt hungry until he added bacon and roast beef fat to it.

The amusing part for me was when, after experimenting for 16 days, the nutritionists showed Hanson figures provided by the National Research Council which said that man can't assimilate more than 35% of fat in his diet, and so, 'proved' to him that he was 'either dead or coasting along on my last reserves of energy.' He says: 'It was a gorgeous battle, especially in view of the fact that I had more "pep" for such purposes as arguing with nutritionists than I remembered ever having had before.' He finally gave up fruitless arguments with the nutritionists when they asked him in despair whether he didn't even believe the National Research Council!

So who should we believe?

I believe Admiral Sir Leopold McClintock had the right approach. He paid no attention to a dietetic theory which happened to be in vogue among the doctors and nutritionists, if he knew that the food condemned by them had been found wholesome and desirable by large numbers of people through long periods. He said he always preferred experience to theory if the two were in conflict. On this, Stefansson suggests a corollary:

> 'When a precept of the nutritionists, like the one against fat in warm weather, is in conflict with the tastes and practices of many people in many countries through many centuries, then it is likely the nutritionists themselves will eventually learn, probably through animal experimentation or by deduction from some recently announced or recently noticed chemical fact, that the opposite of the previously held theory is true.'

Stefansson believed that nutritionists would eventually wake up to the facts in the real world and change their advice. Regrettably, he was wrong; things have not changed – at least not yet. Not surprisingly, perhaps, since the days of Stefansson, Price and the others, the number of degenerative conditions in western 'civilized' societies has multiplied. It is my contention that it is not only the pharmaceutical industry's greed that is responsible for this sorry state of affairs, but a general ignorance, or at least confusion, within the whole 'health industry' about what really constitutes a healthy lifestyle.

There is no doubt in my mind that many of the foods that grace our supermarket shelves are rightly condemned by nutritionists, dieticians and doctors. But it seems to me that the modern concept of 'healthy eating' may not be all that much better.

This is because modern nutritionists simply seem unable to see the evidence all around them, or to learn from past – or even contemporary – experience.

For example, in 2003, British newspapers reported two studies which showed that for weight loss, the so-called Atkins diet, which is low in carbohydrates and high in fats, was far superior to the usual calorie-controlled, low-fat slimming diets. These studies were criticized by nutritional orthodoxy with the claim that the long-term safety of such diets has not been demonstrated. That statement merely serves to illustrate the level of the critics' ignorance. These studies were just two in a vast wealth of such studies that date back as far as 1863 – over a century before Atkins. It is the nutritionists' so-called 'healthy' diet that lacks long-term safety data. And as we have seen obesity, diabetes, heart disease and cancers all increasing at an alarming rate since the introduction of 'healthy eating' in 1984, it is clear that there never will be any. What we – and nutritionists – should remember is that it is the populations who live healthily on their diet who are the experts, not someone with a college degree.

A hieroglyph in an ancient Egyptian tomb reads: 'One-quarter of what you eat keeps you alive. The other three-quarters keeps your doctor alive.' The three-quarters keeping the health industry in business today are the foods that nutritionists advise you to fill most of your plate with.

Nutritional nonsense

Let me give another example. The British Dietetic Association produces an illustration of a plate which is divided up into segments illustrating the proportions of different foods they say we should (or shouldn't) eat. The larger the segment on the plate, the more we should eat of it. One-third of the plate is covered with fruit and vegetables, another third with starchy foods such as bread, pasta, breakfast cereals, rice and potatoes. At the bottom of the plate we are advised: 'cut down on fatty and sugary foods.'

Carbohydrates, whatever their source – fruit, cereals, sugar, pasta, bread, et cetera – are all converted to a simple sugar – either glucose, or fructose (which is later converted into glucose) – when they enter the bloodstream. Fruit sugar enters the bloodstream as fructose; starches enter the body as glucose. Table sugar (*sucrose*) is converted to 50% fructose and 50% glucose. So to put the recommendations in another way, they are telling us to eat lots of foods that supply fructose and glucose, but to cut down on foods that contain fructose and glucose!

Okay, I know that sugar doesn't contain any other nutrients whereas the other foods do; however, those other nutrients can be much better supplied from non-carbohydrate foods. In that way we can avoid the dangers of sugar overload which leads to obesity, diabetes and many other diseases. Perversely, these healthier foods tend to be the foods we are told to eat less of.

Cut calories

Another example of the nonsense is demonstrated when dieticians tell us that lower GI foods are better for us. Because sugar is metabolized to equal parts of glucose and fructose, it has a lower glycaemic index (GI) than starchy foods such as bread and root vegetables. Doesn't that imply that sugar is better for you than bread?

And still with sugar and starch, because of the way sugar and starch are digested and *hydrolyzed*, gram for gram starch puts more calories into the body than sugar does. People are told that they need to cut down on the calories to lose weight. So advice to cut down on sugar to lose weight yet eat starch makes no sense at all.

Fool the public

There are many programmes in which the media also reinforce the 'healthy' message. And as it is impossible to show that 'healthy eating' is healthy, they have to resort to ridiculous scams to 'prove' their case.

The Channel Five TV programme, *Diet Doctors*, screened in Britain on 12 September 2006, wanted to 'prove' that a high-fat diet was fattening. To demonstrate this, they forced the retired show jumper, Oliver Skeet, to eat a pound of cheese (mostly cheddar) a day for two weeks – on top of his normal diet. Oliver Skeet hates cheese. He made it quite clear that there was no way he was going to eat any, let alone a pound of it a day. But the Diet Doctors were adamant: he had to. He also ate that cheese in sandwiches made with thick slices of bread. Not surprisingly, he became quite nauseated after only a day or so. Nevertheless, he was forced to persevere. Despite being quite unwell, after the two weeks Skeet had put on two inches around his waist. This proved, said the Diet Doctors, that a high-fat diet was fattening. They didn't seem to take into account that forcing him to eat a pound of cheddar, which contains about 1850 calories, effectively doubled his calorie intake every day; nor did they take into account all the bread he was also eating.

It's nonsense. I have eaten a high-fat diet all my adult life – and I am not fat. I also love to eat cheddar and other cheeses. But I simply couldn't eat a pound of cheese a day; it would be too much on its own. And, don't forget that Skeet ate this *as well as* all the food he normally ate. He was forced by the programme makers to eat in a way that no-one would normally eat.

There is one other point that is relevant: Oliver Skeet is Afro-Caribbean. His racial background contains no evolutionary history of eating dairy products, so cheese is quite alien to his digestion. This also could well explain why he fared so ill on it.

The programme was a totally ridiculous and futile exercise. All it really demonstrated was the ignorance of the programme makers. Unfortunately, there will be many people who may well have been influenced by this nonsense and whose lives will have been made less healthy as a result.

'Healthy' diet is no longer defensible

All in all, the trend towards a 'healthier diet' has been an unmitigated disaster. I am not the only one who thinks this by any means. There are many others who can see the harm that current dietary policies are causing. One such is Dr Sylvan Lee Weinberg, a former President of the American College of Cardiology, a former President of the American College of Chest Physicians and current editor of *The American Heart Hospital Journal*. In a paper published in the 4 March 2004 edition of the *Journal of the American College of Cardiology*, Dr Weinberg issued a critique of 'healthy eating'. The abstract of his critique reads:[6]

> 'The low-fat "diet heart hypothesis" has been controversial for nearly 100 years. The low-fat, high-carbohydrate diet, promulgated vigorously . . . may well have played an unintended role in the current epidemics of obesity, lipid [blood fat] abnormalities, type II diabetes, and metabolic syndromes. This diet can no longer be defended by appeal to the authority of prestigious medical organizations or by rejecting clinical experience and a growing medical literature suggesting that the much-maligned low-carbohydrate, high-protein diet may have a salutary effect on the epidemics in question.'

Unfortunately, I doubt that the end is nigh for this disastrous experiment that has caused so much hardship and ill-health because too many reputations depend on its continuing. The only way it will be beaten is by us not succumbing to the brainwashing.

'Healthy eating' recommendations

You will remember that in the 1930s we were told to eat more eggs, milk, meat and butter. Today, as a result of the phoney war against cholesterol and fats, those recommendations have been turned upside down. 'Healthy eating' now tells us to:

- reduce our intake of fats to less than 35% of calories
- change from eating 'saturated' fats to eating polyunsaturated vegetable oils and margarines
- base meals and snacks on starchy foods (bread, pasta, breakfast cereals, et cetera)
- eat five portions of fruit and vegetables a day
- eat less salt

- take more exercise.

These recommendations have become regarded and accepted by most as the correct lifestyle for a long and healthy life. But if they are, why are we less healthy now than we were a century ago? And why are we even less healthy now than we were when they were introduced just two decades ago? It is beginning to look as if these recommendations are not in the best interests of our health.

We will look at the individual recommendations in more detail in the next few chapters.

Chapter Five

Fats: from tonic to toxic

For the sake of our hearts, we are told to replace traditional 'saturated' fats with processed, polyunsaturated vegetable oils.

There are three ways in which a substance can increase the risk of cancer: it can cause body cells to become cancerous; it can promote a cancer's growth; it can suppress the immune system. Polyunsaturated vegetable oils have been shown to do all three.

For a modern disease to be related to an old-fashioned food is one of the most ludicrous things I ever heard in my life.

Dr T. L. Cleave

The most far-reaching 'healthy' recommendation to come from government and nutritionists was that we should reduce our intakes of saturated fats – by which they meant animal fats and tropical oils – and change to eating polyunsaturated vegetable margarines and oils.

As a species, we have eaten animal fats and tropical oils, all of which contain a significant amount of saturated fatty acids, for the whole of our existence. Until the 20th century, before which time coronary heart disease (CHD) was either unknown or at least extremely rare, such fats were the only ones we did eat. With that background, why should we change?

The reason we are told to restrict our total fat intake to about 35% of calorie intake is because it is assumed that eating fat makes us fat, and that being fat predisposes us to diseases such as diabetes, heart disease and cancer.

The reason for the specific warning against *saturated* fats is the belief that saturated fats increase the risk of heart disease. Animal fats are sought out particularly for damnation as they not only contain some saturated fatty acids but cholesterol as well – so they must be doubly bad. Polyunsaturated oils, on the other hand, tend to lower our blood cholesterol levels, so they must be healthier. We saw earlier that there is precious little evidence to support these assertions; nevertheless, these are the sole bases for the recommendations.

Fat facts

Fats are important constituents in our diets for many reasons. With the highest amount of calories of any food, they are an important energy source. Our bodies need energy all the time. The amount of energy coming from carbohydrates is stored in our bodies in the form of glucose and glycogen, but that store is very limited: enough for perhaps two days if we take it easy. Our bodies' major energy store is body fat – a 'saturated animal fat', by the way.

But fats are much more than just an energy reserve. Our brains are mostly composed of fats; and fats are building blocks for body cell membranes and a wide range of hormones and hormone-like substances; fats also play an important part in cushioning vital organs.

Fats are also essential if our bodies are to use the fat-soluble vitamins A, D, E and K; they are essential for the conversion of carotene from plant foods to vitamin A.[1] Butter is the best source of these important nutrients, and vitamin A is more easily absorbed and utilized from butter than from any other source.[2] In fact our bodies have great difficulty with the carotene in plants. Our digestive system is not well equipped to convert carotene to vitamin A. Only about one-sixth of the carotene you eat may be converted, and only about one-third of that sixth is actually absorbed into the body. Much of the blindness in developing countries, which is blamed on a lack of vitamin A, is actually due to a lack of fat in the diet, so that what vitamin A there is cannot be metabolized. In an attempt to stop the blindness, rice is genetically modified so that it contains more carotene – but as it doesn't contain fat, what's the point?

Fats are also needed for mineral absorption.

As well as having a wide range of important functions within our bodies, eating fat with any meal slows down the rate at which food is absorbed so that we feel fuller more quickly and can go much longer without feeling hungry. And it is well nigh impossible to eat too much fat.

The 'saturated fat causes heart disease' myth

The idea that saturated fats cause heart disease is based on nothing more than wishful thinking. There is no science behind it. Indeed, there is a lot of work which shows that low-carbohydrate diets that are rich in saturated fat are beneficial in protecting us against cardiovascular diseases.[3] In addition, a major review of several studies into the effects of saturated fats has found that there is a general failure to produce evidence that would justify the recommendation to reduce saturated fat in the population.[4]

Other critical reviews of the evidence have questioned whether health recommendations for reducing saturated fat intake are appropriate at all.[5]

The potential for individual saturated fats to cause atherosclerosis has also been tested. Stearic acid, a major saturated fatty acid found in beef, chicken, and pork, has repeatedly been shown *not* to raise LDL levels.[6] Even the most abundant saturated fatty acid in the diet, palmitic acid, doesn't raise LDL when combined with other fatty acids as it is in meat fats.[7] And a recent report has shown that for women on a relatively low-fat diet, a higher intake of saturated fat slowed down the progression of coronary atherosclerosis.[8]

We also need to consider the relationship of saturated fats to other suggested causes of atherosclerosis apart from LDL. Studies have shown that if carbohydrate is replaced with any type of fat, levels in the blood of triglycerides (which are 'bad') go down and HDL (which is 'good') rises. The rise in HDL is greater with saturated fat than with unsaturated fat.[9] If we reduce saturated fat, the larger and more beneficial HDL_2 molecules are reduced,[10] and, conversely, increases in saturated fat increase this 'anti-heart attack' fraction.[11,12]

The real problem with fats is when they are attacked inappropriately by oxygen, and create 'free radicals'. Our bodies derive energy from fatty acids that are oxidized in a natural, controlled process. But we don't want fatty acids incorporated, for example, in a structural position within cell membranes to be oxidized. So, while oxidation in the right place is beneficial, in the wrong place it can be disastrous. It is the auto-oxidation and free radicals that do the damage, which is the reason we are advised to consume antioxidants.

The reason that unsaturated fats are so unstable is the double bonds which unite some of their carbon atoms. These are double connections between carbon atoms and, despite being double which sounds strong, are actually relatively weak and unstable. Fatty acids can break at these points into smaller molecules. When this happens, the carbon atoms each side of the break have a powerful attraction for any other compound with an opposite charge. The more double bonds a fatty acid has, the weaker and more unstable it is, and the more chances of liberation of abnormal carbon atoms with the subsequent formation of toxic free radicals there is. So you will appreciate that the degree of unsaturation and the number of double bonds a fatty acid has is all-important to our health. *Mono*unsaturated fatty acids have one double bond, *poly*unsaturated have two or more. Saturated fats, which have no double bonds, don't auto-oxidize at all and are completely stable and harmless. There is now considerable evidence that polyunsaturated fats are by far the most toxic fats; and saturated fats which resist auto-oxidation are the healthiest.

The significance of temperature

Have you ever wondered why polyunsaturated margarine has to be kept in a fridge, yet coconut oil can be kept out at room temperature for a year or more without any untoward effects?

All fats and oils in nature are a mixture of saturated, monounsaturated and polyunsaturated fatty acids. The only difference between them is the proportions of each. Whether they are in plant or animal tissues, this is governed by the temperature at which the different fats and oils are designed to operate. This point, which is often neglected when discussing the healthiness or otherwise of fats and oils, is actually a most important consideration. The degree of saturation or unsaturation determines not only a fat's melting point, but also its chemical stability and its likelihood of auto-oxidizing and creating harmful free radicals. The higher the proportion of saturated fatty acids a fat has, the less likely it is to go rancid; the more polyunsaturated fatty acids it contains, the more difficult it is to stop it going bad.

In plants, oils are usually found in their seeds. The degree of saturation of plant oils and fats is entirely dependent on the temperature at which they are grown. These oils provide a store of energy for the seeds' germination, usually in early spring when the weather is cool. For this reason, the energy contained in the oils must be accessible when ambient temperatures are low. Unsaturated oils melt at lower temperatures, and the more unsaturated they are, the lower the temperature at which they are viable. So we find oils that are highly saturated, such as coconut oil, in the tropics; palm oil, which grows slightly further from the equator, is a little less saturated; monounsaturated oils are found in olives grown in Mediterranean regions; and polyunsaturated oils in the seeds of plants grown in cooler climates. It has also been shown that the same plant species grown in a warm climate will be more saturated than if grown in a cooler region.[13]

The same is true of animals. Pigs dressed in sweaters were also found to have more saturated fat than unclothed pigs.[14] Animals must have body fats which are liquid otherwise they would be too stiff to move. So cold-blooded animals such as fish, which also live in cold water, contain highly polyunsaturated fatty acids with many double bonds: the EPA and DHA of fish oils have five and six double bonds respectively. But as body or environmental temperatures rise, so we find fats tending to become more saturated. The fats of all warm-blooded animals contain mixtures of saturated and unsaturated fatty acids, but the degree of saturation is quite high. Human body fat is naturally about 40% saturated, 57% monounsaturated and only 3% polyunsaturated.

This temperature aspect is highly relevant because any fat or oil must be stable at the temperature at which it is going to be used. If it is attacked by oxygen and goes rancid, as polyunsaturated margarines do if they are not refrigerated, then they become unfit for consumption if they are outside the body, and extremely harmful if they are inside it.

All polyunsaturated fatty acids will auto-oxidize at body temperature unless they are protected in some way. Nature makes sure it doesn't happen.

Coconuts are found in equatorial regions where the ambient temperature may be well over 40°C (104°F). Coconut oil contains a small percentage of polyunsaturated fatty acids – but significantly, coconut oil doesn't go rancid at this temperature because the polyunsaturated fatty acids in coconut oil are protected by the very high percentage of saturated fatty acids.

Our body temperature at 37°C (98.6°F) is not really much lower than the coconut's environment. Our fat must also be both liquid and stable at this temperature. So it, too, contains a high proportion of saturated fat and only a small amount of polyunsaturated fat. Just like the coconut, the saturated fatty acids in our bodies protect the polyunsaturated fatty acids from oxidation. However, if we eat a diet that contains high levels of polyunsaturated fats, as 'healthy eating' tells us we should, those fats will be incorporated in our body cells. And that, as we will see later, makes them a recipe for disaster.

In Table 5.1, the figures for food animals are based on animals eating

Table 5.1: Fatty acid composition of selected fats[15]

Fat or oil	Saturated (%)	Monounsat (%)	Polyunsat (%)
Coconut	91	6	3
Palm kernel	83	16	1
Butter	60	34	6
Human milk	**54**	**39**	**8**
Lamb	53	41	5
Beef	45	51	5
Pork	43	48	8
Human (body fat)	**40**	**57**	**3**
Hen's egg	39	47	14
Chicken	35	48	16
Cod	26	16	59
Margarine (polyunsat)	24	21	55
Soy oil	18	24	58
Olive oil	17	74	9
Corn oil	13	24	60
Sunflower oil	5-16	14-40	48-74
Safflower oil	9	12	75
Canola oil	6	67	27

their natural diet as they did when these values were determined. Today, however, many food animals are fed on foods which are more polyunsaturated – and the figures can be very different. For example, pork fat which should be about 8% polyunsaturated, can now be well over 30%.[16]

And as many of our intensively farmed food animals are now fed large amounts of grains and soya, it is no longer accurate to speak of their fats as 'animal fats'; in many cases they are more akin to vegetable oils. In the same way that these are taken up by the animals, when we eat them they are also incorporated in our body cells. That turns what should be a healthy fatty acid profile into a decidedly unhealthy one, with serious implications not only for those animals, but for our health as well.

'Healthy' polyunsaturated fats are the danger

Dr Catherine Shanahan is a doctor of medicine with a PhD in biochemistry/chemistry. She told me: 'Many times I have cured elevated triglycerides and elevated liver enzymes simply by advising canola oil (and other vegetable oil) using patients to switch to butter, olive oil or one of a list I give out of low polyunsaturated fat content oils and fats . . . Patients making the changes experience reversal of the elevated liver enzymes, their triglycerides go down and their HDL goes up. Avoiding canola and all the other high polyunsaturated fat content oils often reduces heartburn symptoms and I am quite sure it saves lives. I have had multiple patients tell me they used canola oil to fry their fish the night before they show up in the ER with anginal chest pain, but never do those who follow my list of good fats have heart problems.'

One of the main points is that polyunsaturated vegetable oils cannot handle the processing; the heat and pressure alone result in shape changes, and the rest of the processes add to the problem. According to a paper published in 2003: 'Heating, pressurization, degumming, neutralization, and bleaching altered the fatty acid profile.'[17] It explains that fatty acids were damaged and *lipid hydroperoxides* were produced. According to the chemistry, lipid hydroperoxides are potentially more toxic than trans-fats. The article continued: 'Deodorization produced substantial quantities of trans-fatty acids (more than 5% of total fatty acids in some bottles) and small amounts of cyclic fatty acid monomers.' These are also toxic.

Of course the real problem with all vegetable oils is that they are not extracted by pressing; heats and solvents are used. Few fatty acids will stand up to that. Olive oil is only healthy because it comes from a super oily seed and can be produced in a healthy manner; squashing fruits under a heavy object at ambient temperature. Olive oil – or any oil – that is extracted with heat and solvents can be expected to be as full of contaminants as the 2003 study shows canola oil to be.

Look in Table 5.1 at the fats our bodies store and those that are found in human milk. These – the fats that our bodies are designed to use – contain very little of the polyunsaturated fatty acids found in vegetable oils. Instead, they are made up of a mixture of saturated and mono-unsaturated fatty acids which are very similar to the fatty acid profiles found in the fats of cattle and sheep. Our bodies haven't evolved to do things that harm themselves. As our natural body fat is nearly half saturated, how did we ever come to believe that such fats can be harmful to us? Human breast milk is 54% saturated. Does anyone believe that this is harmful to a human child? I cannot understand how this ridiculous idea ever got started.

Butter, which is 60% saturated, doesn't need to be refrigerated. The 'spreads straight from the fridge' slogan was coined by a margarine company as a marketing ploy to promote its product. Butter that 'spreads straight from the fridge' today is adulterated with toxic polyunsaturated vegetable oils (they are cheaper and make more profit for the food companies). Real, unadulterated butter can be kept at room temperature – and it will then spread easily.

The evidence of a cancer link

You don't have to look very far to find the evidence that unsaturated fats are dangerous. Studies go right back to 1945, when a scientist named Rausch at the University of Wisconsin noticed that rats whose diets were supplemented with corn oil had more cancers.[18] That observation alone should have ensured that there was a thorough investigation of unsaturated fats before they were applied to humans. Yet no such trials were ever done.

In 1957 an investigator from the Veterans Hospital in San Francisco cautioned against the use of polyunsaturated fats because of the cancer-producing compounds that could result from their susceptibility to attack of free radicals.[19] He also pointed out that the Japanese had many more stomach cancers than were seen in other countries and suggested that the high content of polyunsaturated fats in their fish diet might be a major factor.

Publications on experimental animals began to appear. In 1960, Ershoff found that when fish oil formed 10% of rats' diet, they stopped growing and produced diarrhoea.[20] In 1967, Norkin reported more cirrhosis of the liver in rats fed polyunsaturated corn oil than in those fed saturated coconut oil.[21] In 1968 Carroll in Canada produced more breast cancers in rats fed corn oil than in those fed coconut oil.[22] In the same year the *New England Journal of Medicine* reported seven premature babies suffering from oedema, haemolytic anaemia, and abnormal blood cells.[23] (Because of the propaganda about saturated fats, they had been started on pre-diluted, skimmed cows' milk, vegetable oils and iron.) And a 1971 report in *The Lancet* told of the much greater numbers of deaths from cancer in a heart trial among men on polyunsaturated diets to lower their cholesterol.[24] In this study, the scientists split war veterans into two groups for the study. One group ate their normal diet with animal fats, while the other group's diet was high in polyunsaturated fats. During the study, careful records were kept and autopsies were performed to verify causes of death. The results showed that there were a few more deaths from heart attacks among the men on the saturated fats, but this was unremarkable as variations in numbers of this sort were not unusual. What was far more important was that there were almost twice as many deaths from cancer in the polyunsaturated fats group. This did come as a surprise, for deaths from cancer do not show the variation that is seen with heart attacks. Not surprisingly, this study questioned the advisability of using polyunsaturated fats. But there is another question hanging over this paper: it was not published in an American journal, but an English one. I have to wonder: was it refused publication in the US? And, if so, why?

That first cancer observation in 1945 alone should have been enough for a thorough investigation of the safety of polyunsaturated vegetable oils for human consumption. If similar evidence had been produced concerning a pesticide, a food additive or an environmental pollutant, the authorities would have called for immediate cessation of its use until it was proven safe. That was not the case in 1945. If you did not die within a week from any exposure, the product was safe. Now, over more than half a century later, despite the vast amount of data in the literature indicting polyunsaturated fats in cancer, nothing has been done. In fact, polyunsaturated fats are being thrust upon the public by the press, radio and TV, doctors, nutritionists, dieticians and government and called 'healthy'.

Margarine – a natural food?

What takes up most of the space in the dairy section of every supermarket? Margarine. Yet margarine is not a dairy product; it is not a fresh food; it's a fake food. And, contrary to popular belief, it is not a 'healthier choice'.

The polyunsaturated fats used to make margarine are generally obtained from vegetable sources: sunflower seed, cottonseed and soybean. As such they might be thought of as natural foods. Usually, however, they are pressed on the public in the form of highly processed margarines, spreads and oils and, as such, they are anything but natural.

Look at the difference in the ingredients for butter and margarine.

Table 5.2: Ingredients which may be present in margarine

Edible oils,	tocopherols,
edible fats,	propylene glycol mono- and di-
salt or potassium chloride,	esters,
ascorbyl palmitate,	sucrose esters of fatty acids,
butylated hydroxyanisole,	curcumin,
phospholipids,	annatto extracts,
tert-butylhydroquinone,	tartaric acid,
mono- and di-glycerides of fat-	3,5,trimethylhexanal,
forming fatty acids,	ß-apo-carotenoic acid methyl or
disodium guanylate,	ethyl ester,
diacetyltartaric and fatty acid es-	skim milk powder,
ters of glycerol,	xanthophylls,
propyl, octyl or dodecyl gallate (or	canthaxanthin,
mixtures thereof),	vitamins A and D.

Butter is simple. It is just cream from milk plus a little salt. Margarine, on the other hand is quite different as, Table 5.2 demonstrates.

After extraction from the seeds using petroleum based solvents, the oils go through more than 10 other processes: degumming, bleaching, hydrogenation, neutralization, fractionation, deodorization, emulsification, interesterification . . . that include heat treatment at 140-160°C with a solution of caustic soda; the use of nickel, a metal that is known to cause cancer, as a catalyst, with up to 50 parts per million of the nickel left in the product; the addition of antioxidants such as *butylated hydroxyanisol* (E320), which has been shown to cause cancer in animals.[25]

The hydrogenation process, that solidifies the oils so that they are spreadable, produces *trans*-fatty acids that rarely occur in nature. The heat treatment alone is enough to render these margarines nutritionally inadequate. When the massive chemical treatment and unnatural fats are added, the end product can hardly be called either natural or healthy.

Polyunsaturated fats and cancer risk

There are three ways in which a substance can increase the risk of cancer:

- It can suppress the immune system thus preventing the body from fighting cancer.
- It can cause body cells to become cancerous.
- It can promote an existing cancer's growth.

Polyunsaturated fats have been shown to do all three.

Polyunsaturated fats suppress the immune system

During the early days of kidney transplantation doctors first encountered the problem of tissue rejection as their patients' bodies destroyed the alien transplanted kidneys. If transplantation were to be a success, they had to find a way to suppress the immune system. The first person to suggest that polyunsaturated fats (PUFs) do this was Dr E. A. Newsholme of Oxford University.[26] What Newsholme wrote was that when our bodies get sufficient nutrition, our diet includes immunosuppressive PUFs which make us prone to infection by bacteria and viruses. When we are starved, however, our bodies' stores of PUFs are depleted. This allows our bodies' immune systems to recover which, in turn, allows us to fight existing infection and prevent other infections. He was making the point that the immunosuppressive effects of PUFs in sunflower seeds are useful in treating auto-immune diseases such as multiple sclerosis,[27] and that the same fatty acids could be used to suppress the immune system to prevent rejection of kidney transplants.

Newsholme had said that there was no better way to immunosuppress a renal patient than with sunflower seed oil. So kidney transplant doctors fed their patients linoleic acid,[28] the major polyunsaturated fatty acid in vegetable seed oils. Anything that suppresses the immune system is likely to make a person more susceptible to cancer. Despite such knowledge, the transplant doctors were astonished to see how quickly their patients developed cancers – and the treatment was stopped.

By the early 1980s, we were being exhorted by doctors and nutritionists to eat more PUFs because they were 'good for us' despite the fact that *Oncology Times* carried yet another paper in January 1980 from the University of California at Davis showing that mice fed PUFs were more prone to develop melanoma. In May 1980, the same publication carried a similar report from Oregon State University which also said that PUFs fed to cancer-prone mice increased the numbers of cancers formed.

In 1989 there was a report of a 10-year trial at a Veterans' Administration Hospital in Los Angeles in which half the patients were fed a diet which had twice as much PUFs as saturated fats; the other half ate saturated fats. In the half of patients on the high PUF diet there was a 15% increase in cancer deaths compared with the saturated fat group.[29]

The late American cancer researcher, Wayne Martin, liked to tell a story about just how cancer-causing PUFs are. In 1930 in the US, 80% of men smoked cigarettes and the tar content of cigarettes was much higher than it is today. The death rate at that time from lung cancer was very low. In 1955 doctors decided that PUFs were beneficial in terms of heart disease protection. After this, lung cancer deaths increased dramatically. Other research confirmed this. By 1980 although the number of American men who smoked had dropped to only 30%, three times as much PUF was being eaten – and there were 60 times as many lung cancer deaths.[30]

In 1990, Martin called Newsholme's office but by then Newsholme had retired. Martin spoke to his successor to find that they were still treating auto-immune diseases with PUFs. By then they were using fish oil. The Oxford doctor said the reason for the fish oil was that the degree of immunosuppression increased with the degree of unsaturation and fish oil was much more unsaturated than sunflower oil. Martin asked the doctor why they were not talking about PUFs causing cancer. The doctor replied that if he did, he would be run out of Oxford.

Polyunsaturated fats initiate cancer

Since 1974, the increase in polyunsaturated fats has been blamed for the alarming increase in malignant melanoma (skin cancer) in Australia.[31] We are all told that the sun causes it. Are Australians going out in the sun any more now than they were 50 years ago? It seems they aren't, but they are certainly eating more polyunsaturated oils. When I was in Australia, I noticed that even the cream on milk is removed and replaced with polyunsaturated vegetable oil.

Dr Bruce Mackie found that patients who developed skin cancers were those who had reduced their intakes of saturated fat and replaced it with polyunsaturated fat.

Malignant melanoma is also increasing in Britain. Does the sun cause this? It is not likely since all the significant increase is in the over-75-year-olds, who tend to get very little sun.

That the sun is not to blame is confirmed by other findings:

- Melanoma occurs 10 times as often in Orkney and Shetland than it does on Mediterranean islands.
- It also occurs more frequently on areas that are *not* exposed to the sun – on ovaries, for example.
- In Scotland there are five times as many melanomas on the feet as on the hands.
- In Japan, 40% of melanomas on feet are on the soles of the feet.[32]

Absorption of ultra-violet radiation from the sun causes excitation of, usually followed by conversion of, the absorbed photon of light into heat energy, increasing polyunsaturated oils' vulnerability to attack by an oxygen free radical. This is known to damage a cell's DNA and this can lead to cancer. Saturated fats are stable and safe from such attack.

Polyunsaturated fats promote cancer

Many laboratories have shown that diets high in polyunsaturated fatty acids also promote tumours. Cancer promotion is not the same as cancer causation. The subject is complex; suffice to say that promoters are substances that help to speed up the reproduction of existing cancers.

It has been known since the early 1970s that, again, it is linoleic acid that is the major culprit. In 1987, Professor Raymond Kearney of Sydney University wrote: 'Many laboratories have shown that a greater proportion of polyunsaturated fats are superior to diets rich in saturated fats in promoting the yield of experimental mammary tumours. In such studies, omega-6 linoleic acid appeared to be the crucial fatty acid . . . Vegetable oils (eg corn oil and sunflower oil) which are rich in linoleic acid are potent promoters of tumour growth.'[33]

Polyunsaturated fats and breast cancer

In 1991, two studies, from the US[34] and Canada,[35] found that linoleic acid increased the risk of breast tumours. This, it seems, was responsible for the rise in the cancers noted in previous studies. Experiments with a variety of fats showed that saturated fats did not cause tumours but, when small amounts of polyunsaturated vegetable oil or linoleic acid itself were added, this greatly increased the promotion of breast cancer.

In 1996 a case control study of over 5,000 Italian women looking at diet and breast cancer was published in Italy.[36] Dr Sylvia Franceschi and her team assessed the influence of high intakes of fat and other macronutrients on breast cancer risk. They found that women with the highest intake of fat had significantly *less* breast cancer. The authors concluded: 'The risk of breast cancer decreased with increasing total fat intake . . . the intakes of saturated fatty acids . . . were not significantly associated with breast cancer risk.' In the same year, another team also: 'found no evidence of a positive association between total dietary fat intake and the risk of breast cancer. There was no reduction in risk even among women whose energy intake from fat was less than 20 percent of total energy intake. In the context of the western lifestyle, lowering the total intake of fat in midlife is unlikely to reduce the risk of breast cancer substantially.'[37]

So eating a lot of fat protects against breast cancer – but only, it seems, if those fats are the right sort. A study of 61,471 women aged 40 to 76, conducted in Sweden, looked into the relationship between different types of fat and breast cancer. Like those before it, this study found: 'no positive association between intake of total fat and risk of invasive breast cancer.' What it did find, however, was that PUFs found in vegetable oils and margarines *increased* the risk of breast cancer and monounsaturated fats found in animal fats and olive oil *protected* against breast cancer. Saturated fats were neutral.[38]

In 2002 another Swedish study, the Malmö Diet and Cancer (MDC) cohort study, confirmed the earlier study, finding again that saturated fats were entirely healthy and that only 'specifically high intakes of omega-6 fatty acids were associated with an increased risk'.[39] Omega-6 fatty acids are predominantly found in 'healthy' vegetable oils.

In 2003, two studies which purported to show that an increasing intake of animal fat increased the risk of breast cancer were published just two days apart. The first was an American study of 90,655 women aged 26 to 46, conducted by the Harvard Medical School. It was reported in the American press with the headline: 'ANIMAL FATS LINKED TO INCREASED BREAST CANCER RISK, STUDY FINDS.' But that's not what the figures showed.[40]

The women studied were divided into five 'quintiles' depending on their fat intakes, the first quintile eating the least fat and the fifth quintile the most. There were no absolute risk figures, which makes analysis difficult. However, there were enough data reported to work out the percentages of women who did *not* get breast cancer in each quintile: 99.3, 99.2, 99.2, 99.1, 99.3. If eating animal fat increased the risk of breast cancer, one would expect that the more that was eaten, the more breast cancer there would be. That was clearly not the case. There was no trend of increasing cancer as fat intake increased; both the first and last quintiles are similar.

Another thing that is strange about this study is that this group had published a paper only four months earlier in which they 'found no evidence that intake of meat or fish during mid-life and later was associated with risk of breast cancer.'[41] It refutes their other study.

The second 'animal fat causes breast cancer' study wasn't really looking at that at all. It was a study about the way data are collected, as its title, '*Are imprecise methods obscuring a relation between fat and breast cancer?*' suggests.[42] What it really said, in essence, was: 'We "know" that saturated animal fat causes breast cancer, but we can't prove it in trials. So let's see if we can manipulate the figures to get a result that is acceptable.' This was, I imagine, because all trials published so far – and there had been a lot – had found that animal fats did *not* cause breast cancer, only vegetable fats did, but that finding wasn't politically correct. So this team looked at the way data are gathered to see if they could spin their findings to show what they wanted to see.

They compared a food frequency questionnaire, the usual way to gather information, with a food diary which, they said, was very much more reliable. Using this method they studied 25,630 men and women to look for effects of fat intake and breast cancer.

They, too, split participants into quintiles based on fat intakes. There were 168 cases of breast cancer between January 1993 and September 2002 in participants who had completed both dietary monitoring methods. Unfortunately, the report from this study doesn't break them down into how many ate how much fat, as the Harvard study did. However, 168 cases out of over 25,000 people in 10 years is not very many on which to base reliable findings. And again the data show clearly that the ones who ate the *most* fat had *less* breast cancer than those who ate less. The numbers with cancer in the two highest intakes (fourth and fifth quintiles) were less than the numbers in the third. So their attempt to manipulate the data failed.

These two studies tried to contradict not only all other studies of fats and breast cancer produced to date but our entire evolutionary history; cancer has really only 'taken off' in the last century, yet we have been eating animal fats for millions of years.

The anti-cancer fats

Fortunately there is one form of linoleic acid that is beneficial. *Conjugated* linoleic acid (CLA) differs from the normal form of linoleic acid only in the position of one of the bonds that join its atoms. But this small difference has been shown to give it powerful anti-cancer properties. Scientists at the Department of Surgical Oncology, Roswell Park Cancer Institute, New York,[43] and the Department of Biochemistry and Molecular Biology, New Jersey Medical School,[44] showed that even at concentrations of less than 1% in the diet CLA protects us against several cancers including breast cancer, colorectal cancer and malignant melanoma.

Conjugated linoleic acid has one other difference from the usual form – it is not found only in the fat of ruminant animals. The source with the highest proportion of CLA is kangaroo fat. If you don't live in Australia, the best sources are dairy products and the fat on red meat, principally beef.[45]

As well as CLA, the saturated fatty acids lauric acid and capric acid found in animal fat also have anti-cancer properties.[46]

It has also been suggested that the consumption of red meat increases the risk of colon cancer, yet in Britain there is no evidence to support this.[47] It may be significant that all the evidence purporting to implicate red meat in cancer comes from the US – where they cut the fat off. But beware: there are two types of CLA. One found in animal fats that is protective; the other, manufactured from vegetable oils for the health-food industry and sold in capsules that is not.

Summary on cancer

Saturated fats and animal fats are usually blamed for all manner of diseases in western society. But what all the work in the last half century has demonstrated is that polyunsaturated fatty acids increase cancer risk, monounsaturated fatty acids lower risk and saturated fatty acids are either beneficial or are neutral.

As all fats in Nature are a combination of the three types, let's look at them in a different way:

- The vegetable oils used for cooking oils and margarines are mainly polyunsaturated. These are most likely to increase risk of cancer and other diseases.
- Some vegetable oils, such as olive oil, are mainly monounsaturated, so are likely to reduce cancer risk. But at about 13%, these also contain a significant amount of polyunsaturated fatty acids.
- Tropical oils such as coconut oil, which are over 90% saturated, are neutral.
- Animal fats contain about 50% monounsaturated, reducing risk; just under 45% saturated, which has no effect one way or the other; and a small percentage of polyunsaturated fatty acids, which might increase risk, except that they also contain CLA which is a powerful anti-cancer agent.

Whether the dramatic increase in the numbers of cancers in the last century was a result of a similarly dramatic rise in our intake of polyunsaturated vegetable oils is not proven – but the evidence strongly favours such a conclusion. Look at the facts from history:

- In the 19th century, when animal fats were all that was available, cancers were rare (as was heart disease).
- Polyunsaturated fats and oils are used to suppress the immune system, and have been found to cause cancers to start and to promote cancer.
- In this last century there has been a change in favour of polyunsaturated fats and oils – and cancer rates have soared.

All polyunsaturated margarines, from the brand leader to shops' own brands, are 39% linoleic acid. Cooking oils – sunflower, safflower, soy and corn oils – are between 50% and 78% linoleic acid. Butter, on the other hand, has only a mere 2% and lard around 9%.

We may need about 2% of calories in the form of omega-6 linoleic acid. With a 2,000-calorie intake, that is about a teaspoonful. We may also need about half that amount of omega-3 alpha-linolenic acid. These amounts are readily available from animal fats.

Under the circumstances, it seems prudent to get what linoleic acid we may need from animal sources – or to restrict polyunsaturated oil consumption so that the linoleic acid it contains is no more than 3% of our total fat intake.

Omega-6 vs omega-3

The vegetable oils used for margarines and cooking oils are heavily biased in favour of omega-6 fatty acids, with little or no omega-3. Several recent studies which have increased the omega-3 content of diet by adding flax oil and fish oils have reported health benefits from the change in a variety of conditions. This has led to the suggestion that the unhealthiness of PUFs is because the balance between the two types is all wrong with too much omega-6 and too little omega-3. Omega-6 fatty acids are inflammatory while omega-3 fatty acids are anti-inflammatory. For this reason, fish oils in particular are now being promoted heavily as a panacea for heart disease and a wide range of other conditions.

But as all omega-3 fatty acids have more double bonds (between three and six) which can be attacked by oxygen than the ubiquitous omega-6 linoleic acid, which has just two, is this necessarily a good idea? Might it not be better to redress the balance by reducing the amount of omega-6, rather than increasing the amount of omega-3?

How essential are EFAs

Both omega-3 and omega-6 fatty acids are essential, we are told. Omega-6 linoleic acid and omega-3 alpha-linolenic acid are the two 'essential fatty acids' or EFAs. When we use the word 'essential' in the context of a nutrient such as 'essential fatty acids' we mean that our bodies need it, and that we have to eat it as our bodies can't manufacture it for themselves.

Given that polyunsaturated fatty acids seem to be unhealthy, the question is: just how essential are they really? And if they are essential, how much of each is it safe to eat, and can we eat too much?

The essentiality of some fatty acids was first mooted in 1929 when two scientists named Burr showed that mice with a particular complaint recovered when fed particular fatty acids.[48] This was debunked around 1940 when mice with the same deficiency disease were cured with a fat-free diet containing Vitamin B_6. According to reviewers, pigs and humans have not been shown to require the essential fatty acids.[49]

So, the first point to make is that there is still some debate about whether EFAs are actually essential. The question of essentiality is beyond the scope of this book, but as we know that polyunsaturated fats can have some decidedly unhealthy effects, it is certainly worth considering just how much of these 'essential nutrients' is enough, so that people can minimise their consumption of the dangerous stuff. And in that respect there is agreement: the necessary amount of omega-6 linoleic acid is about 2% of calorie intake and the amount of omega-3 alpha-linolenic acid is about half that amount. Putting that into the context of a 2,000 calorie diet, it means we need about a teaspoon of linoleic acid and half a teaspoon of alpha-linolenic acid. Fortunately, both of these fatty acids, in the right proportions, are found in meat fats, butter, cream, cheeses and eggs. Vegetarians can get their EFAs from unprocessed seeds: about a handful of sunflower seeds for linoleic acid and half that amount of flax seeds for alpha-linolenic, for example.

The essential fatty acids that are found in their natural, unprocessed state are harmless in these quantities without the need for antioxidant supplements. It is the processed products such as margarine, cooking oils, cakes, cookies, and other confectionary that do the damage. EFAs sold in capsules as food supplements are generally extracted from seeds with the use of solvents and heat. These are invariably damaged and should be avoided.

Beware of fish oils?

Recently a new fad has emerged. Nutritionists are now recommending that we get our omega-3s in the form of oily fish (eat two portions a week) and fish oil supplements because of their high levels of omega-3 derivatives, EPA and DHA.

The reasons for eating fish oils, we are told, are to prevent heart problems and cancers. In fact the evidence is that they could actually *increase* the risk of both – and a number of other conditions as well. For example, the form of heart disease that doctors are worried about when they discuss dietary fats is 'ischaemic heart disease' where the coronary arteries become blocked. But the greatest cause of heart death is actually something else entirely: atrial fibrillation. A Danish study showed that Danes who consumed 1.29 grams of omega-3 fish oil per day had a 34% *higher* rate of atrial fibrillation than did those who consumed 0.16 grams of fish oil per day.[50]

There is another point. As the two EFAs are ubiquitous in animal fats and easily obtained from vegetable sources, they are actually difficult to avoid. Under normal conditions, the average adult diet meets all requirements for linoleic acid. In addition, linoleic acid constitutes 8% to 10% of our fatty tissue depot. This can amount to as much as 700 grams in the normal individual. Even in starvation, this stored amount is enough to meet the body's requirements for months, perhaps years. For this reason, deficiency of essential fatty acids is unusual except in a very thin patient after prolonged starvation, in newborn infants, and in patients receiving fat-free total intravenous nutrition.

There appears to be little benefit from taking the EFA derivatives such as gamma-linolenic acid (GLA), eicosapentanoic acid (EPA) or docosahexaenoic acid (DHA).

Dr Broda Barnes wrote in 1976:

> 'Everyone should have the privilege of playing Russian Roulette if it is desired, but it is only fair to have the warning that with the use of polyunsaturated fats the gun probably contains live ammunition.'

I think it is fair to say now that the word 'probably' can be deleted; there is no doubt that eating polyunsaturated margarines and cooking oils is risky.

Trans-fats = toxic fats

There is one class of fats that everyone agrees is harmful: they are called *trans*-fats.

To make a solid margarine from the liquid vegetable oils they must be *hydrogenated* to change the double bond(s) from bent to straight. This process involves heating the fat with hydrogen and a catalyst under pressure. Unfortunately, the conversion in this process is not complete. A small proportion of the unsaturated fatty acid is not hydrogenated but converted to a trans-fatty acid (TFA). For example, the TFA arising from oleic acid is still unsaturated, with a double bond in the same place, but with a different spatial arrangement around the double bond. This change gives the new molecule a different shape and property. Partially hydrogenated vegetable fat is used primarily in fast food and other commercially manufactured fried and baked foods to boost their shelf life; TFAs are found in thousands of products on supermarket shelves.[51] A diet high in frozen meals, pies, crackers, biscuits, chips, muffins, doughnuts, snack bars, margarine or cooking oil, is likely to contain high levels of TFAs.

There is no argument by either side of the fat debate that fats containing such TFAs are unhealthy. TFAs inflame the arteries and accelerate heart disease.[52] Despite this, margarine manufacturers claim that margarine is healthier than butter because they class saturated fatty acids and TFAs in margarine together, and then show that the two combined in margarine are less than the total saturated fatty acid content of butter. This, of course, is based on the totally untrue assumption that saturated fatty acids are harmful.

If we were wise, we would ban this harmful ingredient from our food supply. Denmark banned these commercial fats in 2004 with no adverse effect on taste or price of affected food, including fast food and even their famous Danish pastries.[53]

But even then the message can still go wrong. In a recent issue of the *New York Times* there were samples of new FDA food labels that included TFA levels in foods. But conjugated linoleic acid (CLA), which is entirely healthy and beneficial as it has been shown to reduce cancer and heart disease risk and help with overweight, is a trans-fat. So now butter, which contains about 0.5 grams per serving of CLA, has to be labelled as containing trans-fat. This makes butter look unhealthy when the truth is actually exactly the opposite.

So let me put the record straight: trans-fats in vegetable margarines, cooking oils and commercially baked products are harmful; the trans-fats that occur naturally in animal fats are good for you.

Companies are swapping trans-fats for another dangerous fat

Man-made trans-fatty acids are now being abandoned by many manufacturers. Instead, a new type of fat, called *interesterified* fat, has been developed. Interesterified fat is hydrogenated and then rearranged at the molecular level, a process which hardens fat in much the same way as trans-fatty acids. New research published in a recent issue of *Nutrition & Metabolism* suggests that interesterified fats may be even more unhealthy than the trans-fats they replace.[54] Two key results from the study, which compared diets containing natural saturated palm oil with partially hydrogenated soybean oil and interesterified soybean oil, stood out. Firstly, HDL levels dropped in participants on the interesterified fat diet; and secondly, while blood glucose levels remained relatively stable for eight hours on the palm oil and partially hydrogenated soybean oil diets, the interesterified fat diet suppressed insulin production allowing blood glucose levels to rise by an alarming 20%.

So why are we told to eat polyunsaturated fats?

You might expect that before we were advised to eat such potentially harmful things as polyunsaturated margarines, they had been extensively tested to ensure they were safe. They weren't! They weren't even tested on animals. Those who would have us eat polyunsaturated margarines were so convinced that saturated fats were to blame for heart disease that they couldn't be bothered to wait for proof. In 1970, a Harvard nutritionist, Dr Frederick Stare, refereed a symposium on Diet and Cardiovascular Disease.[55] The members concluded that, if they waited for proof that lowering the blood cholesterol with polyunsaturated fats prevented coronary disease, it would cost up to one million human lives in the US alone over the following five to seven years. Despite the fact that there had been many reports by this time of the toxicity of polyunsaturated fats and the report acknowledging the dangers they posed, these were dismissed out of hand.

Conclusion

Dr T. L. Cleave wrote: 'For a modern disease to be related to an old-fashioned food is one of the most ludicrous things I ever heard in my life.'

Natural fats and oils found in both animal fats and tropical oils, as well as cold-pressed oils such as olive oil, are entirely natural parts of our diet, and entirely healthy. By changing, or allowing a change of, dietary fat intakes from these healthy sources to processed vegetable margarines and cooking oils, nutritionists have changed our diets from tonic to toxic.

Chapter Six

The seeds of ill health

Base meals on starches, we are told. Eat bread, pasta, rice, breakfast cereals. Indeed, we eat more cereals than any other foodstuff. But all cereal grains pose significant health risks to humans. Wheat, on which we depend the most, is probably the worst of them all. And legumes (beans) are almost as bad.

All cereal grains have significant nutritional shortcomings which are apparent upon analysis.

Professor Loren Cordain

As fat became a 'four-letter word' and we cut down the amount we ate, the energy from the fats lost had to be replaced by energy from something else or we would have starved. As a consequence, we were advised to base meals and snacks on starchy foods. In effect this meant eating considerably more cereal-based foods such as bread, breakfast cereals, rice and pasta. Today, worldwide, cereals supply more food calories than all other foods combined as is shown in Table 6.1 opposite.

Yet, while cereal grains like wheat, maize (corn) and rice provide over half the world's energy and protein needs,[1] there is considerable evidence that their use is not without significant health risks.

Professor Loren Cordain of Colorado State University points out that cereal grains are something of a double-edged sword. On the one hand, the agricultural revolution could probably never have happened without them; we would not be able to sustain the enormous present-day human population; we wouldn't have the industrial culture in which we live; the enormous increase in human knowledge would probably never have taken place; and we would not have our understanding of medicine, science and technology. But on the other hand, neither would we have most of humanity's chronic ills including whole-scale warfare, starvation, tyranny, infectious epidemics and a wide range of chronic degenerative diseases.[2]

Table 6.1: World food supplies

Food group	**Totals** (million tonnes) (estimated edible dry matter)
Cereals	1,545
Tubers (potatoes, etc)	136
Pulses (beans, lentils)	127
Meats, milk and eggs	119
Sugar	101
Fruits	34

Despite the risks inherent in consuming cereals, it is clear that humanity has now become dependent upon them for the majority of its food supply, that 'cereal grains literally stand between mankind and starvation.'[3] In view of this fact, it is essential that we fully understand the nutritional implications of milling, processing, refining and eating cereal grains on our health and well-being – and, perhaps, modify our reliance on them as best we can to minimize their adverse effects.

Cereal grain domestication

The cereals we eat today were all derived from wild grasses, found worldwide. The first Agricultural Revolution began as a domestication of animals about 10,000 years ago in the Near East, a move that spread to northern Europe over the following 5,000 years or so, and to other countries and peoples as recently as the present day.[4,5] In their wild form, these seeds would have been of little use to us because, being similar to present-day grass seeds, they would have been small and difficult to harvest.[6] They also would have needed a considerable amount of processing before they could have been eaten: they would have had to be cut and collected, and winnowed to separate the seeds from the rest of the plants. That in itself would have been very time-consuming, and would certainly have used more energy than the small seeds would have provided. There is also the problem that, even today, our gut is not equipped with the enzymes required to derive energy from the types of starch and fibre which predominate in grasses. Consequently, unless cereal grains were milled to break down the cell walls and cooked to gelatinize or break down the starch granules and make them more digestible, the proteins and carbohydrates the seeds contained were largely unavailable for absorption and assimilation. For these reasons, it would have been well nigh impossible for our ancestors to exploit this food source.

It is almost certain, therefore, that grains were not originally cultivated as a food for humans, but used only as animal feed. Only by selective breeding would the seeds of the grasses have gradually increased in size to make their exploitation by humans a feasible proposition. Even then, in view of the substantial amount of energy required to harvest, process, and eat cereal grains, it is very unlikely that they would have been eaten except under conditions of severe shortage of other foods.[7]

This is confirmed by observations that very few of the world's recently studied hunter-gatherer populations consume cereal grains. Even amongst those who did eat grass seeds – modern hunter-gatherers such as the Australian Aborigine and the American Great Basin Indians – those seeds still represented only a small percentage of their total caloric intake and were eaten for only a few weeks of the year.[5]

Nutritional shortcomings

Essential amino acids

No cereal grains can be called complete foods as they all have significant deficiencies in the essential amino acids. Maize is deficient in trypto-phan; wheat and most other cereals are low in lysine and threonine. Taurine, considered a conditionally essential amino acid as there is in-creasing recognition that humans have limited ability to synthesize it, is not detectable in any cereal.

Essential fatty acids

Cereal grains are low in fats. They average only 3.6% fat for their total caloric content, their fatty acid profile is heavily weighted towards omega-6,[8] and their omega-3 content is almost non-existent. Conse-quently, cereal-based diets, particularly if they are supplemented with vegetable oils, all have an unhealthily high ratio of polyunsaturated to saturated fatty acids, and of omega-6 to omega-3. Compounding this is that the omega-3 alpha-linolenic acid from plants is very poorly metabo-lized to EPA and DHA (see Glossary), making it far less desirable.

Vitamins

Vitamin A. Cereals contain no vitamin A and, except for yellow maize, neither do they contain its metabolic precursor, beta-carotene. Vitamin A deficiency is a major nutritional health problem in the Third World.[9] As many as 40 million children worldwide are estimated to have at least mild vitamin A deficiency.[10] It is a leading cause of blindness among children and also a major determinant of childhood growth and suscepti-bility to disease.[11] Where infectious diseases are contracted, vitamin A deficiency results in greater frequency, severity and higher death rates.[12] An analysis of 20 trials of vitamin A supplementation in Third World children showed a 30-38% reduction in deaths in those given vitamin A supplements.[13] It is clear that excessive consumption of cereal grains plays a major role in the high levels of ill health in many parts of the underdeveloped world.

B Vitamins. Many nutritionists consider cereal grains to be good sources of all of the B vitamins except for vitamin B_{12}. And it is true that cereals do contain adequate amounts – at least in terms of the percentage of Recommended Daily Allowances. However, what should concern us is not how much they contain, but how much of what they contain is actually available after milling, processing and cooking. It is somewhat ironic that two of the major B vitamin deficiency diseases which have plagued agricultural man – beriberi and pellagra – are almost exclusively caused by excessive consumption of cereal grains: a deficiency of thiamine in the case of beriberi and of niacin in the case of pellagra.[14] Pellagra occurs almost exclusively in peoples whose staple food is maize (corn). The first half of the 20th century witnessed a pellagra epidemic in the southern states of the US. Approximately three million people were affected and there were over 100,000 deaths.[15] There have also been similar epidemics in India and Europe,[16] and even today, pellagra is still found in some parts of Africa.[17] Maize, like all cereal grains, is rich in lectins, chemicals which are known to decrease intestinal absorption of many key nutrients.[18,19]

Vitamin B_6, arguably the most important of the B vitamins in prevention of cardiovascular diseases, is another vitamin that looks to be plentiful in cereals, apart from oats, but whose bioavailability is poor. While almost all of the vitamin B_6 in foods of animal origin is absorbed, the amount our bodies actually absorb from cereal grains tends to be very low.[20] B_6 deficiency is common in populations utilizing cereals and pulses as their staple diet.[21,22]

Vitamin B_7, usually known as *Biotin*, has not been much studied in humans. However, animal studies have shown that, with the exception of maize, most cereal grains have very low levels of available biotin.[23] Biotin is highly available from animal sources.

Vitamin B_{12}. As vitamin B_{12} is found only in foods of animal origin, diets based primarily or wholly upon plant food sources are either low or deficient in vitamin B_{12}.[24] Vitamin B_{12} deficiency causes megaloblastic anaemia, which causes irreversible damage to the brain and nervous system. This ultimately results in death. Vitamin B_{12} deficiencies are common in countries such as India and Mexico where diets are mainly cereal and pulse based, even when small amounts of animal foods are also eaten.[25,26]

Vitamin C. Cereals contain no vitamin C, yet vitamin C is essential for us to metabolize the carbohydrates which form the major part of all cereals. High usage of cereals depletes the body of the vitamin C it has. Although scurvy is blamed on insufficient fruit intake, the disease was only rife in sailors eating ship's biscuits; scurvy was unknown in sailors or explorers eating only meat and fish.

Vitamin D. Not only do cereals contain no vitamin D; they can indirectly adversely affect vitamin D metabolism. Animal studies have shown that excessive consumption of cereal grains can induce vitamin D deficiencies in many animal species including primates.[27] Vitamin D deficiency is widespread in human populations consuming high levels of unleavened whole grain breads.[28,29] This may be due to insufficient sunlight (see Chapter 11), but a clinical study of humans consuming 60 grams of wheat bran per day for 30 days clearly demonstrated an increased loss of vitamin D through the intestine.[30]

Minerals
Cereals appear to provide adequate amounts of most minerals needed for health, but again we have to consider their bioavailability. The phytic acid that all cereals contain chelates (binds with) several key minerals to form insoluble *phytates* which are not digestible.[31] As the phytic acid is found almost exclusively in the outer husks of the cereal grains – bran – we have the situation where B vitamins and proteins are lost from white bread, and minerals are not available from wholemeal bread.

Calcium, phosphorus and magnesium. Cereals have a naturally low level of calcium, and calcium is also one of the minerals chelated by the phytic acid. This low calcium intake from cereal grains does not normally represent a problem since full-fat dairy products are good sources of calcium, if they are included in the diet. However, if the dairy is replaced with soya milk and other sources of calcium are replaced by cereals, this can be a recipe for disaster. The ideal ratio of calcium to phosphorus is 1:1. However, cereals contain much higher levels of phosphorus, compared with calcium. This relationship has a negative impact on bone growth and metabolism. Consumption of a large excess of dietary phosphorus, when calcium intake is adequate or low, leads to secondary hyperparathyroidism and progressive bone loss.[32] In addition to the adverse ratio of phosphorus to calcium, cereal grains also have a low ratio of calcium to magnesium. This decreases the intestinal absorption of calcium and also leads to calcium excretion.[33]

The net effect of a low calcium content and low bioavailability of calcium due to the phytic acid, combined with disproportionate amounts of potassium and magnesium, is to induce bone diseases such as rickets, osteomalacia and osteoporosis in populations where cereal grains provide the major source of calories.[34-36]

Iron. In addition to their deleterious influence upon calcium metabolism, cereal grains when consumed in quantity can adversely influence the bioavailability of iron. Iron deficiency is probably the most prevalent nutritional deficiency in the world today. It affects 2.15 billion people throughout the world and is severe enough to cause anaemia in 1.2 billion people.[37,38] The causative factor has been clearly demonstrated to be the poor bioavailability of iron from cereal-based diets, the staple food in many developing countries.[39]

Zinc. Zinc absorption is also impaired by whole grains such as wheat, rye, barley, oats and triticale.[40] Again it is the phytic acid that is mainly to blame. In human populations, zinc deficiency results in a characteristic syndrome called *hypogonadal dwarfism* in which there is arrested growth, small and undeveloped gonads and delayed onset of puberty.[41] This is despite the fact that the zinc intake of these populations exceeds our recommended daily intakes by a substantial margin.[42]

Other minerals. The absorption of chromium, manganese and selenium from cereals is not affected,[43] but the bioavailablity of copper in cereal grains is poor.[31]

Up to the middle of the 20th century, the adverse effects of phytic acid were lessened by processing methods such as malting, soaking, scalding, fermentation, germination and sourdough baking. But these processes take time and, today, time is money. So they are no longer used in large-scale cereal processing.

Natural toxins in cereals

Like all living things, plants have no desire to become the food source of another species. Their whole *raison d'être* is to survive and reproduce. They have evolved to do this with the development of defence mechanisms which deter insects and animals that would eat them.[44] Many plants also provide their seeds with substances which ensure the survival of the seed and subsequent seedling until it can synthesize its own protective compounds.

Cereal grains are no exception. They contain a whole cocktail of chemical protectants that may be either outright toxic, antinutritional or uncomfortable to a predatory animal – including us. For example, the fact that wheat grains can lie buried in the soil for several years before they finally sprout demonstrates how very successful are the toxic properties of the bran coating in warding off soil microbes. Bran is extremely durable and resistant to breakdown by organic action.

Of course, these defences don't always work. Insects, birds, and other animals have evolved to cope with these substances and, by so doing, are able to consume cereals with few if any adverse effects. We, unfortunately, have not. Like all primates, our species evolved in the tropical forest; our food would have been from broad-leafed plants, and that is what our gut was initially adapted to cope with. Cereals are quite different.[45] Although a few species of primates have been seen to eat grass and grass seeds under certain conditions, this behaviour is rare. We, like all other primates, have had little time to develop a resistance to the toxic compounds found in cereal grains. For this reason, when the energy from cereal grains reaches 50% or more of the daily energy intake, many of us suffer severe health consequences.

The main sources of ill health due to higher levels of cereals are:

- **Phytic acid** found in bran, which binds to minerals, inhibiting their absorption.
- **Lectins**, which also reduce intestinal absorption of many key nutrients.
- **Protease inhibitors**, which inhibit the metabolism of dietary proteins.
- **Alpha-amylase inhibitors**, which prevent starch digestion and are known to be prominent allergens.
- **Alkylrescorcinols**, which suppress growth and cause kidney damage.
- **Molecular-mimicking proteins**: amino acid sequences that have the same structural form as a variety of amino acid sequences in body tissue and can cause auto-immune diseases.

Genetic changes to the human gut

But, you might suggest, we have been eating cereals for several thousand years. Isn't it possible that we could have adapted to their use by now?

The time-frame since we began to cultivate cereals is actually very short in evolutionary terms. It is possible that some adaptation could have taken place in the 500 or so generations since grains were first used in northern Africa, but time-frames within northern Eurasia are of the order of no more than 100 generations, and in some others – Inuit, northern Scandinavians, Icelanders, Siberians, Native Americans – as few as three or even one generation. If those who have had more time to adapt had been able to do so, there should have indeed been measurable differences between their guts and enzyme systems and those with a more recent history of grain use. But anatomical and physiological studies among and between various racial groups indicate that there are few differences in the basic structure and function of the gut. Thus it is reasonable to assume that there has been insufficient evolutionary experience since the advent of agriculture to create large genetic differences among human populations in their ability to digest and assimilate various foods.

The complete re-arrangement of the gut and the evolution of new enzyme systems capable of handling such new food types is, therefore, quite unlikely to have occurred in humans in the short time since the advent of agriculture.

Where there has been some adaptation, is in an increased ability to digest *disaccharides*: the milk sugar, lactose, and sucrose (table sugar). Although insulin is not a direct component of the gastrointestinal tract, there is substantial evidence to indicate that populations without a long history of carbohydrate use are more prone to high levels of insulin in the blood as a result of unaccustomed high intakes of carbohydrates and the resultant high blood glucose levels. These peoples are much more prone to the consequences: type-2 diabetes mellitus, obesity, hypertension and coronary heart disease.[46]

So while there has been some adaptation to dietary sugars, the same is not true of the starches found in cereals. There is no apparent difference between human groups in their ability to deal with the harmful effects of the antinutrients in cereals regardless of their genetic background. And no human can digest and assimilate the energy contained in bran.

Early hunter-gatherers' bodies did not have biological mechanisms that recognize the wheat protein, gluten, as a viable protein; and many individuals today still have problems with it. This is because of the similarity of some gluten peptides with several pathogenic viruses. Wheat can set off a complex defence mechanism that searches for these non-existent pathogens and when it does not find them, ends up activating an autoimmune response which damages the intestines and other organs.[47]

What all this means is that the human gut remains relatively unchanged from Palaeolithic times – when we did not eat cereals. And that, in turn, means that we should be very circumspect about how much of them we eat today.

Similar problems apply to legumes

If that weren't enough, most of the above is also applicable to legumes: beans, particularly soy, and other pulses.

Last but not least, some cereals are dirty

Scientists connected with the flour industry have for many years published articles in trade journals not seen by the general public which describe in detail the filth found in flour.

The wheat grain from which flour is made has a groove on one side which is so deep that it goes more than half way through the grain. This groove naturally contains dirt and microbes that have accumulated while the plant was growing. And it is such a deep and tight groove that the grain cannot be thoroughly cleaned.

After harvest, the grain is stored in huge silos until it is required for use. These silos are frequently the homes of insects, mice and rats. For these reasons, by the time grain reaches the mills, it is infested with insects, and droppings, urine and hair from rats and mice. Although the grain will have been sprayed with insecticides and anti-fungal chemicals to help preserve them (the chemicals themselves being an unwelcome trespass on our health), there will still be insects, grubs and their droppings inside the wheat grains, which cannot be separated out easily.

The mills do what they can to clean the grain but it's a daunting task, and flour has to be such a cheap product that they cannot afford to do very much. Inevitably, dirty grain goes through the mills to be ground into flour. Microscopic examination of flour commonly reveals ground up fragments of insects and rat hair, and traces of rat dung and urine. Bacteriological tests of flour have indicated an extremely high content of microbes. For this reason, the flour from which our daily bread is made is probably more highly contaminated than anything else to be found in the food industry.

To this can be added:

- a plethora of insecticides, herbicides and fungicides such as disulphoton (Di-Syston) while growing
- 'protectants' such as chlorpyrifos-methyl and pyrethrins which are added to grain to protect it against insects
- fumigation in the form of methyl bromide, aluminium phosphide and magnesium phosphide during storage and as the grains are being treated.

And when the wheat is made into bread and similar products:

- overheating, which often denatures the protein
- dough conditioners and preservatives, partially hydrogenated vegetable oils and toxic soya flour
- chemical preservatives to extend the shelf life far beyond the few days it would take to spoil naturally.

Conclusion

As you go to buy your bread, you might ponder the problem that the whole enterprise of agriculture, which first emerged 10,000 years ago, may be harmful to your health. When you started this chapter, such an idea might have seemed absurd. After all, when inhabitants of what is now the north-eastern coast of Africa began cultivating naturally occurring grasses they were laying the foundation for what would become the first permanent human settlements. But that agriculture introduced Mankind to unnatural dietary habits for which millions of years of evolution had not prepared us.

I'm not talking merely about that bloated feeling that so many complain of after eating bread. Dr Staffan Lindeberg, a Swedish physician and scholar of evolutionary nutrition, points out that a typical European gets at least three-quarters of his or her calories from foods that were practically unavailable during human evolution: milk products, most oils, refined sugar, processed foods like margarine and, of course, cereals. There is little doubt that modern European diets rely far too heavily on grain-based foods, whether it be wholewheat bread or handmade pasta.

Like Lindberg, Professor Loren Cordain teaches that the widely accepted notion that cereal grains are the foundation of a healthy diet leaves people woefully short of nutrients and vitamins better provided by meat, vegetables, and fruit.

So, while we are taught that bread is the 'staff of life', we should look at the facts. Cereals, and the bread and other products made from them, are a very recent addition to our diet. And even today, there are many parts of the world, particularly in the Far East, tropical Africa, Arctic regions and South America where bread is not eaten at all. Since there are millions of well-fed, healthy people living today who do *not* eat cereals, it is very clear that they are not necessary. And they are not my idea of a suitable food on which to base a 'healthy' diet.

So what is the answer? Well, there is no doubt that we cannot now do without cereals – there are just too many of us. But we could at least limit the amount of them we eat.

Chapter Seven

Climb off the bran wagon

With cereals comes bran (cereal fibre). We have been urged for generations to eat fibre to prevent and cure many bowel and other health conditions. However, research shows that, while vegetable fibre may be relatively harmless, bran increases the risk of many of the conditions it is promoted to prevent and cure – and a lot more as well.

The tragedy of science is the slaying of a beautiful hypothesis by an ugly fact.

T. H. Huxley

The belief that regular bowel movement is important for health is very ancient. In 1932 a 'New Health' movement was promoted in which people were urged to include plenty of roughage in their diets and it was hoped then that the prompt passing of stools after each substantial meal would reduce the incidence of intestinal diseases.[1] Thirty years later Dr Dennis Burkitt, while working as a doctor in Africa, discovered that there were far fewer cases of colon cancer among rural black Africans than among Europeans and Americans. He attributed this to the Africans' relatively crude diet.[2] The theory was that fibre – that part of a vegetable which passes undigested through the human gastrointestinal tract – hastened the passage of the bowel contents thus allowing less time for cancer-inducing agents to form. This, of course, presupposed that food became carcinogenic in the gut; there was no evidence that it did. Neither was there any evidence that moving food through the intestine at a faster rate decreased the risk of cancer.

So the theory was unsubstantiated at the time and it was to be disproved later when the rural Africans moved into towns and adopted a western-style, low fibre diet, and it was noticed that they continued to have a low incidence of colon cancer. This pattern has also continued with the second generation. It should also be noted that the rural Africans' lifestyle is quite different from that of the western city dweller: their diet is different in that their energy intake is lower and they eat less protein, fat and sugar; they are also not exposed to so many pollutants, toxins or mental stresses and any of these factors could be responsible for the difference in disease patterns. Other studies have also shown that there are western communities (the Mormons of Utah, for example) who also enjoy a low incidence of colon cancer but eat a low fibre diet.[3] Nevertheless, the later findings were not publicized; Burkitt's theories caught the attention of the media who, always ready to exploit a good story, expanded what was at best a very weak hypothesis into a treatment dogma which teaches that fibre is a panacea for all manner of illnesses.[4]

Commercial interests were quick to see the potential in the recommendation. Although Burkitt's recommendations were based on vegetable fibre, bran has a far higher fibre content than vegetables and bran was a practically worthless by-product of the milling process which, until then, had been thrown away. Bran is quite inedible – there is no known enzyme in the human body that can digest it; nevertheless, backed by Burkitt's fibre hypothesis, commercial interests could now promote it as a valuable food. Virtually overnight, it became a highly priced profit maker. The late Dr John Yudkin, Professor of Nutrition and Dietetics at London University, pointed out that 'perhaps one reason for the wide acceptance of the suggestion that fibre is an important, if not essential, dietary component is that it had the enthusiastic support of commercial interests.'[5]

Dr Hugh Trowell, Burkitt's partner and another strong advocate of dietary fibre, confirmed this in 1974, saying that: 'a serious confusion of thought is produced by referring to the dietary fibre hypothesis as the bran hypothesis, for many Africans do not consume cereal or bran but remain almost free of constipation, irritable bowel syndrome and diverticular disease.'[6]

Bran is the tough outer covering of cereal grains. Every civilization in history has devised methods and implements solely for the purpose of separating bran from the grain so that they would not have to eat it.

Fibre and colon cancer

Animal studies have variably suggested that dietary fibre reduces risks, increases risks, or has no effect on bowel cancers. Epidemiological studies on humans have also found that intakes of dietary fibre are either protective, or have no effect; there is also a growing scepticism in the US that lack of fibre causes cancer; some studies have even suggested that a fibre-enhanced diet may increase the risk of colon cancer.[7]

In the mid-1980s dietary fibre was shown to increase the risk of colon cancers.[8] In 1990 the British Nutrition Foundation admitted that the hypotheses that irritable bowel syndrome (IBS), diverticulosis and colorectal cancer were caused by a deficiency of fibre had not been substantiated; and neither had claims that fibre might protect against diabetes, obesity and CHD.[9] The Seventh King's Fund Forum on Cancer of The Colon and Rectum commented that: 'cereal fibre does not offer protection against cancer.'[10]

In 1995 Dr M. Inoue and colleagues published an investigation of cancers at several colorectal subsites: ascending, transverse, descending, sigmoid, and rectum, within a Japanese hospital environment. They concluded that loose or soft faeces are a significant risk factor for cancer at these sites.[11] But bran loosens and softens faeces – that's why it is recommended.

The following year Drs H. S. Wasan and R. A. Goodlad of the Imperial Cancer Research Fund showed that bran can increase the risk of colorectal cancers.[12] 'Many carbohydrates,' they said, 'can stimulate epithelial-cell proliferation throughout the gastrointestinal tract,' and concluded: 'Until individual constituents of fibre have been shown to have, at the very least, a non-detrimental effect in prospective human trials, we urge that restraint should be shown in adding fibre supplements to foods, and that unsubstantiated health claims be restricted . . . Specific dietary fibre supplements, embraced as nutriceuticals or functional foods, are an unknown and potentially damaging way to influence modern dietary habits of the general population.' This study spawned several critical letters. It comes as no surprise that half were from people connected with the breakfast cereal industry.[13]

The results of a very large, long-term trial also suggest that, contrary to popular belief, high dietary fibre intake does not protect against colorectal cancer.[14] Researchers at Harvard Medical School and the Dana-Farber Cancer Institute, both in Boston, Massachusetts, studied 88,757 women over 16 years. They say: 'no significant association between fiber intake and the risk of colorectal adenoma was found.' But there was what they call an 'unexpected' finding, in that, according to their data, a high consumption of vegetable-derived fibre was actually 'associated with a significant increase (35%) in the risk of colorectal cancer'.

That fibre increased the risk of colon cancer was confirmed six years later by a large analysis of 17 studies of the effect of dietary fibre on colorectal cancer.[15] Although the abstract of the study said that people with the highest intakes of fibre had a reduced risk of colon cancer, that was exactly the opposite of what the study data showed. Using the study's Table 3, dividing the number of cases of colorectal cancer by person-years of exposure, and multiplying by 10 to obtain number of cases per 10-person-years, since the mean study length was about 10 years, the

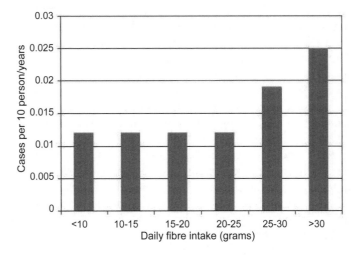

Figure 7.1: Colorectal cancer and fibre intake

effect was not a reduction in cancers as fibre intake increased but an increase. This is graphically illustrated in Figure 7.1. Lead researcher, Yikyung Park, said that 'There are more questions to be answered but clearly this adds to the growing body of evidence finding that high fiber intake does not lower the risk of colorectal cancer.'

Fibre and heart disease

The idea that fibre could protect against coronary heart disease was hypothesized by Dr Trowell in 1973,[16] again based on research on rural Africans. But while pectin, guar gum, fruit and vegetables lowered blood cholesterol levels, they were not lowered by wheat fibre (bran), or a diet containing wheat and whole maize. There is little evidence that fibre of any type is effective in reducing levels in the blood of triglycerides or other fats.

The paucity of evidence, however, did not stop COMA (the Committee on the Medical Aspects of Food Policy) seeing advantages in compensating for a reduced fat intake with increased fibre-rich carbohydrates, although it makes no specific recommendations. On dietary fibre, the report at paragraph 4.3.3 says: 'However, epidemiological data suggest that cereal fibre is protective against coronary heart disease.' Yet COMA's own reference for that statement says: 'However, wheat fibre appears to have no consistent effect on plasma cholesterol or triglycerides in man.' The report also says at 4.3.5 that: 'the protective effect in relation to coronary heart disease has not been adequately tested.'

Oat bran – the wonder fibre?

Oat bran is regarded as a 'healthy' cholesterol-lowering food. It is advertised with statements such as 'recent medical research shows that oat bran could actually lower your cholesterol level.' This is based, apparently, on an experiment conducted at Northwestern University, Evanston, Illinois, in 1986, which involved only 208 subjects, lasted just six weeks and whose results were not statistically significant.[17] Despite this, an oat bran campaign in the US saw sales of oat bran cereals increase 240% by 1989.

More recent medical research has come up with very different findings. Results of an American study into the effects of oat bran showed that oat bran was not the cure-all it had been claimed to be – just another example of dietary advice that is 'without foundation' and 'verging on quackery'.[18] In this test, people were fed 100 grams of oat bran per day (three times the recommended dose), the placebo (control) group having 100 grams of a white flour, low-fibre placebo. There was no appreciable difference in blood cholesterol levels between the two groups. The authors said: 'Some dietary fibres do bind bile acids and thus may have a cholesterol-lowering effect similar to that of the bile-acid-sequestrant drugs. However, many experiments, both in outpatients and in metabolic wards, have failed to demonstrate that wheat bran does, in fact lower plasma cholesterol levels.' They then said that: 'oat bran had no effect over and above that of the wheat placebo. It did, however, produce gastrointestinal rumbling and some discomfort.'

Another American study published the same year also had similar findings, and concluded: 'As we also found, low-fibre products can achieve the same result with fewer gastrointestinal side effects.'[19]

The following year oat bran was tested in people with high blood cholesterol levels.[20] Using 30, 60 and 90 grams of oat bran per day, they found that it made not the slightest difference either to total cholesterol levels or to levels of low density lipoprotein (LDL).

That rules out cereal fibre. Could other plants that also contain fibre be better?

Fruit and vegetables contain quite small amounts of fibre (see Table 7.1) so that if a significantly larger amount is to be eaten, this will have a dramatic effect on the volume of food consumed. Thus the advice to increase fibre in the diet, if we are to use 'natural' sources, must involve a substantial change to the diet as a whole. And that is likely to be unpopular or we would be eating it already.

We know, then, that an increase of the right kind of fibre in the diet may lower blood cholesterol. The important question is: will it also lower the risk of heart disease? The various multifactoral intervention

Table 7.1: Amounts of fibre in typical foods

Food	Fibre g/100 grams	Fibre g/100 kilocalories
Apples, raw	2.0	4.3
Beans, haricot, boiled	7.4	8.0
Cabbage, winter, boiled	2.8	18.7
Carrots, young, boiled	3.0	15.0
Potatoes, new, boiled	2.5	2.6
Plums, raw	2.9	8.0

trials tested this and all had to conclude that increasing dietary fibre had no effect on heart disease. In addition, there is really no direct evidence that an increase of fibre by itself will prevent or cure any of the other diseases.

Clearly there are two sides to this debate and claims of benefit are by no means proven. That, of course, does not stop a variety of commercial interests from jumping on a very lucrative 'bran wagon'.

When the American Heart Association published its dietary recommendations in 1982, the US National Cancer Institute (NCI) and Kellogg's got together to promote All-Bran.[21] But by making such health claims, Kellogg's effectively turned All-Bran from a food into a drug – and drugs must be approved by the Food and Drugs Administration (FDA). This gave the FDA a problem as the NCI had already given its blessing to All-Bran. They have an even bigger problem now because of the lack of evidence that fibre protects against cancer.

Fibre pills for obesity

In Boots, the chemist, I saw fibre pills which, their label claimed, would reduce obesity. Each pill contained 0.2 grams of fibre and the recommended dose was four to six pills before each meal or when one feels hungry. Its makers claimed that fibre stays in the stomach longer and so wards off the pangs of hunger. There are two points to be made here: firstly, that the theory on which the fibre hypothesis is based is that it does *not* stay in the gut longer but that it moves through quickly and, secondly, that even if it did stay in the stomach, around one gram (five pills) would have no effect whatsoever. It is about the amount of fibre one would find in one dried prune.

Fibre and mineral absorption

The fibre hypothesis was based on the fact that an increase in dietary fibre moved food through the gut faster. However, all the nutrients in food are absorbed through the gut wall and this takes time. If the food travels through faster, there is less time for its absorption and consequently less is absorbed. Because of this, *all* fibre, whether it is from fruit, vegetables or cereals, inhibits the absorption of such nutrients as zinc,[22] iron, calcium, phosphorus, magnesium, energy, proteins, fats and vitamins A, D, E and K.[23] Now this doesn't matter too much if you eat a good nutrient-dense diet which contains plenty of these nutrients. But there is another problem with cereal fibre (bran): its phytate content.

Phytate

The *American Journal of Clinical Nutrition* is arguably the most important journal of nutrition. In 1992 Professor Harold Sandsted, its Editor-in-Chief, noted that:

> 'the evidence seems overwhelming that high intakes of fiber sources that are also rich in phytate can have adverse effects on mineral nutrition of humans . . . In view of the data, it appears that some health promoters who suggest that [we] should consume 30-35 g dietary fiber daily either have not done their homework or have simply ignored carefully done research on this topic.'[24]

What he was talking about was the phytic acid that cereals, soya and other legumes have in their husks. It is well known that by this mechanism wholegrain cereals decrease the absorption of minerals and that this leads to a variety of deficiency diseases in both developed and undeveloped countries.

The minerals mostly affected by phytic acid are calcium, iron[25] and zinc.[26] For example, subjects absorbed more iron from white bread than from wholemeal bread even though their intakes of iron were 50% higher with the wholemeal bread.[23] And while white bread must have added calcium, the law does not require it of wholemeal bread.

Bran fibre has also been shown to cause faecal losses,[27] and what the medical profession calls 'negative balances', of calcium,[28] iron, zinc, phosphorus,[29] nitrogen, fats, fatty acids and sterols. A negative balance is where more is lost from the body than is absorbed. What this means is that bran causes a loss of these nutrients from your body.[30]

Dr E. J. Moynahan suggested that: 'Any substantial return to a high-fibre diet may lead to a reversal to the situation that obtained a century ago . . . Apparently, therefore, the amount of fiber must be strictly limited or the cereals fortified not only with calcium but also with iron and zinc as well, if this is to be avoided.'[31]

This prophecy turned out to be well founded as tests soon showed that there could be harmful side effects; since the advent of 'healthy eating', we have seen the re-emergence of many previously rare deficiency diseases.

Although most of the experimental studies conducted using fibre consumption of 30-40 grams/person/day and with supplements added in the range 10 to 30 grams/day (which are broadly around the levels recommended) showed little adverse effect, tests on mineral availability did suggest that excessive consumption would have significant undesirable effects on mineral status. It would appear, therefore, that although a modest increase in vegetable fibre would probably not have any significant adverse effects, provided that there were adequate amounts of proteins, minerals, etc in the diet, any advice must be given in such a way as to prevent the excessive intake of phytate associated with cereal fibre (bran). Incidentally, as a breaker of teeth, granary bread, made with whole wheat seeds, is second only to a punch in the mouth.

So why on earth are we still told the opposite?

Burkitt and Trowell were firmly committed to the United States' McGovern Committee's dietary goals, namely the replacement of animal products with grains as a way to 'prevent cancer and heart disease' and to 'forestall world hunger'. Burkitt's writings on dietary fibre led to calls for increased amounts of whole grains in the American diet in order to prevent colon cancer and other diseases of the intestinal tract. Dietary fibre soon became a household word, and America embraced the oat bran fad.

What Americans failed to recognize was that Africans do not eat their grain foods as we do in the West, in the form of quick-rise breads, cold cereals, energy bars and pasta; they eat them as a sour or acid porridge. Throughout Africa, these porridges are prepared by the fermentation of maize, sorghum, millet or cassava. Preparation in the home begins with washing the grains, then steeping them in water for up to three days. The grain is then drained and the water discarded. Soaked grains are wet milled and passed through a sieve. Whatever is left in the sieve is discarded. In other words, *the Africans throw away the bran*. The smooth paste that passes through the sieve may undergo further fermentation. Soaking water that rises to the top is discarded and the slurry is boiled to make a sour porridge. Sometimes the slurry is allowed to drain and ferment further to form a gel-like substance that is wrapped in banana leaves, making a convenient energy bar that can easily be carried into the fields and consumed without further preparation.[32] Often sour porridges are consumed raw as 'sorghum beer', a thin, slightly alcoholic slurry that provides lactic acid and many beneficial enzymes.

Acid porridges made from grains are far superior to western grain preparations. Fermentation increases mineral availability by neutralizing the phytic acid, it increases vitamin content, predigests starches and neutralizes enzyme inhibitors. Insoluble fibre can cause pathogenic changes in the intestinal tract unless properly soaked in an acid medium.[33] Oat bran, which is high in phytic acid as well as related bran products, can cause numerous problems with digestion and assimilation, leading to mineral deficiencies, irritable bowel syndrome and auto-immune conditions such as Crohn's disease. Case control studies indicate that consumption of cereal fibre can be linked to *detrimental* effects related to colon cancer formation.[34]

Another fermented food consumed throughout Africa, and universally ignored by most investigators, is a paste made from dried shrimp and hot peppers. This strong, spicy condiment is a rich source of fat-soluble vitamins. Shrimp has ten times more vitamin D than organ meats, and vitamin D protects against cancer of the colon and rectum, neurological disorders such as multiple sclerosis, and osteoporosis [35] – all of which are extremely rare among Africans.

Several researchers have noted that, along with sugar, tea and white flour, vegetable oils made from peanuts, cottonseed or soya have made inroads into the African diet. What these oils replace is highly saturated palm oil, which has been a staple in Africa for millennia. This has resulted in overall decline in the consumption of saturated fat in Africa. Like vitamin D, saturated fats play a role in protecting the intestinal tract from cancer and other diseases, and in preventing osteoporosis.

Doctors who write about diet are severely limited by their lack of familiarity with basic cooking methods. One gets the distinct impression in reading Dr Burkitt's book that none of the authors had actually tasted traditional African food, let alone observed its preparation. Otherwise they would have known that Africans customarily cook calves' feet to make broth for soups and stews. Often dried fish and shrimp are added to these stews, along with meat, peanuts and vegetables. Pieces of gristly calves' feet go into the pot along with everything else and are eaten with relish. Americans are just beginning to discover the health benefits of beef cartilage; Africans have enjoyed such benefits for centuries.

Men only

Professor David Southgate is a world-renowned expert on dietary fibre. He concluded that the effects of excessive intakes of dietary fibre on calcium, iron and zinc absorption would be particularly undesirable for infants, children and young adolescents, and recommended that dietary fibre intakes in those groups should be separated from those for the general adult population and given on a body-weight basis.[36] To them should be added pregnant women and post-menopausal women whose mineral needs are greater and who should also be protected from excessive consumption of fibre.

The advice given by dieticians, nutritionists and doctors appears to include no caveats concerning age, sex or body weight. Indeed, the impression given by them all is that we should all eat as much fibre as we can tolerate. The British Medical Association in its publication *The Slimmers' Guide*, even recommended bran as a good source of calcium![37] Not unnaturally, the makers of breakfast cereals and wholemeal breads stress the goodness contained in their products by virtue of the high bran content. Yet the only members of the population who may eat these in any quantity with relative impunity are adult men.

Can ripping intestinal cells really be beneficial?

Although they have pushing bran for many years to facilitate the movement of faecal material through the gut, nutritionists had no idea how it worked until scientists at the Medical College of Georgia found the answer in 2006.[38] It seems that as the rough, bulky bran makes its way down the gastrointestinal tract, it scratches and tears cells in the gut wall. According to cell biologist, Dr Paul L. McNeil: 'What we are saying is this banging and tearing increases the level of lubricating mucus. It's a good thing.'

That consuming roughage increased mucus production was known years ago; Dr McNeil discovered that cell injuries and repairs occur when we eat. The new research tied the two together. 'These cells are a biological boundary that separates the inside world, if you will, from this nasty outside world. On the cellular scale, roughage, such as grains and fibers that can't be completely digested, are a mechanical challenge for these cells,' said Dr McNeil. In what he and colleague, Dr Katsuya Miyake, view as an adaptive response, most of these cells rapidly repair the damage and, in the process, excrete even more mucus, which provides some cell protection as it eases food down the gut. The scientists aren't certain how many times cells can take this punishment, but they suspect turnover must be high because of the constant injury. Acidic substances, such as alcohol and aspirin, can produce so much damage that natural recovery mechanisms can't keep up. But they doubt a roughage overdose is possible.

However, why would you want your intestinal lining stripped in such a sandpaper-like manner, potentially exposing the underlying, immature cells to the assaults they may not cope with well? Inflammation can start a cancer. Could this abrasion possibly start colon cancer? Or, perhaps, cause pre-cancerous changes under stress from bacterial metabolites or 'toxins'?

I would have thought that mucus cells could play their normal role without being ripped to shreds. And this benefit of bran (if it can be called a benefit) applies only to the large intestine (colon). What adverse effects would such rough treatment do to the delicate villi which line the small intestine or the wall of the stomach?

Incidentally, I haven't eaten any cereal fibre, and very little vegetable fibre either, for many years. I have no trouble at all keeping 'regular.'

Conclusion

What we have is evidence that some forms of vegetable fibre – but not bran – have been found to lower blood cholesterol levels, but that this has had no effect on heart disease mortality or morbidity rates (which is not surprising, as lowering blood cholesterol levels in the general public by any means has not proved beneficial); and that the consumption of fibre – and bran in particular – may be hazardous.

There is a very real danger that mothers of growing families, perhaps already obsessed with slimming, will spend much of their limited food budgets on heavily advertised, expensive, fibre-rich breakfast cereals and biscuits. With the balance tipped away from nutrients, their children could well suffer in terms of growth which can have serious long-term consequences apart from those already mentioned.

There is also a similar danger of malnutrition in the elderly who are also at risk from hypothermia. On both sides of the debate there is agreement that the recommendations on both fibre and fats will not benefit the over-60s. But one only has to look in the supermarket shopping trolleys of elderly women to see packets of highly priced, nutrient poor commodities such as bran flakes, when their pensions would be better spent on highly nutritious and energy-rich food such as eggs.

It seems unlikely that eating bran is of benefit to any section of society. There is a limit under which bran may not be harmful – but no ready way to know what that limit is. Therefore, it is much safer for you to avoid bran than to try to gauge what your safe limit might be. And if you do suffer from constipation, you would be better advised to drink more water. About four pints a day should do it.

As a postscript, I am informed that, ironically, Dr Burkitt died of colon cancer.[39]

Chapter Eight

Why 'five portions'?

The mantra that everyone will know is 'eat five portions of fruit and veg a day'. Yet there is little evidence of benefit over about two portions a week; and eating as much as five a day could have serious adverse effects on health. Growing them is also a wasteful use of land.

> The public is completely unaware that the strength of the message is not matched by the strength of the evidence.
>
> *Dr Barnett Kramer*

Some time ago I was making a documentary video. The then-current craze for low-carbohydrate diets, sparked by a sudden upsurge of interest in the 'Atkins diet', was causing all kinds of confusion. The idea of the documentary was to sort out the truth from the hype and give some useful advice. We interviewed several dieters about their experiences on various slimming regimes; they reported on the benefits of low-carb, high-fat diets. But wanting to be unbiased and put both sides of the debate, we also interviewed general medical practitioners, nutritionists and dieticians.

One of the dieticians – I'll call her Jane – came to be interviewed directly from the headquarters of a national dietetic authority in London. During the interview, I asked Jane why the British Dietetic Association (BDA) recommended five portions of fruit and vegetables a day. 'Because that's healthy eating,' she told me. 'Yes,' I said, 'but what is the basis for the recommendation – what is the evidence for it?'

Jane told me that it was government advice. 'But,' I persisted, 'that isn't evidence.' I asked again on what evidence the recommendations were based; which study or studies had shown that 'five portions' was healthy.

'It's healthy eating,' she replied.

I tried another tack. The BDA and American Dietetic Association base their recommendations on findings from the Framingham Heart Study. I knew that this study had been misrepresented so I decided to ask for her comments on the various pronouncements from Framingham that did not agree with the BDA's recommendations. I started by asking: 'Would you agree with me that the Framingham Heart Study is the world's most respected and influential study into the dietary causes of heart disease?'

'What's the Framingham Study?' she asked. That stopped me in my tracks and, although I did ask further questions, it effectively finished the interview.

Jane was paid her fee and left. A week later her cheque was returned with a solicitor's letter warning us that action would be taken if we used any part of her interview in the video.

Jane's was not an isolated case. In the end, although we used material from all the doctors we interviewed, we couldn't in all conscience use material from any of the nutritionists or dieticians without compromising their careers (although we would have liked to do just that!). It was obvious even to our camera crew that none of them knew their subject.

The science is flawed

It's not difficult to see that the science behind the '5 portions' recommendations is flawed if you compare the wide discrepancies between the recommendations and portion sizes as defined by US and UK governments. If the recommendations were made on the basis of a rational analysis of a coherent body of data, you might expect the advice on both sides of the Atlantic to be similar. It isn't. In Table 8.1 opposite, is a comparison of official US[1] and UK[2] recommendations.

First, take a look at the numbers of portions and their sizes: note that portion size can vary by quite a large amount between the US and UK. Also, in the UK, dietary components such as fruit juice, legumes and dried fruit only work their magic on the first portion; extra portions are not counted as far as the '5 portions' rule is concerned. In the US it all counts. Another anomaly is that, in the US, raw vegetables count just as much as cooked ones, even though the bioavailability of the nutrients in raw vegetables is much lower than in cooked vegetables.

So what is the evidence for '5 portions' a day?

This was a question I had hoped that Jane could answer because there simply didn't seem to be any evidence when the recommendations were first drawn up. But there is now – and it doesn't support the recommendations.

But first things first. We are told that we should eat '5 portions' to prevent cancer and cardiovascular disease. If there is a dose-response whereby

Table 8.1: Comparison of US and UK '5 portions' recommendations

	Serving sizes US	Serving sizes UK	US : UK Ratio
Fruit or vegetables	8 tbs (1/2 cup)	3 tbs	2.67 : 1
Whole fruit	One medium-size fruit	One medium-size fruit	1 : 1
Dried fruit	4 tbs (1/4 cup)	'1 heaped tbs'*	4? : 1
Fruit juice	3/4 cup (6 fl oz)	'one small glass 150 ml'*	1.2 : 1
Canned or frozen legumes	8 tbs (1/2 cup)	Unclear ††	?
Raw, leafy vegetables	16 tbs (1 cup)	1 cereal bowl (However much that is)	? *

*(http://www.bbc.co.uk/health/healthy_living/nutrition/dietary_cvd.shtml)
† only one portion per day counts
†† although no portion size is given, only one portion counts.

four portions, say, aren't good enough, then surely the size and number of portions would be important. Yet neither seems to matter. Other scientists must have wondered about this as well, because over the last few years several studies into the five-a-day claim have been conducted to test the advice.

The prestigious CARDIO2000 study published its results in 2003.[3] This study was looking at intakes of fruit and vegetables specifically in relation to acute heart disease. They found that vegetables did reduce the risk of heart disease. But, significantly, it didn't need '5 portions a day' for the maximum effect. In their conclusions the researchers say:

> 'Our findings support that even low consumption of fruits and vegetables (1–2 servings per week) is associated with about 45% lower coronary risk. Consumption of *2 or more servings per week* is associated with about 70% reduction in relative risk.' [emphasis added]

The *Daily Mail* reported the study's results.[4] The *Mail* interviewed Professor Sir Charles George, medical director of the British Heart Foundation, about the obvious conflict with the five-a-day guidelines. Sir Charles answered: 'There is some argument about how much you need; I think five may be an arbitrary figure' – and, by so doing, admitted that this was yet another example of dietary advice which was based on nothing more than guesswork. So we don't need to eat five a day to derive benefits in terms of heart disease.

But is there a benefit in terms of the other major disease it is aimed at: cancer? This was considered in another study of over 100,000 people conducted by the Harvard School of Public Health and published in 2004.[5] This showed that: 'Increased fruit and vegetable consumption was associated with a modest *although not statistically significant* reduction in the development of major chronic disease' [emphasis added]. It continued: 'The benefits appeared to be primarily for cardiovascular disease and not for cancer.' And concluded: 'Consumption of five or more servings of fruits and vegetables has been recommended . . . but the protective effect of fruit and vegetable intake may have been overstated.'

Not surprisingly, supporters of the '5-a-day' campaign were outraged by the findings, repeating their mantra that eating the recommended number of fruit and vegetables has numerous health benefits – without specifying what those benefits might be.

So you won't be surprised to learn that a very large study found no benefit in breast cancer from eating 'five portions.' In this study, 20 named researchers investigated 7,377 incidents of invasive breast cancers and a wide variety of fruit and vegetable intakes among 351,825 women at 17 cancer research centres in the US, Germany, the Netherlands, and Sweden. They found no association for green leafy vegetables, eight botanical groups, and 17 specific fruits and vegetables. They concluded: 'These results suggest that fruit and vegetable consumption during adulthood is not significantly associated with reduced breast cancer risk.'[6]

Whenever studies such as these are reported, the diet police repeat their dogma that eating the recommended number of helpings of fruit and vegetables has numerous health benefits; they say that the evidence is 'overwhelming'. But they never seem able to quote any of that evidence or to specify exactly what the benefits are. In view of the above studies, that will probably come as no real surprise. The point is that, just like almost all the health advice we have had forced down our throats and come to believe over the last few decades, there is practically no scientific basis for the 'five portions' advice.

Dr Barnett Kramer, of the National Institutes of Health in the US, said of the healthy eating message: 'Over time, the messages on diet and cancer have been ratcheted up until they are almost co-equal with the smoking messages . . . a lot of the public is completely unaware that the strength of the message is not matched by the strength of the evidence.'

Fructose: the harmful sugar in fruit

We are told over and over again about 'good' and 'bad' fats. Now it is becoming clear that there are also good and bad sugars. New evidence suggests that one sugar may be particularly harmful. That sugar turns out to be fructose – the sugar found in the fruit we are told to eat more of.

Fructose, obesity and diabetes

Fears that fructose is fuelling the obesity epidemic and leading to diabetes have been circulating for years, but human data were scarce. So Dr Peter Havel at the University of California, Davis, persuaded 33 overweight and obese adults to go on a diet that contained either pure fructose or glucose. He presented the results at a meeting of the Endocrine Society in San Francisco in June 2008.[7]

The differences between the two groups were staggering. In those given fructose, there was an increase in the amount of intra-abdominal fat, which wraps around internal organs, causes a pot belly and has been linked to an increased risk of diabetes and cardiovascular disease. The fructose group also became more insulin resistant. Glucose appeared to have no effect on these measures.

Although pure fructose was used in this trial, sucrose (table sugar) and high fructose corn syrup were also implicated.

Fructose and heart disease

Too much fruit may also be a cause of heart disease. Recently the *American Journal of Clinical Nutrition* published a review article which revisited an old hypothesis where sugar, particularly excessive fructose intake, expressed a critical role in the epidemic of heart and kidney diseases. The authors of this review presented evidence of fructose's unique ability to induce an increase in uric acid. This, they suggested, may be a major mechanism by which fructose can cause cardio-renal disease.[8] This added weight to a much older study which found that various sugars had different effects which were related to differences in the rapidity of combustion of the sugar or differences in the rate at which sugars were transformed into fat.[9] Fructose was the worst.

Hypertension is another suggested risk factor for cardiovascular disease. In 2008 another study also implicated fructose, this time mainly from soft drinks, as a cause of high blood pressure.[10] The worrying aspect of this study was that the blood pressure rises were seen in young adults.

Fructose and cancer

In recent years, there has also been growing concern that dietary fructose increases the risk of cancer, particularly the deadly pancreatic cancer.[11] But this is really not all that new. Dr John Beard, Professor of Embryology at Edinburgh University, had shown that fructose might be responsible for cancers as long ago as 1911.[12]

Fructose summary

Fruits bred today are nothing like natural fruit. They are bred for sweetness, and are generally little more than sugared water. Unfortunately, that sugar is pure fructose. Pure fructose is found in fresh fruit, fruit juice, and preserves. It is also found in table sugar, maple syrup, and corn syrup, and in 'healthy' foods such as honey, and many vegetables.

Sugars and starches lower our immunity to infectious diseases

Have you noticed how many cases of meningitis there seem to be, these days? I don't recollect hearing the word in my youth. There are also many other infectious diseases that seem to have started only in the late 20th century: lots of acronyms like SARS, AIDS, and MRSA; the exotically named *necrotising fasciitis* which has a nasty habit of eating us alive; *Clostridium difficile*, which has taken over from MRSA as the major killer hospital disease; a different flu every year . . . I won't go on. Why? What is happening?

We are told that medical science has been able to prevent diphtheria and smallpox by vaccination. But has it? According to Dr Abram Hoffer, 'The role played by vaccinations over the past 100 years has been grossly exaggerated and the harm that this has done and still does has been carefully hidden from public view . . . In brief the vaccine industry has not been honest with the public.'[13] We supposedly reduced tuberculosis by pasteurizing milk and improving general hygiene – but it is returning. A clean water supply and proper sewage disposal prevented typhoid and cholera. Today, we in Britain and the US are protected from these diseases because we have been artificially immunized against them and cocooned from them; *not* because our bodies' inherent ability to prevent infection has been strengthened. And therein lies the problem.

The microbiologist, Rene Dubos, wrote half a century ago in his book, *Mirage of Health*, that plants, animals and humans can live healthily side by side with their most notorious microbial enemies. 'The world is obsessed by the fact that poliomyelitis can kill and maim several thousand unfortunate victims every year. But more extraordinary is the fact that millions upon millions of young people become infected by polio viruses, yet suffer no harm from the infection,' he wrote.[14]

Dubos' remarks might seem extraordinary but it is a fact that infection can occur without producing disease. In a community properly endowed with health, the *extraordinary* event would be somebody getting sick at all. This is ably demonstrated in cultures other than ours (although they are becoming fewer as they succumb to western dietary assaults).

We in the 'civilized' countries are aware that we can no longer rely on antibiotics to treat our illnesses. As we've seen from the increasing spread of 'superbugs', antibiotics are fast losing the battle against infections. This is because the overuse of antibiotics has led to certain strains of bacteria developing a resistance to their action. In response, doctors have been forced to develop stronger and more toxic antibiotics to fight infections. This can lead to increased side effects such as diarrhoea, vomiting, rashes, ringing in the ears, jaundice and, in rare cases, epileptic fits. At the same time, the bugs will continue to adapt and we progressively lose the battle.

There is a much better way to combat the bugs that would harm us.

In the constant fight against infectious diseases, our bodies have a sophisticated defence mechanism – our immune system. When it is functioning properly, our immune system is far more effective than you might imagine: it can dismantle and rid the body of a transplanted kidney very quickly. It can do the same to invading bacteria and viruses if it is kept in good condition. Unfortunately, in our society the general level of health and, therefore, the general level of our immunity is marginal. We accept high numbers of all kinds of infections, particularly colds, influenza, herpes, hepatitis, candida and so on, as normal events we have to put up with. They aren't.

A major part of our immunity relies on cells called *neutrophils*, a type of *leukocyte* or white blood cell. These circulate in our blood streams and mop up any bacteria, viruses or other foreign bodies they come across. This process is called *phagocytosis* (from the Greek *phagein* = eat). While this process is an energy requiring mechanism that needs an adequate supply of the blood sugar, glucose, too much glucose has the effect of reducing the neutrophils' ability to ingest and kill off invading bacteria.

The measure of how many organisms one leukocyte can eat in an hour is called the '*leukocytic index*' (LI). It is a simple measure: if a leukocyte eats 10 organisms in an hour, its leukocytic index is 10.

The neutrophils that we rely on to kill any invading bacteria and viruses form 60 to 70% of the white blood cells in our bodies. They are generally much more active than any other blood cell. It can be disastrous to our health, therefore, if their effectiveness is compromised in any way. Of all the factors in our modern world that are working against our immune defences, our diet is the worst, for this is exactly what happens if we eat too much carbohydrate and too much sugar in particular.

By 'sugar' I do not mean just the white, granulated stuff we serve from a bowl on the table. That is *sucrose*; the term 'sugar' applies also to glucose, fructose (fruit sugar), maltose (grain sugar), lactose (milk sugar) and honey (a mix of glucose, fructose, sucrose and dextrin).

Test results

Forty years ago researchers carried out a series of studies that examined how the sugar we eat weakens the ability of white blood cells to destroy bacteria. The results of the study, in Table 8:2 below, showed that if a person ate no sugar for 12 hours, each white blood cell could destroy an average of 14 bacteria. As sugar intake was increased, so the numbers of bacteria consumed lessened until, by the time 24 teaspoons of sugar were consumed, the white blood cells were so compromised that they could only destroy an average of one bacterium each.[15] The implications of this study are obvious. Eat white sugar and you severely compromise your body's ability to fight infection.

But white granulated sugar is only one form of 'sugar' that we eat. In 1973 another study was performed to check the effects of a range of sugars on our immune system. After an overnight fast and their leukocytic index (LI) had been recorded, 10 people were fed 100 grams of a specific sugar or starch.[16] Table 8.3 shows that all forms of carbohydrate – starch as well as sugars – reduced the white blood cells' effectiveness at destroying bacteria and other micro-organisms (the figures are averages across all subjects). This study also found that leukocytes' effectiveness was compromised as blood glucose rose.

Consequences

Based on these studies, any person who eats largely carbohydrate-based meals, particularly those containing sugars, and snacks with carbohydrate-based meals spread throughout the day, could lose up to half their immunity to disease for much of the waking day.

It is important to note that, again, the worst sugar was fructose.

Fructose is harmful for several reasons.[17] Unbound fructose can interfere with the heart's use of vital minerals such as magnesium, copper and chromium; it reduces the affinity of insulin for its receptor, which is the principle characteristic of insulin resistance and type-2 diabetes; it has been implicated in raising blood cholesterol levels; and it has been found to inhibit the action of white blood cells in the immune system. So if you want to live a healthy life, free from infection, 'five portions of fruit' may not be such a good idea, even if vegetables are.

Table 8.2: How sugar affects our white blood cells' ability to destroy bacteria

Teaspoons of sugar	Number of bacteria destroyed	This amount of sugar can be found in:
0	14.0	–
6	10.0	1 scoop of ice cream
12	5.5	1 can of fizzy drink
18	2.0	Less than half a malted drink
24	1.0	1 milk shake

Table 8.3: Reduction in immune function with different carbohydrates

	Fasting LI	Lowest LI	Decline %	Time before returning to normal
Fructose	15.5	8.5	45.1	more than 5 hours
Sucrose	15.2	8.6	44.0	more than 5 hours
Orange juice	16.6	9.6	42.1	more than 5 hours
Glucose	16.2	9.6	40.5	more than 5 hours
Honey	15.9	9.7	39.0	more than 5 hours
Starch	15.7	13.6	13.4	more than 5 hours

When doing nothing is better than taking an antibiotic

Around 15 million antibiotic prescriptions are written every year in the US for children with the ear infection, *acute otitis media*.

When people get such an infection, they often hurry off to their doctors and are put on a course of antibiotics. A recent American study showed that you might be better off doing nothing.[18] In this study, children with the ear infection were split into two groups: one given an antibiotic immediately, the other told to 'wait and see' for 48 hours before taking the drug. There was no difference between the two groups in terms of either fever or ear pain. But when a sub-group of those in the 'wait-and-see' group did finally take an antibiotic, they experienced worse fevers and more ear pain.

On top of that, antibiotics have a nasty habit of creating resistance while doing very little to cure the problem.

Vaccination may also help to create more resistant 'superbugs.' In November 2007, came a report of a variant of antibiotic resistant *Streptococcus pneumoniae* which causes cases of acute otitis media in children. So far, nine cases have been reported by doctors in America, but researchers fear that many more children have been affected. Of those nine cases, four could be treated only by surgery. This new strain emerged following the introduction of a vaccination programme in 2000.[19]

Antibiotic resistance

MRSA, the bug that thrives in hospitals, was a bigger killer than AIDS in the US in 2005 and experts believe the MRSA infection rate has increased dramatically since then.[20]

But have you noticed that it is only hospital *patients* who are harmed by or die from MRSA? Doctors, nurses, porters, cleaners as well as the patients' visitors don't seem to be affected by this nasty bug. Could that be because of some way patients are fed? If you are unfortunate enough to need hospital treatment that involves intravenous feeding, that feed will be heavily glucose-based. So, with a condition in which your immune system is probably already compromised by your illness, the hospital will feed you a concoction that could damage it still further.

It is important to understand that it is not easy to boost the immune system artificially; but given the right conditions, principally the right nutrients through a correct diet, it can regenerate of its own accord.

Vaccinations

It's the same story with vaccination. I'll only give one example. At a time when health officials are quietly admitting that there could be a link between the MMR (measles-mumps-rubella) vaccine and autism, a new study has also discovered that the MMR vaccine doesn't always work.[21] Researchers investigating a large outbreak of mumps in 2006, when 6,584 cases were reported among college students, discovered that almost every sufferer had been vaccinated against the disease – twice.

Diabetics and infection

We have known for over 70 years that diabetes is caused by excessive intake of carbohydrates.[22] Excessive carbohydrate intake may also be why diabetics have been found to have impaired phagocytic activity when compared with healthy people, and are thus at significantly greater risk from infections.[23,24] Current dietary advice should be reviewed to ensure that diabetics are even more careful not to consume a carbohydrate- and particularly a fruit-based diet.

Infections and cancer

Every day we are all attacked by things that could start a cancer: particles in the air we breathe, the water we drink and the food we eat. It is estimated that at any one time we have thousands of potentially cancerous cells circulating in our bodies. But in a healthy body these are mopped up by our immune system before they can get a foothold. You will see, therefore, that just as healthy leukocytes can stop us catching a cold, they might also stop us from getting cancer.

According to Dr Donald Maxwell Parkin, from the University of Oxford, an estimated 18% of cancer worldwide is caused by infections.[25] The worst culprit is the ubiquitous peptic ulcer-causing bacterium *Helicobacter pylori*, which is associated with the development of 5.5% of all cancers, particularly stomach cancer and gastric lymphoma. This is closely followed by the *human papilloma virus*, which is specifically associated with the development of cervical cancer. Other cancers with an infectious cause include liver cancer, Hodgkin's and non-Hodgkin's lymphomas, leukaemia and Kaposi's sarcoma.

Dr Parkin explains that if such infections could be prevented, it would significantly reduce the number of cancer deaths and the burden placed by the disease on worldwide health resources.

Unfortunately, this is an area where nearly everyone is still in massive denial over the influence of sugars on cancer. Even though a Nobel Prize was awarded to the German physician, Dr Otto Warburg, in 1931 for recognizing this, three-quarters of a century later very few physicians have applied this basic concept.

Infections and heart disease

The popular belief that a fatty diet causes heart disease is untenable because the process that creates atherosclerotic plaques is not, as we are led to believe, fatty formations in the arteries themselves, but the intrusion of LDL particles into the walls of the arteries. Yet there is no obvious way in which LDL can get through the lining of artery walls (*endothelium*) in an otherwise healthy person because the endothelium is a barrier to LDL.[26]

The only way LDL can get through the lining and into the artery wall is if that lining is damaged in some way, by either a cut, shear stress or disease. This means that anything that can damage the endothelium or promote the formation of a clot may have a serious impact on plaque formation, growth and rupture. What is attributed merely to cholesterol is actually a combination of damage to the endothelium followed by the formation of a clot (*thrombus*), which contains cholesterol, over the area to repair the damage. The endothelium then grows over the thrombus, effectively drawing it into the arterial wall – a natural inflammatory, healing process. This process, repeated, causes plaques to grow and eventually rupture, causing a blockage in an artery.

A cut or similar damage is unlikely in the coronary arteries: they are buried too deep in the body. But what about, for example, a bacterial or viral attack which damages the endothelium? This seems more likely and it is seriously considered as a likely cause: a large number of studies have reported associations between human coronary heart disease and certain persistent bacterial and viral infections. Particularly implicated are *Chlamydia pneumoniae*, a bacterium that commonly causes respiratory infections, and *Helicobacter pylori*.[27] Other equally ubiquitous *herpesviruses* and *cytomegalovirus* are also candidates. According to Drs Kei Namuzaki, Assistant Professor of Paediatrics, and Shunzo Chiba, Professor and Chairman, Sapporo Medical University, Japan: 'Endothelial cells are one of the main targets of the cytomegalovirus infection.'[28]

Such an effect is very likely, as atherosclerosis, the condition thought to lead to heart attacks, and sepsis, the putrefactive destruction of body tissues by bacteria, share several similarities, including immune dysfunction, increased formation of blood clots, and systemic inflammation.

In mid-2007 scientists at the Atherosclerosis Research Laboratory, Texas Heart Institute in Houston, demonstrated for the first time that systemic infections can themselves trigger heart attacks.[29]

Thus, by reducing the body's ability to fight infections, a 'healthy diet', based on carbohydrates, particularly sugars and fruit juices, provides several avenues which may precipitate a heart attack.

Fruit and vegetables as antioxidants

Many of the conditions we experience today occur when the fats and cholesterol in our bodies are attacked by oxygen. This is why we are told to eat fruit and vegetables: they contain antioxidants. But there isn't much point in eating foods that contain antioxidants unless those antioxidants are absorbed into the body.

In 2004, scientists at the University of Oslo, Norway, set up a study to determine the contribution of various food groups to total antioxidant intake, and to assess just how much of these antioxidants was actually absorbed into the bloodstream from each of the various food groups. [30]

Figure 8.1 shows these levels. As you can clearly see, fruit and vegetables play very little part. Wine and tea, which we are told are great suppliers of antioxidants, are also actually very poor suppliers. With 11.1 mmols in the bloodstream, coffee supplied over twice as much usable antioxidant as all the rest put together.

So, should we drink lots of coffee? A review published in 2001 reported the dismal findings of several sizeable randomized trials of antioxidant vitamins. These showed that not only did they not help to decrease death rates, but in two studies of the antioxidant, beta-carotene, there was a possible increased risk of heart attacks.[31] This was confirmed in a report of 2002 when the huge Heart Protection Study was forced to conclude that:

> 'Despite assessing the combined effects of several years of substantial daily doses of different antioxidant vitamins (including 600 mg of vitamin E) in a large number of high-risk people, the Heart Protection Study has not been able to demonstrate any benefits from such supplementation.'[32]

But those taking part in the trials may not have been drinking coffee; it wasn't tested. In a critical review of the actual value of antioxidants, scientists from the University of Bern, Switzerland, the University of Southern California, Los Angeles, and King's College, London, pointed out

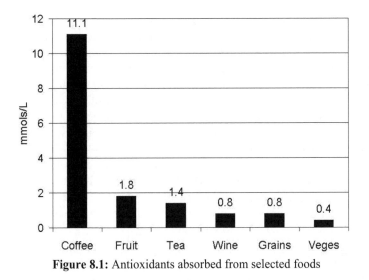

Figure 8.1: Antioxidants absorbed from selected foods

that there are several problems with chemicals that are considered to be antioxidants.[33] Firstly, many antioxidants are not absorbed into the body from the gut and so can do no good; secondly, chemicals that have anti-oxidant activity when tested in laboratory dishes, as most are, may have an entirely different effect or no effect at all when ingested into the body; and thirdly, the 'antioxidants' are not always beneficial and may actually be harmful. They conclude that after a period of flourishing research on oxidants and antioxidants:

> 'It is time . . . to critically reflect on the field. Speculation that many (if not all) diseases are related to radical damage needs to be supported by more secure data. The hope that antioxidants can prevent or cure a number of pathological situations also requires reconsideration . . .'

Is there a biological need for vegetables or fruit?

'Everybody knows' that scurvy, the blight of ancient mariners, is caused by a lack of vitamin C, that vitamin C is found in fruit and vegetables, and that British sailors were called 'limeys' because British ships carried supplies of lemons and limes to ward off scurvy. This belief suggests hard evidence that we do need to eat fruit and vegetables.

The Icelandic-born anthropologist and explorer, Dr Vilhjalmur Stefansson, spent many years in the early 20th century living with the Eskimos of Northern Canada and Alaska, eating as they did. He also mounted several sea- and land-borne expeditions and conducted much research on the North American Indians as well as on European-born trappers and hunters. All of them ate a diet completely devoid of all fruits and vegetables – and none of them developed scurvy, or any other degenerative disease.[34] The same is true of many other cultures around the world: the traditional diet of the Maasai and Samburu tribes of East Africa, for example, is composed entirely of milk, blood and meat from their cattle, and they are also untroubled by any of the degenerative diseases that plague us. But we shouldn't be too surprised at this. Contrary to popular belief, plants aren't the only source of vitamin C; foods of animal origin also contain it.

The story below illustrates just how unimportant fruit and vegetables are if the underlying diet is correct. On the other hand, fruit and vegetables are essential as a greater source of vitamin C if cereals are eaten. This is because vitamin C is needed for the metabolism of carbohydrates – and cereal grains contain no vitamin C.

Case history

Lord Strathcona – the Donald Smith of Mount Sir Donald, Smith's Landing, and countless towns and natural features throughout Canada – was not only one of the richest men in the British Empire, he was Canada's High Commissioner in London in the late 19th and early 20th century. Vilhjalmur Stefansson, in his autobiography, *Discovery*, gives a detailed account of Lord Strathcona's dietary habits which illustrate well how a restricted diet can be eminently healthy. After Stefansson had told Lord Strathcona what he had learned from the Eskimos, His Lordship told Stefansson that years ago in Canada he had begun a regimen all his own. He told how he had begun to wonder why, since he liked some things better than others, he should bother to eat something different on one day when he had liked what he had eaten the previous day better. 'This led,' recounts Stefansson, 'to his questioning what he really did like and, when he got the answer, eating nothing else – eggs, milk, and butter.' Stefansson was frequently a guest at Lord Strathcona's home in Grosvenor Square, and so had plenty of opportunity to observe him. He wrote: 'Strathcona, a broad-shouldered man taller than six feet, would be seated at one end of the long table, Lady Strathcona at the other. As course after course was served to the rest of us, he would converse, drinking a sip or two of each wine as it was poured. Sometime during the middle of the dinner, his tray was brought: several medium-soft boiled eggs broken into a large bowl, with plenty of butter and with extra butter in a side dish, and, I believe, a quart of whole milk, or perhaps half-and-half.'

Lord Strathcona must have been doing something right because he lived entirely healthily to the ripe old age of 93.

The humble egg is not only one of the healthiest, cheapest and easiest-to-use foods, it has also been shown to reduce, yes reduce, the risk of a heart attack.[35] I know eggs are supposed to be 'unhealthy', but study shows that eggs actually have anti-inflammatory properties, possibly due, so the study says: 'to the presence of cholesterol, which increases HDL, and to the antioxidant lutein which modulates certain inflammatory responses.'

Economic considerations

There is one other consideration as far as vegetables are concerned. It's a purely economic one. The sheer bulk and the absence of calories in vegetables make them impractical and wasteful to cultivate in comparison to animal products like eggs, dairy produce and meat. Only a society which has a surplus of calories readily and cheaply available can afford to waste time, effort and cultivable land growing high-waste, low-calorie foods like vegetables.

Conclusion

Although there is a small amount of evidence which suggests that a few vegetables may confer a degree of protection against heart disease in the context of our industrialized society, with its generally unhealthy 'healthy diet', there seems little or no evidence that fruit does. There is also precious little evidence that either fruit or vegetables confer any protection against cancer, and that fruit and some veges may increase the risk.

You will die without protein and fats which are essential to build and maintain the body. But, scientifically, carbohydrates should not be classified as a macronutrient as they are not essential for life or even good health. Indeed, the sugars contained in fruit in particular could be considered a significant hazard to health.

Under the circumstances, you may be wiser to compromise and eat one or two portions of vegetables a day, if there is land surplus on which to grow them, but go easy on fruit.

Incidentally, the only sailors who got scurvy were those who ate ships' biscuits.

Chapter Nine

The phoney war on salt

Salt was so valuable that Roman soldiers were paid with it. Today, salt is the subject of the latest health scare. However, if the evidence against the 'diet/heart' hypothesis is flimsy, the evidence against salt is practically non-existent. While salt has been shown to increase blood pressure in a small proportion of people, in others it lowers blood pressure and in most it makes not the slightest difference. Current strictures against salt are increasing health problems.

The heart attack fatality rate among those on low-sodium diets was 20% higher that those on normal diets.

Dr Helen Whalley

The human heart is nothing more than a muscular pump. When it contracts, it forces blood through the arteries. At this point blood pressure is at its highest. Between heartbeats, the heart relaxes and pressure drops.

When blood pressure is measured, the cuff is usually wrapped around the arm just above the elbow, level in height with the heart, and a stethoscope or electronic sensor is placed over the brachial artery. The cuff is then inflated with air to such a pressure that the brachial artery is closed and no blood flows down the arm. Then the air is allowed to escape slowly from the cuff. When the pressure is just less than the pressure in the artery, a jet of blood will spurt through the artery and be detected by the sensor. This is the *systolic* measurement. As more air is allowed to escape, the pressure falls until the point at which the blood flow is continuous between heartbeats. This is the *diastolic* pressure. These numbers are the pressure needed to raise a column of mercury to a height in millimetres (mm Hg); blood pressure is expressed as the systolic pressure over the diastolic pressure, e.g. 125 over 70 or 125/70.

High blood pressure (*hypertension*) has been variously defined as a systolic pressure higher than: 100 plus your age, then 100 plus half your age, then a fixed figure incorporating both systolic and diastolic: 160/100, then 140/90, and currently it's 130/80, although by the time you read this it might well be lower still as numbers have been steadily decreasing over the years. I have even heard of people with perfectly normal blood pressure described as 'pre-hypertensive', which has the 'benefit' of turning practically everybody into a patient.

Whatever the measurement, it can be misleading, particularly among the elderly. As arteries become stiffer, usually with age, a greater pressure in the cuff of the sphygmomanometer is required to close them, giving the impression of a higher blood pressure than is, in fact, present. Blood pressure is also affected by your physical condition at the time it is measured. If you are working hard, your muscles use up more nutrients and oxygen, and produce more waste products. Blood, which carries all nutrients throughout the body and removes waste from muscles, must be pumped round faster. Under these conditions a raised blood pressure is quite normal. Similarly, when you rest, your blood pressure falls. Even asleep in bed, if you turn over there will be a change in blood pressure. There are also significant variations dependent upon where you are when your blood pressure is measured. When you are at home with your family, it will be at its lowest. With friends it will be higher, and when you are with strangers it will be higher still.[1]

Interarm blood pressure differences are common

If you have had your blood pressure measured in one arm, and your doctor said it was high, did he also measure it in your other arm too? Or in your legs? A large difference between limb measurements is generally believed to indicate the possibility of disease involving the major arteries and their tributaries in the upper part of the body. For this reason measuring blood pressure at several sites is thought essential; a single measurement tells only part of the story.

In 1997, researchers at the State University of New York reported that large differences in blood pressure between the right and left arms are actually quite common.[2] Measuring both arms either simultaneously or sequentially (right arm first followed immediately by the left arm), the researchers discovered that the mean systolic blood pressure difference was about 10 while the mean diastolic pressure difference was 8.5 and 6.7 for sequential and simultaneous measurements respectively. They suggest that initial blood pressure measurements should be made in both arms and follow-up measurements should always be made in the same arm. The researchers also found that patients with known coronary heart disease tended to have a greater interarm systolic pressure difference than did people with no heart disease (14.5 mm Hg compared with 10.4 mm Hg). They did, however, conclude that even a difference as large as 20 may not be indicative of a problem.

High blood pressure and heart disease

People with high blood pressure do seem to suffer a greater degree of heart disease, but it is quite obvious if one looks at the history of both those conditions that the forces responsible for each are different and independent of each other: a comparison of hypertension with coronary heart disease in the US shows that death rates from the latter decreased in log-linear fashion after 1950 while deaths from the former were still rising.[3]

Why blame salt?

As in other 'diseases of civilization', hypertension is generally blamed on an item of food we eat: in this case, salt. In fact, salt was one of the first dietary items to be indicted by the 'healthy eating' faddists. We saw in Chapter Three how weak the argument against fat is; in the case against salt, it's even weaker: none of the 17,000 studies published on salt and blood pressure since 1966 has shown population-wide health benefits from low-salt diets.

For centuries, salt, or to give it its scientific name, *sodium chloride* (NaCl), has been regarded as essential for health. Salt was so important that people were paid in salt; the Roman soldiers' *salarium* is the origin of our word 'salary'. The word 'soldier' comes from the Latin (*sal dare*), which means 'to give salt'. Salt was also used extensively as a valuable commodity for bartering: in ancient Greece, slaves were traded for salt; it's the origin of the phrase 'not worth his salt'. In Biblical times, salt was also used to seal an agreement or contract. When Jesus called his disciples 'the salt of the earth' he meant they were people on whom he could rely. Participants at medieval feasts were seated in order of importance based on the location of the salt dishes. Distinguished guests dined at an elegant elevated banquet table 'above the salt'. Common people sat 'below the salt'. And there are many more examples through-out the world demonstrating that salt was regarded as a very valuable, purifying and healthy commodity.

Then, suddenly, in the late 20th century salt became a killer, indicted as a cause of hypertension and, thence, of stroke and of heart disease. The evidence on which this was based arose from poorly controlled, cross-cultural studies carried out earlier in the century.

Salt is a naturally occurring chemical that is vital to the body. It is an essential constituent of secretions such as perspiration and tears, and it plays a major part in the regulation of fluids within the body. We don't know why some people have permanently high blood pressure but the mechanisms which regulate and stabilize blood pressure in the body are many and extremely complex. They are also very efficient: when people eat more salt than is required by the body, it is excreted in the urine and, if they eat less than the body needs, the kidneys conserve it.[4] People living in the tropics, particularly in desert conditions, know only too well the value of salt. Deaths from sunstroke and dehydration are not usually caused by loss of water but by loss of salt.

Hypertension is rare in primitive cultures out of contact with civilization, untouched by western living stresses and eating little salt. When these people move into a western situation their blood pressure tends to rise. Comparing cultures in an attempt to pin the cause of disease on just one difference is notoriously unreliable. If we look at individuals in any one country or culture, we find that salt plays not the slightest part in hypertension: those with the condition have not been shown to eat more salt than those without it. We also find that if hypertensives do reduce their salt intake, in some their blood pressure goes down while in others it goes up.

Studies on rats show that salt restriction is associated with an increased susceptibility to haemorrhage and kidney problems and the long-term effects of salt restriction on humans are unknown[5] – although it is known that even moderate reductions of sodium can cause problems with erection in men, and fatigue in men and women.[6]

Clinical, placebo controlled studies using drugs on people with mild to moderate hypertension have shown no benefit in terms of total mortality, there being a similar number of deaths in the drug intervention groups as in the group taking the placebo.[7] But those taking the drugs, *propranolol*, a beta blocker, and *bendrofluazide*, a diuretic, had to endure such side-effects as gout, diabetes and impotence.[8]

Diagnosis is harmful

Strangely, in these trials, the placebo groups also suffered similar side-effects, although to a lesser degree, and this points to another side-effect of this and similar interventions. It is recognized by most that diagnosis itself increases stress as it focuses the patient's mind on the possibility of not recovering and of having to be careful what he or she does; it adds uncertainty; and it adds reliance on others. It also sets the patient apart from the normal and healthy: when people who feel well are told that they have a life-threatening condition it alters their whole attitude to life in ways which have serious consequences, affecting their psychological well-being, their attitude to work, and their marital and social relationships.[9] People treated for hypertension are more likely to complain of more symptoms and are more depressed than untreated hypertensives; also they are more prone to absenteeism and they lose the ability to enjoy social and recreational activities.[10]

So a recent trend is particularly worrying. A friend of mine, an apparently healthy man aged 84, has normal blood pressure. When he tried to arrange insurance for a holiday abroad in 2004, his insurance company asked for medical details, which were duly supplied by his doctor. They then refused to insure him because he was 'hypertensive'. But he knew he wasn't. He contacted his doctor to clarify the situation. It turned out that, although he did *not* have high blood pressure, without his knowledge or consent, his doctor had put him on a blood-pressure lowering drug, a beta-blocker 'so that he didn't become hypertensive'!

Even today (2008), the long-term safety of low-salt diets has not been tested. Nevertheless, several committees recommended in the early 1980s that we should reduce our intake of dietary salt. In Britain the two most influential committees were, again, NACNE and COMA (see Glossary).

The bizarre reference

NACNE's report stated that a comparison between western and primitive societies appeared to show that raised blood pressure was due to an excess consumption of salt. Its reference for this statement, one purporting to demonstrate the benefit of a reduction in salt, was *Abstracts of the 18th annual conference of cardiovascular epidemiology 1978,* in the *Cardiovascular Disease Newsletter No. 28.* The choice of such a reference is bizarre to say the least. Many thousands of papers have been published in medical journals over the years which failed to show any benefit from reducing salt intake. These are not mentioned. Perhaps the committee had too much difficulty finding one that would support their recommendations. NACNE's choice of so obscure a reference provoked a storm of complaints from leading scientists from Scotland, England, the US, Sweden and New Zealand who wrote in *The Lancet*:

> 'We are concerned with the way in which this important issue is currently being handled. The idea (or likelihood) that salt in the diet has some positive value is totally ignored. The usual scientific standards for weighing evidence and giving advice which are now well established . . . seem to have been forgotten in an evangelical crusade to present a simplistic view of the evidence which will prove attractive to the media.' [11]

Professor Swales of Leicester University also pointed out:

> 'Such a citation would not even get into the bibliography of hypertension. The use of such a publication to support a major recommendation is not acceptable scientific practice . . . it is fairly apparent that an enormous superstructure is being built on extremely weak foundations.'[12]

The COMA report stated: 'We believe that the intake of salt in the United Kingdom diet (approximately 7-10 g per day) is needlessly high.' But the reference they used as evidence in support of this states: 'but a mechanism whereby salt could lead to the development of essential hypertension has not been established.' Also 'detailed investigations within a single community frequently fail to demonstrate such a relationship.'

Not that a lack of evidence has ever stopped the diet dictocrats from proclaiming the gospel, or the food industry from capitalizing on yet another golden opportunity for them to increase their very profitable range of 'healthy' foodstuffs sold to an unsuspecting public, this time 'with no added salt'.

Reduce hypertension – but increase heart disease?

With regard to heart disease, there is a confounding factor in that, in Japan, where hypertensive diseases are much more common, studies have shown that an increased consumption of saturated fats and cholesterol have led to a reduction in hypertension.[13,14] So, if the twin hypotheses that both dietary fat and high blood pressure can cause heart disease are correct, how can one be reduced without aggravating the other?

Where risk factors for both heart disease and hypertension do seem to run in parallel is in birth weight. Low weight at birth and high placenta weight, particularly if the two go together, have been shown to be a common factor in 50-year-old men with high blood pressure.[15] Similarly, a larger head circumference in relation to body length at birth, seems to mean higher systolic blood pressure.

In a study testing the relationship between diet towards the end of the first trimester of gestation and subsequent birth-weights, mothers of low birth-weight babies were found to be consuming a diet significantly lower in some essential nutrients than mothers of larger babies.[16] Particularly mentioned were sodium and chlorine (the two elements which make up salt). The authors of this study recommend that expectant mothers should *increase* salt intake.

The first National Health and Nutrition Examination Survey (NHANES I) established baseline information during 1971-75 in a representative sample of 20,729 American adults aged 25 to 75.[17] Of these, 11,348 underwent medical and nutritional examination. They were rechecked on 30 June 1992. By then there had been 3,923 deaths, of which 1,970 were due to a cardiovascular disease. Comparing salt intakes, this study found that those who ate the most salt had the *fewest* deaths – from any cause. And the same was found for cardiovascular deaths.

Dr Helen Whalley, writing a feature in *The Lancet*, talked of the continuing debate on the supposed association between salt and hypertension. She pointed out that an analysis of the NHANES I survey showed that 'the heart attack fatality rate among those on low-sodium diets was 20% higher that those on normal diets.'[18] She went on to report a study of the impact of long-term salt reduction. It found 'a four-fold increase in heart attacks among those on low-salt diets.'

The following year a large meta-analysis was published in an attempt to resolve the controversy.[19] Fifty-eight trials published between 1966 and the end of 1997 were reviewed to estimate the effects of reduced sodium intake on systolic and diastolic blood pressure, particularly as in recent years the debate has been extended by studies indicating that reducing sodium intake has adverse effects. This review found that reducing salt intake did reduce blood pressure slightly, but that it increased LDL. The authors concluded that: 'These results do not support a general recommendation to reduce sodium intake.'

And in May 2005, Dr Hillel W. Cohen, Assistant Professor of Epidemiology and Population Health, Albert Einstein College of Medicine, New York, presented study results to an American Heart Association meeting in Washington, DC. In their study, Cohen's team collected data on 7,278 men and women who participated in the Second National Health and Nutrition Examination Survey (NHANES II). During a follow-up over more than 13 years, the researchers looked for the number of deaths from heart disease and the number of deaths from any other cause. According to Cohen, they found that an intake of less than 6 grams of salt a day was associated with a 50% *higher* risk of heart disease; they also found that as the intake of salt went down, all-cause mortality and cardiovascular disease mortality went up.

These controversial findings challenge recommendations that people consume no more than 2.4 grams of sodium ion, which represents 6 grams, or about one teaspoon of table salt, a day.

Cohen told delegates: 'We are urging those who make these guidelines to go back to their data and look at additional data prior to making universal recommendations.'

Cohen also believes that the amount of salt that's right for one person may not be right for another. 'It is likely that there are differences between individuals with regard to sodium intake,' he said. 'And it's clear that the data do not support the current recommendations.'

According to Cohen, some people cannot tolerate high levels of salt, while others can. 'From a biological standpoint, if one's kidneys are working reasonably well, sodium within the usual range of intakes shouldn't be a problem.'

Not surprisingly, the findings were challenged by at least one expert, who called them unreliable.

There may be no need to cut your salt intake

In 2005, scientists across Europe completed the independent Rotterdam Study which involved almost 8,000 people in their 50s and above. The findings showed that as long as their salt intake was no more than 16 grams a day it had no significant effect on blood pressure. Stroke risk only increased with an intake over 21 grams. And even then, it had no detrimental effect on cardiovascular problems such as heart failure. This flatly contradicts government health warnings that people should cut their intake to 6 grams a day.

Professor Deiderick Grobbee, a cardiovascular specialist, said: 'If people stick within a range of moderate sodium intake, which we normally get from salt in our food, there is no material variation to the risk of mortality.' And by 'moderate', he was talking of the equivalent of up to 16 grams or 3½ teaspoonfuls a day. Other scientists went further, saying that the guidance to reduce salt intake could be dangerous to two significant sections of the population: Professor Markus Mohaupt, from the Inselspital Academic Health Centre, Switzerland, found that pregnant women with pre-eclampsia, a condition that affects about one in 12 pregnant women, and causes high blood pressure and can lead to still birth, benefited from up to 20 grams of salt a day; the other group that are at risk if they eat a low-salt diet, according to Professor Ingo Füsgen, a cardiovascular specialist from Kliniken St Antonius in Germany, are the elderly. Professor Füsgen's findings showed that one in 10 elderly people suffered from sodium deficiency which could result in nervous disposition, hallucinations, muscle cramps and hip fractures.

Once again, the results, which were presented at a conference in Brussels in May 2005, were condemned by supporters of salt reduction. But the Rotterdam Study had confirmed other earlier work: the huge Intersalt Study, which found no evidence of benefit in cutting down on salt,[20] and a Scandinavian study which showed that 10-fold variations of salt intake, either up or down from a starting point of 10 grams a day – in other words, from 1 gram to 100 grams – produced on average only marginal changes in blood pressure.[21]

Blood pressure drugs increase ill-health

It is generally accepted practice to treat people with high blood pressure with antihypertensive drugs in order to prevent heart attacks. This is despite the fact that clinical trials and recent population studies have both raised serious questions about the effectiveness of antihypertensive drugs in this regard. Nevertheless, the prescription of antihypertensive drugs for the prevention of heart attacks continues and there is an increasing trend to prescribe them for people whose blood pressure is only just above normal. Now Swedish researchers report that treating elderly men who have a diastolic blood pressure less than 90 mm Hg with antihypertensive drugs increases their risk of having a heart attack by a factor of four.[22] This may be because such medical therapy can induce or contribute to nutritional deficiencies. Diuretic drugs, commonly used in cases of hypertension, are the most widely known group of drugs to cause loss of minerals in urine.

And there are other side effects. The drugs are not comfortable to take. An indication of the severity of this is the fact that half of the users of antihypertensive drugs discontinue them within a year.[23] Side effects range from chronic coughing, mental confusion and dizziness to increased blood glucose, kidney failure, kidney stones, muscle paralysis, and interference with red blood cell production.[24]

Blood pressure levels are dropping without drugs

Antihypertensive drugs represent one of the most lucrative sectors for the pharmaceutical companies, who suggest they are effective because blood pressure levels are reducing in industrialized countries.

But a World Health Organization (WHO) study which monitored blood pressure levels in 38 populations from 21 countries across four continents from 1985 to 1995, found that blood pressure levels are declining among people who have never been prescribed a hypertensive drug; and they were already falling across populations before the drugs were being so readily prescribed.[25] This suggests that these drugs are taking credit for a phenomenon that is more down to lifestyle changes. Despite this, antihypertensive drugs account for 20% of all prescriptions made out by family doctors.

Doctors should be encouraging people with high blood pressure to adopt healthier lifestyles – and this alone should be enough to improve the problem – without reaching for their prescription pads. But will the drug companies be prepared to stand back and watch their revenues decline?

The case of salt and hypertension is a good illustration of the harm that ill-conceived and unsupported hypotheses can do. Yet, despite the vast amount of evidence that screening the population to identify people with high blood pressure, and vilifying salt, does more harm than good, it is being advocated more and more widely.

It's better to cut carbohydrate

Despite the many studies that have shown that salt appears *not* to be the primary culprit, many still insist that it is. In these circumstances, could it be that another dietary item is confusing the issue?

A strong association between diabetes and hypertension has been recognized for over 80 years.[26] In patients with diabetes and impaired glucose tolerance, systolic blood pressure correlates significantly with both fasting blood glucose and glucose levels measured two hours after eating glucose.[27]

Dr W. L. Bloom noticed that salt excretion was greater during fasting than when on a low-salt diet. This suggested either that food in general, or some constituent in food, might be involved in the regulation of salt excretion. In 1962 he conducted a study which showed that salt excretion in urine dropped to low levels immediately after carbohydrate was eaten.[28] Fat and protein, as well as salt, on the other hand, increased the salt excretion of fasting.

What Dr Bloom suggested was that salt is important in cases of hypertension, but that *eating carbohydrates prevents the body from ridding itself of any excess salt*. For this reason, current 'healthy' dietary guidelines that we should eat more carbohydrates could contribute to hypertension.

Obesity may cause hypertension

A study of 1,031 people in Oakland, California, who developed hypertension over a six-year period, showed clearly that obesity and weight gain were clear precursors of hypertension.[29] As I argue throughout this book, obesity is caused by a carbohydrate-based diet.

Dairy products reduce hypertension

The risk of developing hypertension in African Americans is more than twice that of their white counterparts, and thus they are at dramatically increased risk of excessive mortality from cardiovascular disease.[30] This greater risk is evident in all age groups and both sexes. While being overweight and sensitivity to dietary salt are often thought to contribute to this excessive risk, neither fully explains this relation:

- In groups with similar weights and body mass indexes, African Americans have higher mean blood pressure than whites.
- Salt sensitivity is more prevalent in African Americans, but there is no evidence that salt intake is notably greater in this population.

Over a decade in the late 1980s and early 1990s, a credible body of evidence emerged supporting the concept that maintaining an adequate dietary mineral intake, specifically of calcium, magnesium and potassium, protects against high blood pressure in humans. Observational and interventional studies in humans and extensive use of laboratory models showed that a significant portion of blood pressure variability in response to salt could be linked to the adequacy of the mineral content of the diet. In particular, a report published in 1998 provided valuable evidence that adequate dietary calcium intake was essential for optimal blood pressure regulation in humans.[31] This beneficial effect was greatest when dairy products were added to the diets of individuals whose diets were deficient in calcium and the other minerals.[32]

Analysis of NHANES I also showed in 1994 for the first time that there were important, relevant dietary intake patterns that predicted blood pressure in Americans,[33] and confirmed an earlier observation that hypertension was associated with a diet poor in dairy products and calcium, potassium and magnesium.[34] This analysis showed that the cardiovascular benefits of calcium and potassium were continuous across the age range from 18 to 75 years of age and were evident in both men and women as well as across racial groups. The benefits appeared to have a dose-response relation with a threshold at less than 600-700 mg of calcium per day. Below that, blood pressure and the risk of being hypertensive were greater.

The benefits of calcium are even greater among pregnant women. Controlled trials showed that women who eat some 1,500 and 2,000 mg/day of calcium reduce their risk of developing pregnancy-induced hypertension by as much as 50%. It has also been shown that maternal calcium intake directly affects the infant's blood pressure. Women with a high calcium intake gave birth to babies with higher birth weights and lower blood pressures. This lower pressure persisted throughout at least the first five years of life.

These findings have been confirmed many times since. The evidence is clear that food sources that contain dietary calcium rather than supplements are more effective. The best source of calcium by far is a hard cheese. Parmesan and similar Italian cheeses are best, with Swiss cheeses a close second. The best British cheese is cheddar.

It is important to note that low calcium can be the result of a diet high in 'healthy' cereal fibre and also associated with a lack of vitamin D (see Chapters Seven and Eleven).

Conclusion

Over the years the level of blood pressure considered 'normal' has been progressively lowered until now practically everyone is a potential patient – and a 'customer' for the drugs industry. At the same time, the general population has been exhorted to undertake dietary changes which are unsupported by any coherent body of evidence. When the hoped for reductions are not achieved by salt restriction, these 'patients' are prescribed drugs which may be harmful. This is despite the undoubted fact that salt restriction has not been shown to be beneficial in terms of either morbidity or mortality: most people who suffer strokes today have blood pressures that are well within the normal range.

Dr James LeFanu, a General Practitioner in London, wrote that: 'The important question that emerges from these papers is why the combined intellects of so many distinguished epidemiologists should maintain that the evidence incriminating salt in hypertension is so convincing when clearly it adds up to very little.'[35]

Let me leave the last words to Dr Michael Alderman, President of the American Society of Hypertension, Department of Epidemiology and Social Medicine, Albert Einstein College of Medicine, New York, who wrote in 1997:

> 'Public health recommendations must be based on proof of safety and benefit. Even if a low sodium diet could lower the blood pressure of most people (probably not true) and both the diet and the change in blood pressure could be sustained (not established), this alone would not justify a recommendation to reduce sodium intake.'[36]

Six grams of salt a day may, indeed, be all that is necessary for health. But there can be little doubt that the strident exhortations to reduce salt are driving people to consume less than this amount. And that could be decidedly unhealthy.

Incidentally, only about 5% to 10% of salt consumed occurs in natural foods such as meat. While more may be added during cooking or at the table, by far the greatest amount is found in processed foods. Foods normally thought of as being excessively salty (e.g. potato crisps) usually contain much less salt than foods with 'hidden' salt. The worst foods seem to be 'healthy' ones such as bread and canned vegetables and soups.

It seems clear that advice to reduce sodium intake should be taken with a pinch of salt.

Chapter Ten

Soy, fluoride and the thyroid

The thyroid gland controls many functions within the body, including the rate at which we use energy. When its action is suppressed, weight gain is an inevitable result. Soya and fluoride, widely promoted as 'healthy', both have such an effect.

There is abundant evidence that some of the isoflavones found in soy demonstrate toxicity in oestrogen sensitive tissues and in the thyroid.

Dr Daniel Doerge

There are two other factors that must be considered when thinking about a healthier way to eat: both have a reputation for being healthy that is not justified; and they both adversely affect the thyroid gland and other body systems that control how our bodies deal with dietary nutrients and energy expenditure. They are the legume, soy, and the chemical element, fluorine.

You will remember from Chapter Three that when Anitschkow fed rabbits an experimental, cholesterol-rich diet, the result was to produce atherosclerosis in the rabbits' arteries. In 1965, Dr Malasheva at Anitschkow's laboratory published an explanation for these observations.[1] The rabbits' high levels of cholesterol, he said, were symptoms of thyroid deficiency. Thyroid deficiency, or *hypothyroidism*, is also a well-known cause of high blood cholesterol levels in humans.[2]

Soy

Whether or not soy is healthy for you is a hotly debated issue. The debate stems largely from the fact that the health benefits of fermented soy have been misconstrued as being applicable to non-fermented soy as well. As you will see, this is simply not the case.

Vegetarians have long used soy products as a replacement for meat, as it has a high protein content. Low in carbohydrate and high in protein, soy seems an ideal food. Soy is also being increasingly used in a wide variety of foodstuffs from meat sausages and fish fingers to salad dressings, breakfast cereals and bread. BSE and other health scares related to meat have also led to rocketing sales of soy-related products in Britain.

Read any American weight loss book's recipes and see the number that incorporate soy in one form or another: in breakfast cereals, soy breads, convenience foods, smoothies, protein shakes, low-carb meal replacements, meat substitutes and so on. Soy is promoted as being a very healthy food. Each year, research on the health effects of soy seems to increase exponentially with suggestions that soy has potential benefits not only for low-carb dieting for weight loss but also for diseases such as cancer, heart disease and osteoporosis.

But soy has a dark side which needs to be considered very carefully, for soy is not the perfect food it might appear at first sight. Modern soy products contain antinutrients and toxins that not only reduce the absorption of vitamins and minerals, but also have other systemic, adverse effects. These include reduction in thyroid activity, which affects our whole metabolism.

A brief history of soy

Soy is a legume, a bean, which hails from southeast Asia. Originally, the Chinese did not eat it, but merely used it to fix nitrogen in the soil.[3] This was for a very good reason: soybeans, like many other plants, contain large quantities of natural toxins to help them ward off potential predators. That made the beans uncomfortable and unsafe to eat. Toxins include:

- **Protease inhibitors** that block the action of trypsin and other enzymes needed for protein digestion. These inhibitors are not completely deactivated during ordinary cooking. They produce serious gastric distress and reduce protein digestion to cause chronic deficiencies in amino acid uptake. In test animals, diets high in trypsin inhibitors have caused enlargement and pathological conditions of the pancreas, including cancer.[4]
- **Phytic acid**, which inhibits the absorption from the gut of important minerals.
- **Phytoestrogens and isoflavones**, which mimic the female sex hormone, oestrogen. These are heavily promoted as an alternative to hormone replacement therapy (HRT) for menopausal women.
- **Goitregens**, which inhibit thyroid activity.

Fermentation and precipitation

Fermented soybeans have been a tradition in Japanese cuisine for more than 1,000 years. The nutritive value of natto, for example, was so high that Samurai consumed it daily, and even fed it to their horses to increase their speed and strength. However, non-fermented soy products are *not* health foods, even though manufacturers of soy products have been allowed to label them 'heart healthy' in the US since 1999.[5]

Fermentation of soy destroys or neutralizes the many toxins, making soy safe to eat. It was only after this discovery, during the Chinese Chou dynasty (1134-246 BC), that soy was eaten – but always in fermented form. The first fermented soy foods were products like tempeh, natto, miso and soy sauce. The use of fermented and precipitated soy products soon spread from China to other parts of the Orient, notably Japan and Indonesia.

Some soy products – tofu and bean curd – are precipitated rather than fermented. This concentrates enzyme inhibitors in the liquid in which the beans are soaked rather than in the curd. While this reduces growth depressants, it does not completely eliminate them. Soy milk, originally a waste product of tofu production, is about as healthy as you would expect a waste product to be.

Phytic acid and mineral status

Many nutritionists condemn low-carb diets because, they say, they are unbalanced, leading to deficiencies in some nutrients. That doesn't happen with a properly constituted low-carb diet. But with a dietary regime in which soy features, deficiencies could well occur because soybeans have one of the highest phytate levels of any grain or legume that has been studied.[6] With wheat and other grains, long slow cooking and fermentation will neutralize the phytate they contain. But the phytates in soy are highly resistant to these techniques.[7] Only a very long period of fermentation will significantly reduce soy's phytate content. And in most of the foods which contain soy today that simply doesn't happen. When precipitated soy products like tofu are consumed with meat, the mineral-blocking effects of the phytates are reduced, but that is all.[8][9] Vegetarians who consume tofu and bean curd as a substitute for meat and dairy products risk severe mineral deficiencies.

Soy inhibits the absorption of zinc the most (for a summary of the effects of phytic acid on zinc absorption, see Leviton, 1982).[10] Soy-based infant formula is particularly harmful because zinc is needed for proper development of the brain and nervous system. It also plays a part in protein synthesis and collagen formation; it is involved in the blood-sugar control and thus protects against diabetes; and it is needed for a healthy reproductive system. Zinc is a key component in many vital enzymes and has an important role in the immune system.

One 12-ounce tub of tofu has 100 milligrams or so of magnesium. That's 25% of the recommended daily intake of magnesium. But only about 10 milligrams is absorbed into your body. Magnesium deficiency is common in schizophrenia.[11] The stress of the disease makes the victim lose even more magnesium leading to more anxiety, fear, hallucinations and physical complaints.

A very worrying 25-year study of individuals consuming a diet containing tofu in middle-age and brain damage in later life was reported in 2000.[12] It found a strong association with brain atrophy and cognitive impairment in mid-life tofu eaters at all levels of intake. Brain atrophy was determined by MRI scans and autopsy results. Low brain weight was seen in 12% of men consuming the lowest amount of tofu and 40% consuming the highest amount. 'Highest' was defined as a mere two or more servings a week. The dose-response effect, whereby the more an individual ate, the greater the brain damage seen, made a very strong case for tofu being harmful to the brain.

To make matters worse, there is some discussion in the nutrition literature that the phytic acid in soy may make soy protein less useable for our bodies.

Soy and the thyroid gland

The thyroid gland produces hormones that have a profound effect on many body functions as they control our bodies' metabolism. This in turn has implications for the cause and treatment of obesity. It also affects such seemingly unrelated things as blood cholesterol levels.

Hypothyroidism – underactive thyroid – is a condition where the thyroid gland does not produce enough thyroid hormone, thyroxin. As this condition progresses, the thyroid increases in size in an attempt to make more thyroxin, producing an unsightly swelling in the neck called a *goitre*. The most important cause of goitre is a lack of iodine and goitres are endemic in parts of the world that are deficient in iodine. But these are now rare in the West, where other causes of hypothyroidism and goitre are more prevalent. Here it is chemicals called *goitrogens* which suppress thyroid function that are more important. One such is fluoride, which will be discussed later in this chapter; soy also contains goitrogens.

In 1991, Japanese researchers reported that consumption of as little as 30 grams – about two tablespoons – of soybeans per day for just one month caused a significant increase in thyroid-stimulating hormone (TSH), the hormone which instructs the thyroid to produce more thyroxin.[13] This

caused goitre and hypothyroidism to appear in some of their trial participants, and many complained of constipation, fatigue and lethargy, even
though they had an adequate intake of iodine. In 1997, researchers from
the US Food and Drug Administration's (FDA) National Center for
Toxicological Research made the embarrassing discovery that the goitrogenic components of soy were the very same isoflavones that were
being promoted to help women through the menopause.[14]

Phytoestogens

Soy contains *phytoestrogens* in the form of isoflavones such as *genistein*
and *diadzen*, which are similar to natural oestrogen. These are used by
many women to stave off the effects of the menopause, despite a British
Government assessment which failed to find evidence of benefit and
warned against potential adverse effects.[15] Today you will be hard
pressed to find any bread that doesn't contain soy flour; indeed, the advertising for a new soy-enriched loaf from Allied Bakeries was targeted
at menopausal women seeking relief from hot flushes in the 1990s. It
was so successful that sales in 1997 were running at 250,000 loaves per
week.[16]

Twenty-five grams of soy protein isolate contains 50-70 milligrams of
isoflavones. Yet it took only 45 milligrams of isoflavones in premenopausal women to exert significant biological effects, including a
reduction in hormones needed for adequate thyroid function. These effects continued for three months after they stopped eating the soy.[17] In
1992, the Swiss health service estimated that 100 grams of soy protein
provided the oestrogenic equivalent of 'the Pill'.[18]

And with that in mind, what of its effects on children and men?

Soy consumption has been linked to numerous disorders, including infertility, increased cancer and infantile leukaemia; and studies dating back
to the 1950s showed that genistein in soy disrupted hormone production in
animals.[19] Laboratory studies have also suggested that isoflavones inhibit
the synthesis of oestradiol and other steroid hormones.[20,21] Several species
of animals including mice, cheetah, quail, pigs, rats, sturgeon and sheep
have displayed reproductive problems, infertility, thyroid disease and liver
disease due to dietary isoflavones.[22-27]

Isoflavones in infancy are probably the greatest cause for concern as
they are likely to affect the way a child develops. In 1998, investigators
reported that circulating concentrations of isoflavones in infants fed soy-
based baby formula were 13,000 to 22,000 times higher than oestradiol
concentrations in the blood of infants fed baby formula made with cow's
milk.[28] An infant exclusively fed on soy formula receives the oestrogenic
equivalent (based on body weight) of at least five birth control pills per

day.[29] By contrast, almost no phytoestrogens have been detected in dairy-based infant formula or in human milk, even when the mother consumes soy products.

An example of these effects is that the age of puberty has been falling significantly for several decades. Girls, for example, used to reach puberty in their teens; the average age has now dropped to around 10 to 11 years of age. What is more alarming is the number of girls who are entering puberty at an even earlier age: in a study reported in 1997 one girl in every hundred seen had started to develop breasts or pubic hair before the age of three; by the age of eight, almost one in six white girls and one in two African-American girls had one or both of these characteristics.[30]

The effect on boys is potentially far more serious. During the first few months of life boys have testosterone levels that may be as high as those of an adult male. Although long before puberty, this is the period when a boy is programmed to express male characteristics after puberty, including not only in the development of his sexual organs and other masculine physical traits, but also patterns in the brain which are characteristic of male behaviour. Little experimentation seems to have been done on human babies; however, a deficiency of male hormones in monkeys has been shown to impair the development of spatial perception, which is normally more acute in men than in women, as well as learning ability, and of visual discrimination tasks such as are required for reading.[31] Learning disabilities, especially in male children, have reached epidemic proportions. The inference is clear.

The FDA's two key experts on soy at the time, Dr Daniel Doerge of the Division of Biochemical Toxicology at the National Center for Toxicological Research, and Daniel Sheehan, disputed the health claims approved by the FDA for soy products, in an official letter of protest to the FDA dated 18 February 1999, saying:

> 'there is abundant evidence that some of the isoflavones found in soy, including genistein and equol, a metabolite of daidzen, demonstrate toxicity in estrogen sensitive tissues and in the thyroid. . . . There exists a significant body of animal data that demonstrates goitrogenic and even carcinogenic effects of soy products. Moreover, there are significant reports of goitrogenic effects from soy consumption in human infants and adults.'

In 2002, Doerge published the results of follow-up research which looked at the goitrogenic and oestrogenic effects of soy in greater depth.[32] Research had already shown that soy consumption is linked to increased risk of goitre. When iodine is deficient, the antithyroid effects of soy are intensified. Soy's ability to affect the thyroid, therefore, depends on the relationship between iodine status and thyroid function. In animal studies, rats given genistein-fortified diets showed an increase in thyroid antibodies, while other measures of thyroid function apparently remained normal. These findings led Dr Doerge to conclude that additional factors appeared necessary for soy to cause overt thyroid toxicity. These factors included: iodine deficiency, consumption of other soy components, other goitrogens in the diet, and other physiological problems in synthesizing thyroid hormones.

Dr Doerge concluded: 'Although safety testing of natural products, including soy products, is not required, the possibility that widely consumed soy products may cause harm in the human population via either or both estrogenic and goitrogenic activities is of concern.'

Soy and cancer

The food industry touts soy products for their cancer-preventing properties. This is because the isoflavone, *aglycone*, contained in fermented soy does have an anti-cancer effect. However, in *non*-fermented soy products such as tofu and soy milk, as well as the raw beans and protein powders, these isoflavones are present in an altered form which does *not* have an anti-cancer effect,[33] but may be responsible for the rapid increase in liver and pancreatic cancer seen in Africa since the introduction of soy products there.[3]

Soy is promoted as a preventative of breast cancer. Yet a review of 18 studies of research carried out at several medical centres in the US found no statistical benefit. The authors say that inconsistencies and limitations among the studies cast doubt on the potential protective effects of the foodstuff in preventing breast cancer.[34]

Soy-related reproductive problems

Experts warn that women who consume soy products for health reasons could be damaging their ability to conceive. A study published in 2006 found that even tiny amounts of genistein could prevent natural fertilization in the female reproductive tract.[35] Another study added a possible reason: Lynne Fraser, Professor in Reproductive Biology at King's College, London, found that genistein causes sperm to 'burn out' before they have a chance to penetrate the wall of the egg.[36] A sperm has a tiny cap on its head called the *acrosome*, which acts as a kind of warhead. At precisely the right time, it is supposed to burst open and release enzymes that allow the sperm to drill through the wall of the egg. However, genistein made the acrosome rupture much too soon, and thereby prevented fertilization taking place. Professor Fraser had previously shown that certain oestrogenic chemicals could affect the functioning of mouse sperm;[37] however, its impact was much more powerful in humans than in mice.

Professor Fraser advised that women hoping to conceive should avoid soy in order not to expose sperm to the compound in their bodies. She said: 'If you drank a carton of soy milk I would think that would give you a reasonable dose of genistein.'

The strange case of 'veggie viagra'

Persistent sexual arousal syndrome is an uncommon sexual complaint. Patients with this disorder can be distressed by the escalation of tension in the pelvic region and the prevailing necessity to diminish the pressure by self-stimulation. Patients frequently suffer from guilt or shame and often do not seek medical care.

In 2005, scientists at the Division of Gynecology, Memorial Sloan-Kettering Cancer Center, in New York reported an unusual case involving soy.[38] It concerned a 44-year-old woman who came for evaluation of painful and heavy periods. During interview, she reported five to six months of increased pelvic tension. It was not associated with an increase in desire, but did require her to self-stimulate to orgasm approximately 15 times a day. Upon further inquiry, she disclosed that her diet included a large intake of soy that began approximately one month prior to the onset of symptoms. She was advised to cut the soy out of her diet, and three months later all her menstrual problems and sexual complaints had resolved.

The authors say: 'Although no known cause or cure of persistent sexual arousal syndrome has been identified to date, the success of reducing dietary phytoestrogens in this patient may provide insight into the etiology of the disorder and suggest potential treatments.'

Soy processors have worked hard to get soy's antinutrients out of the finished product, particularly out of the soy protein isolate which is the key ingredient in most soy foods that imitate meat, dairy products and the protein powders used in commercial low-carb meal replacements so beloved of American low-carb diet gurus. But it is not enough.

It is true that a large proportion of the trypsin inhibitors can be removed through high-temperature processing. But not all is, and there may be as much as a five-fold difference between the trypsin inhibitor content of one soy protein isolate and another.[4] And there is one last problem: the high-temperature processing needed to neutralize these toxins has the unfortunate side-effect of so denaturing the other proteins in soy that they are rendered largely ineffective.[39] While fermented soy provides the least harmful soy products, why bother eating something that even after all that work is still unhealthy? (For references to soy's toxicity, see the FDA Poisonous Plant Database.)[40]

Today, most of our soy comes from the US, where some 72 million acres of the bean are grown. It is a very cheap product for food manufacturers to use if not fermented so you won't be surprised to learn that over 60% of the products sold from supermarket shelves contain unfermented soy flour and soy milk.

Fluoride

The other 'healthy' 'nutrient' that disrupts the thyroid is the ion, fluoride. Fluorine is so reactive that it is never found on its own in nature, but is always compounded with other elements to form 'fluorides'. Fluorides are promoted to help prevent decay in teeth. But they are powerful enzyme disruptors with the potential to affect every cell in our bodies.

Up to the middle of the last century, fluoridated water was used to treat people with an over-active thyroid (*hyper*-thyroid).[41] It was very effective. But for a person with a healthy thyroid function, ingestion or absorption of fluoride produces *hypo*-thyroidism – under-active thyroid.

Many studies confirm this. For example, a study designed to evaluate adverse health effects in adolescents from chronic exposure to various water fluoride concentrations was conducted in three communities located in northern Mexico: Ciudad Juarez, Samalayuca and Villa Ahumada.[42] In these communities the fluoride concentration in water averaged 0.3, 1.0, and 5.3 milligrams per litre (mg/L) respectively (the 'optimal' level recommended for water fluoridation is 1.0 mg/L, also written as one part per million (1.0 ppm)). The study evaluated the effect of fluoride on dental fluorosis (brown staining of teeth), growth, thyroid hormones, liver function, blood fats, uric acid, and electrolytes in 15- to 20-year-olds of both sexes. In Villa Ahumada, 97% of all adolescents had dental fluorosis, and 18% of them had serious damage to their teeth. In Samalayuca, 53% of all adolescents had mild dental fluorosis; 15% had moderate dental fluorosis, and 2% showed serious damage in their teeth. In Villa Ahumada a significant inverse relationship was found between fluoride levels in drinking water and stature: the more fluoride, the more growth was retarded; this association suggested that fluoride exposure didn't affect just the teeth but also the adolescents' growth. Blood samples taken from these individuals suggested that high fluoride ingestion had a definite effect on the prevalence and severity of dental fluorosis, decrease of stature and decrease of thyroid hormone secretion.

Fluoride-related hypothyroidism is also associated with higher body weight, diastolic hypertension, higher total cholesterol and triglyceride levels and higher total cholesterol/HDL (high density lipoprotein) ratio.[43] Before the introduction of the diet-heart hypothesis, if a doctor found high levels of cholesterol in a blood test, his first thought would be to check his patient's thyroid; today, no such checks are done, just an automatic prescription for an expensive cholesterol-lowering statin drug – which, of course, merely treats a symptom while doing absolutely nothing to rectify the underlying condition. A recent Japanese study has confirmed that thyroxin replacement could reduce low density lipoprotein (LDL) in patients with hypothyroidism.[44]

Do you live in a fluoridated area?

Fluorides are not just found in toothpaste; this toxic chemical may also be in your water supply. You can call your water company to find out. If you do live in a fluoridated area, then you should not use aluminium cookware. In January 1987, experiments performed at the Medical Research Endocrinology Department, Newcastle upon Tyne, England, and the Physics Department of the University of Ruhana, Sri Lanka, showed that water 'optimally' fluoridated at one part per million (1.0 ppm), when used in cooking with aluminium cookware, concentrated the aluminium to up to 600 ppm.[45] In 1990 a test of fluoridated tap water in Antigo, Wisconsin, in conjunction with aluminium cookware, showed that aluminium concentration in the water was increased by 833 times and the fluoride content doubled. During the period of fluoridation in Antigo there was a seven-fold increase in the annual cardiac death rate from five deaths per 100,000 in 1949, to 35 deaths per 100,000 population in 1960. Then fluoridation was stopped.[46]

Strangely, in the US, the FDA has required a warning label on toothpaste to prevent fluoride poisoning since 1997. But what about foods and beverages? According to Dr Hardy Limeback, Professor of Preventive Dentistry at the University of Toronto, and one of the 12 panel members of the summary of the National Research Council's review of fluoride's toxicology published on 22 March 2006, to be consistent with the FDA toothpaste warning, you should really contact a poison control centre immediately if you swallow:

- One cup (250 mL) of fluoridated tap water, or
- One third of a cup of tea made with fluoridated tap water, or
- One quarter of a can (335 mL) of iced tea, or
- Two thirds of a can of soda pop made in a fluoridated city, or
- A small bottle (335 mL) of beer made in a fluoridated city, or
- 250 mL of 'from concentrate' fruit juice, or
- One litre of naturally fluoridated spring water (containing 0.25 ppm fluoride), or
- One half of a bottle of formula (500 mL) made with fluoridated tap water (depending on the brand).

So, how can you avoid fluoridated water? The answer is: with great difficulty. There is little point in drinking unfluoridated, bottled water, as fluoride is absorbed through the skin. So, if you bath, wash or swim in fluoridated water you get an unhealthy overdose.[41] You could try to stop your tap water being fluoridated, but it's a vain hope unless you can persuade many people to join you and write to your water supplier. The only practical way is to buy and use a still or a reverse osmosis filter. That will filter out fluoride, where the usual filter jugs do not. But it is expensive and wastes about five times as much water as the drinkable water it produces. The only other way is to move to an unfluoridated part of the country.

The US and Ireland are about 66% fluoridated. In the UK, only about 9% of England is fluoridated; Scotland, Northern Ireland and Wales are not fluoridated. Other English-speaking countries tend also to have some. If you are unsure, call your water supplier, who will normally be quite willing to tell you.

Conclusion

Both soy and fluoride have a serious, harmful impact on the thyroid gland as well as other serious adverse health effects. They should be avoided at all costs. This is a particularly important consideration for children.

Chapter Eleven

Our irrational fear of sunlight

Keep out of the midday sun, cover up and wear a sunscreen, we are told. But the sun is nature's great healer. Sunlight is our only reliable source of vitamin D. It is increasingly recognised that people who sunbathe have less cancer. Sun creams may increase the risk of cancer.

The simplistic idea of a sun/melanoma relationship is based more on a belief than science.

Dr Peter Karnauchow

For the past few decades the numbers of skin cancers have risen dramatically among pale-skinned, Caucasian populations throughout the world. Melanoma is the seventh most commonly diagnosed cancer in the US with an incidence of 14.2 cases per 100,000 population;[1] Queensland, Australia, had the world's highest incidence at 55.8 cases per 100,000 in 1987.[2] The numbers of skin cancers in the general British population have been increasing at an annual rate of 2% to 8% over the past two decades.[3] The risk factors seem to be a combination of being light-skinned, of a northern European descent and living in an area of high ambient sunlight. There is also a seasonal incidence of the disease – there are more cases reported in summer than in winter.

Not surprisingly perhaps, clinicians, physicians, national media and health gurus have warned us to stay out of the sun to prevent the most serious form of skin cancer: melanoma. Yet in spite of the ever-increasing use of sunscreens and intentional reduction of sun exposure, the number of cases of this cancer has continued to rise.

This may be because several aspects of melanoma are anomalous compared with other sunlight-associated skin cancers. For example, people with the greatest risk of melanoma are *not* those with the greatest cumulative exposure to the sun; the areas of the body that receive the most exposure to the sun are *not* the most affected; and not all light-skinned people suffer the same: albino Africans who have no pigmentation, for example, are likely to get sunburn and other skin complaints as a result of exposure to the sun, but they don't get melanomas.[4]

In the 1960s I lived in Singapore, which was almost on the Equator. I have blond hair, fair skin and blue eyes. It is a combination not believed to be suited to the harsh sun of the tropics. Nevertheless, I regularly went on the beach, to the swimming pool, or sailing on the South China Sea, with little or nothing on, in the heat of the midday sun. I don't tan easily. I remember, in an effort to deepen my tan, I would lie out for hours with the sun to one side of me and its reflection in a mirror of cooking foil on the other to increase my exposure. Like everyone else in the ex-patriot Singapore community, I didn't give skin cancer a thought; in those days the phrase 'malignant melanoma' was unheard of.

Nobody used a sunscreen. If we used anything at all – which most of the time we did not – it was a well-shaken mixture of coconut oil and vinegar, a concoction used at the time by naturists. We smelled like a fried fish shop, but my skin never burnt while I lived there.

Today, it seems, all that has changed. Why? What has happened in the last 40 years?

Skin cancers

There are three major forms of skin cancer:

- **Basal cell carcinoma (BCC)** is the most common form of skin cancer. It occurs most frequently in men who spend a great deal of time outdoors and is usually found on the head and neck.[5] BCC is not dangerous as it rarely spreads, although it can extend below the skin to the bone.

- **Squamous cell carcinoma (SCC)** is the second most common skin cancer. It usually affects people who sunburn easily, tan poorly, and have blue eyes and red or blond hair. SCC often develops from *actinic keratoses*, which are rather like warts, and can metastasize (spread) if left untreated.[6]

- **Malignant melanoma (MM)** is the rarest form of skin cancer but the most deadly. It originates in the *melanocytes* – the cells that produce the skin colouring or pigment known as melanin – and can be recognized by its black or grey colour. It often grows from an existing mole, which may enlarge, become lumpy, bleed, change colour, develop a spreading black edge, turn into a scab, or begin to itch. It is more prevalent among city and office workers than among people who work out of doors and is thought to be linked to brief, intense periods of sun exposure such as one might get on annual holidays on sunny beaches, and to a history of severe sunburn in childhood or adolescence. MM metastasizes readily and is almost always fatal if not caught in time[7] as it responds poorly to conventional therapy.[8] Malignant melanoma incidence is growing at a rate of 7% per year in the US. In Canada, melanoma incidence rose by 6% per year for men and by 4.6% per year for women during the period 1970 to 1986.[9] In Australia the incidence for men doubled between 1980 and 1987 and for women it increased by more than 50%.[10]

Ultraviolet radiation

The ultraviolet (UV) part of the spectrum of sunlight is blamed for skin cancers. UV is classified into three distinct wavebands: A, B and C.[5] All are blamed for cancer.

- **UVA** constitutes between 90% and 95% of the ultraviolet light that reaches the earth as it is not absorbed by the ozone layer. UVA light penetrates furthest into the skin and is involved in the initial stages of sun-tanning. UVA tends to suppress the immune function and is implicated in premature aging of the skin.[5, 11]
- **UVB** is partially absorbed by the ozone layer and by the atmosphere. It does not penetrate the skin as far as the UVA rays but it is the primary cause of sunburn. UVB is blamed for cataract formation.[5] It is also our primary source of Vitamin D.
- **UVC** is the most harmful, but UVC is almost completely absorbed by the ozone layer and little or none reaches the Earth.

How strong is the evidence linking exposure to sunlight with melanoma?

During the 1980s and early 1990s more than a dozen studies compared histories of sunburn in patients with melanoma and people without it. The most complete data on melanoma and sunburn came in six studies from Australia, Europe and North America.[12] They found the sunlight/melanoma link was unconvincing: while there was a suggestion of an association, the effect was modest; and they emphasized that brief periods of exposure seemed more risky than constant exposure.

Other clinicians agree. Pointing out that melanoma can be found on ovaries, occurs *less* frequently on sun-exposed areas, that there is five times more melanoma in Scotland on the feet than on the hands, that in Japan 40% of melanomas on the feet are on the soles of the feet, and that there is 10 times more melanoma in Orkney and Shetland than in the Mediterranean islands, Karnauchow wrote: 'The simplistic idea of a sun/melanoma relationship is based more on a belief than science. . . . As with other neoplasms [cancers], the cause of melanoma remains an enigma and most probably the sun has little, if anything, to do with it.'[13]

Newcastle Dermatology Professor, Sam Shuster, wasn't convinced either. He stated that the main reason for the supposed increase in melanomas was a change in diagnostic beliefs: lesions previously regarded as benign became classified first as dubious then as malignant. 'Melanomas are being invented, not found,' he said, 'Exposure to screening and pigmented lesion clinics is a greater cause of melanoma than sun exposure.'[14]

Dr Anne Kricker and colleagues, looking at studies into skin cancer other than malignant melanoma and exposure to sunlight, also found that the evidence linking skin cancers with sun exposure was weak. They noted that most studies had not found statistically significant positive associations, while the few that had lacked empirical evidence that sun exposure was the cause.[15]

The sunscreen connection

So why has there been such an enormous increase in skin cancer over the last quarter of a century?

The Australian experience might provide the first clue. Queensland doctors have vigorously promoted the use of sunscreens for many years and, today, Queensland has more cases of melanoma per head of population than any other place in the world.

The number of cases of melanoma has risen especially steeply since the mid-1970s. The two principal strategies for reduction of risk of skin cancers since this time have been sun avoidance and use of chemical sunscreens. Rising trends in the incidence of and mortality from melanoma have continued since the 1970s and 1980s, when sunscreens with high sun protection factors became widely used.

Drs Cedric and Frank Garland of the University of California are the foremost opponents of the use of chemical sunscreens. They pointed out as long ago as 1992 that the greatest rises in melanoma had been in countries where chemical sunscreens had been heavily promoted.[16] They added that, while sunscreens do protect against sunburn, there is no scientific proof that they protect against melanoma or basal cell carcinoma in humans. Indeed, the Garland brothers strongly believe that the increased use of chemical sunscreens is the primary *cause* of the skin cancer epidemic. Studies by them showed a higher rate of melanoma among men who regularly used sunscreens and a higher rate of basal cell carcinoma among women using sunscreens.[17] This was confirmed by another study group who found that 'always users' of sunscreens had 3.7

times as many malignant melanomas as those 'never using'.

The reasons why chemical sunscreens may be dangerous are several:

- Chemical sunscreens do not stop UVA rays. UVA penetrates deeper into the skin where it is strongly absorbed by the melanocytes which are involved not only in the production of the skin-tanning pigment, melanin, but also in the formation of melanoma.

- More importantly, however, may be the fact that most chemical sunscreens contain up to 5% of *benzophenone* or its derivatives, *oxybenzone* or *benzophenone-3*, as their active ingredient. Benzophenone, used in industrial processes to initiate chemical reactions and promote cross-linking,[18] is one of the most powerful free radical generators known to man. Moreover, benzophenone is activated by ultraviolet light.

- Harvard Medical School researchers also have discovered that *psoralen*, another UV-activated free radical generator, is an extremely efficient carcinogen. The rate of SCC among patients with psoriasis, who had been repeatedly treated with UVA light after an application of psoralen to their skin, was 83 times higher than among the general population.[19] This added weight to a study in 1991-2, in which scientists at the European Organization for Research and Treatment of Cancer (EORTC) found that regular use of sunscreens increased cancer risk by 50% but sunscreens containing psoralen multiplied the risk by 228%. They also showed that in people with a poor ability to tan, psoralen users had almost four-and-a-half times the risk of melanoma compared with regular sunscreen users.[20]

No one believes that exposure to UV leads to skin cancer more ardently than do dermatologists. Dr Roger Ceilley, a leading American dermatologist, proclaimed in 1998: 'We're going to have millions more cases of skin cancer in the next decade if people forgo [sunscreen].'[21] In fact, of course, that is exactly what we are seeing – but in people who *do* use sunscreens.

There is, however, some evidence that regular use of sunscreens helps prevent the formation of actinic keratoses.[22] But so does eating meat. US scientists at the Arizona Cancer Center, University of Arizona, noted that a previous study had shown that vitamin A supplements significantly reduced the risk of squamous cell skin cancer in patients with moderately severe actinic keratoses.[23] Natural sources of Vitamin A are better than supplements. Fruits and vegetables with orange and yellow colouring, and green leafy vegetables contain beta-carotene, a precursor of vitamin A, but the body poorly converts beta-carotene into vitamin A. The best dietary sources of vitamin A are animal products, such as eggs and liver; cod liver oil is also an excellent natural source of vitamin A.

New sunscreens can cause brain damage

There is now a new range of sunscreens that contain tiny nanoparticles of zinc oxide or titanium dioxide. Nanoparticles of these compounds are used in sunscreens because the normally white compounds, which absorb UV radiation, become transparent when the particles are nano-sized. But these seem to widen the range of dangers.[24] Products which contain nanoparticles have caused long-term neurological damage in studies on mice. Scientists say the tiny particles may have different chemical compositions, and because nanoparticles are so small they are more easily absorbed through the skin. It will be years before the safety of nanotechnology can be proven, yet the particles are already being put into use in sunscreens, toothpaste, makeup and other products. You probably won't see the term 'nano' on product labels; however, all eight sunscreens which contained either compound, tested by ConsumerReports.com, contained nanoparticles.

The polyunsaturated fat connection

Since the 1960s, linoleic acid and vegetable margarines and cooking oils that contain it, have been shown time and again to increase the risk of many types of cancer, including skin cancers.

Drs B. S. and L. E. Mackie, working on Australia's Sunshine Coast, have a great deal of experience in skin cancers. As long ago as 1988 they said: 'In view of the work of Black and Erickson in mice and our own work in humans, we believe that human subjects who are at high risk of melanomas and other solar-induced forms of skin cancer should be advised to be moderate in their intake of dietary polyunsaturated fats.'[25]

Patricia Holborrow also pointed out that the increase in melanomas could be a result of Australians' dietary changes to polyunsaturated fats. 'Recently,' she wrote, 'I followed up four families that started in 1976 to use a diet with preferred oils as safflower and sunflower oil and low in salicylates and additives (that interfere with the metabolic pathway of these fats). There had been three cases of cancer resulting in two deaths in these families.'[26]

The Australians are as paranoid about heart disease as are the Americans. I was in Australia in 1995 and noticed that it was even their custom to remove the cream from milk and replace it with polyunsaturated vegetable oil.

Speak against current guidelines – and lose your job?

Johnathan Rees, when Professor of Dermatology, University Department of Dermatology, Newcastle upon Tyne, appraised the melanoma 'epidemic' in 1996, saying:

'There is after all no robust empirical evidence to defend most health promotion in this area. It has been suggested that the antithesis of science is not art but politics; melanoma is perhaps an example of the two having become mistakenly intertwined.'[27]

Professor Rees is lucky that he still has a job. Michael F. Holick, a professor at Boston University, was asked to resign in April 2004 from the university's Department of Dermatology because of his book, *The UV Advantage*, in which he described the importance of sunlight in boosting vitamin D levels; and for simply advocating a few minutes of sunlight exposure per week. The Department chairman, Barbara Gilchrest, MD, told the *Boston Globe* that the book: 'is an embarrassment for this institution and an embarrassment for him.'[28] Gilchrest's disapproval of Holick stemmed from the fact that his statements, superficially at least, seemed to be at odds with the medical profession's consensus on the damaging effects of sunlight. Dermatologists have been warning the public for years that sunlight is a cause of melanoma. Some of them, possibly frustrated at the failure of most of their treatments to reverse advanced melanoma, now regard sun exposure without sunblock as analogous to promiscuous sex without condoms. But sunlight (particularly UVB) has essential functions. And Boston is in the far north of the US, where usable sunlight is scarce and vitamin D is hard to come by.

If there is debate about this subject, isn't a university the right place for such debate to be conducted? Unfortunately, examples such as this where dissidents are summarily dismissed or reviled by their peers are actually common in the medical world.

In addition, Henry H. Bauer, Professor Emeritus of Chemistry & Science Studies, Virginia State University, has said:

'Minority views on technical issues are largely absent from the public arena. Increasingly corporate organization of science has led to knowledge monopolies, which, with the unwitting help of uncritical mass media, effect a kind of censorship. Since corporate scientific organizations also control the funding of research, by denying funds for unorthodox work they function as research cartels as well as knowledge monopolies. A related aspect of contemporary science is commercialization . . .'[29]

What is vitamin D?

Vitamin D is unique among vitamins for several reasons. Firstly, it is not really a vitamin. Vitamins are compounds which the body doesn't sythesize, and which must be obtained from food. But our bodies can make vitamin D through the action of sunlight on cholesterol in our skin, and there is very little found in food unless you eat large amounts of oily fish a day as traditional Inuit do.

Also, most vitamins are catalysts for chemical reactions or antioxidants; vitamin D is neither of these, but the only known precursor of a steroid hormone, *calcitriol*, whose function, like all steroid hormones, is to turn protein production on and off as the body requires. This action means it has a profound influence over a wide range of body processes.

How much D do we need?

Today, most light-skinned people in the UK and northern US only make about 1,000 IU (International Units) of vitamin D a day from sun exposure; many people, particularly the elderly or those with darker skins, make much less than that. Compare that with a single, 20-minute, full body exposure to summer sun at this latitude which could deliver some 20,000 IU (International Units) of vitamin D into the circulation of most people within 48 hours. Yet the recommended daily amount is a paltry and totally inadequate 400 IU.

There is no escaping the fact that our species evolved naked in sub-Equatorial Africa, where the sun shines directly overhead much of the year and where our species must have obtained tens of thousands of IU of vitamin D every day.

As we spread away to higher latitudes, natural selection lightened our skin in colour to compensate for the lower levels of UVB, but we would still have worked outdoors in sunlight. With the coming of the Industrial Revolution, however, we began to work indoors; in the last century we started to travel inside cars; in the last few decades, we began to lather on sunblock and consciously avoid sunlight. As well as sunscreens, increased skin pigmentation, aging and clothing have a dramatic effect on vitamin D production in the skin.

There is no doubt now that vitamin D levels in modern humans are not just low – they are disastrously and unhealthily low.

Vitamin D prevents cancer

In 1941, an American physician, Frank Apperly, compared cancer death incidences in cities at different latitudes across the North American continent, and found a clear pattern: the further people were from the Equator – and thus the lower the amount of sunshine they received – the more cancer there was.[30] Compared with cities between 10° and 30° latitude, cities between 30° and 40° had 85% higher incidence of cancer deaths; cities between 40° and 50° averaged 118% higher incidence of cancer deaths, and cities between 50° and 60° averaged 150% higher incidence of cancer deaths.

Studies of US Naval personnel during 1974-1984 showed that those working indoors had 10.6 cases of melanoma per 100,000 while those who worked both indoors and outdoors had the lower rate of 7.0 per 100,000. Findings from this study suggested a protective role for regular exposure to sunlight and agreed with laboratory studies that showed that vitamin D suppressed the growth of melanoma cells in tissue culture.

The same team found that lack of exposure to UV sunlight could place some populations at higher risk of breast cancer. Annual age-adjusted mortality rates for breast cancer varied from 17-19 per 100,000 in the south and south-west US to 33 per 100,000 in the north-east. Risk of fatal breast cancer in the major urban areas of the US increased as intensity of local sunlight decreased.[31] They found the same pattern across the USSR.[32]

A low blood level of vitamin D is known to be associated with an increased risk of developing breast and colon cancer,[33] pancreatic cancer,[34] and may also accelerate the growth of melanoma.[35] A 2007 study also found that levels of vitamin D above 80 nmol/L in the blood reduced the numbers of colorectal cancers by as much as 72% compared with levels of 50 mmol/L.[36] Worldwide, the United Nations estimated that there are 500,000 deaths from colorectal cancer each year.[37] A 72% reduction would mean 360,000 lives saved annually. That's a lot of lives saved and a lot of misery avoided! All these cancers are far more prevalent than melanoma.

Because of figures such as these, Dr Gordon Ainsleigh in California believes that sunscreens cause more cancer deaths than they prevent.[35]

Insufficient exposure to ultraviolet radiation may also be an important risk factor for other cancers in the US and in western Europe. Dr William Grant found that deaths from a range of cancers of the reproductive and digestive systems were approximately twice as high in New England as in the south-west, despite a diet that varied little between regions. According to Dr Grant's study, northern parts of the United States may be dark enough in winter that vitamin D synthesis actually shuts down completely. Based on his US findings, Dr Grant estimated that a quarter of breast cancer deaths in the UK are a result of vitamin D deficiency.[38]

Although this study focused on white Americans, the same geographical trend affects black Americans, whose overall cancer rates are significantly higher. This should come as no surprise as darker skinned people require more sunlight to synthesize vitamin D. Most people who have skin that is deeply pigmented should seek more sunlight for health reasons.

Sunlight reduces cancer death rates

Many papers have reported that solar UVB radiation and vitamin D reduce cancer death rates.[38-43] There is also increasing evidence that vitamin D increases survival rates once a cancer has been discovered. Two studies from Norway found that those people whose cancer was discovered in summer or autumn lived longer than those whose cancer was discovered in winter or spring.[44,45] A US study of those diagnosed with non small-cell lung cancer found a much higher five-year survival rate with high levels of vitamin D.[46]

So, by how much could higher levels of vitamin D in the UK reduce cancer mortality rates? An analysis of the geographic variation of cancer mortality rates in the US indicates that there are about 50,000-60,000 premature cancer deaths per year due to insufficient UVB and/or vitamin D.[47] These numbers represent about one-tenth of all cancer deaths. By looking at the latitudinal variation of vitamin D-sensitive cancer mortality rates for the eastern US, Canada, France, Germany, Ireland and the UK, it is estimated that as many as a quarter of all cancer deaths in the UK could be considered to be due to insufficient sunlight and vitamin D.

There are 13 types of cancer that definitely benefit from sunlight. They are mostly reproductive and digestive cancers. The strongest benefits are with breast, colon, and ovarian cancer. Other cancers which benefit from sunlight include the really big killers: tumours of the bladder, uterus, oesophagus, rectum, pancreas, stomach and non-Hodgkin's lymphoma. It is even well known that vitamin D protects skin cells from pre-cancerous changes.

It must be midday sunshine

UVB is the only band of light capable of producing vitamin D. It is significantly present only around midday during the summer months in most of Britain. That's the time we are told to stay out of the sun! It's no wonder we have an international disaster in progress due to a misunderstanding of the nature of and need for UVB and vitamin D. A study some years ago looked at the position in Edmonton, Alberta, Canada, at latitude 52°N.[48] It found that vitamin D could only be made from April to September and, even then, only if people went out in the sun for the two hours each side of noon. For the rest of the day and during the rest of the year, the angle of the sun was too low in the sky to allow adequate UVB to reach the earth.

A study in 2003 during the first 10 days of April,[49] showed that one in three children in Edmonton, Alberta, between two and 16 years of age had levels of circulating vitamin D less than half the amount that is now considered to be the lower limit of normal. It is impossible to make sufficient D during Alberta's winter.

The amount of sunlight is roughly the same in the UK as it is in Alberta, as the UK mainland lies between 50° and 59°N. For this reason, no vitamin D is made in the skin in London (latitude 52°N) from about October to April. And, of course, there is even less the further north you live. Yet, we are told to stay out of the sun during the periods that do us any good.

It's clear that two weeks' holiday a year on the Spanish costas or the Bahamas just doesn't cut it. In the UK, you really need *regular* sun exposure, *in the middle of the day* when the sun is high enough to allow UVB to penetrate to ground level, all through the summer – and then to take your holidays in the winter months in sunnier climes to top up.

Some need more sunshine than others

In all populations across the world, females are lighter skinned than males. Women's skin is lighter because their need for vitamin D_3 is particularly important when pregnant or lactating. Natural selection arranged for this higher need to be met by lightening women's skin to permit synthesis of the relatively higher amounts of the necessary vitamin D.[50]

Darker skinned people in Britain and similar latitudes require 10 to 20 times the length of sun exposure compared with lighter skinned people to build up the same amount of vitamin D.

And the use of sunscreen with a sun protection factor of as little as SPF8 inhibits more than 95% of vitamin D production in the skin.[51]

Vitamin D supplements are not the answer

It is obvious from the literature that Vitamin D is one of the essential nutrients most lacking in the average westerner's body. This is due to a combination of high latitude with weak sunshine, a predominantly indoor lifestyle, and current 'healthy' advice to stay out of the sun or cover up while in it. But, you might ask, couldn't we merely eat more vitamin D-rich foods or take supplements?

It is very important to realize that the recommended daily allowance (RDA) of vitamin D of 400 IUs is totally inadequate for most people who do not have exposure to regular sunshine. Many people may need up to 10,000 IUs per day for a short time to build their vitamin D levels up to healthy levels. And there are very few foods that contain significant amounts of vitamin D naturally. A supplement of cod liver oil does, but you would need to drink quite a lot to get sufficient D. And there is a danger of overdosing. Vitamin D is a fat-soluble vitamin; any excess is not flushed out of the body as are excess water-soluble vitamins. If you take too much it can cause calcium to build up in soft tissues and kidneys.

There is also another problem which relates to the type of chemical used for supplementation, whether in supplemented foods or in pills. The 'vitamin D' used for this purpose is *ergocalciferol*, a synthetic vitamin known as vitamin D_2. D_2 is not nearly as good as *cholecalciferol*, the vitamin D_3 which our bodies make with sunlight or obtain from natural food sources like fish oils. There is no doubt that the best – and healthiest – way to get vitamin D is the natural way: from sunlight.

There is another benefit with sunlight: there is no risk of overdosing. The skin does an amazing thing with cholecalciferol. Once you make about 20,000 IU, the same ultraviolet light that created cholecalciferol begins to degrade it. The more you make, the more is destroyed. So a steady state is reached that prevents the skin from making too much cholecalciferol. No-one has ever been reported to develop vitamin D toxicity from sunbathing – but they can when taking it by mouth. Dr Trevor Marshall of the School of Biological Sciences and Biotechnology, Murdoch University, Western Australia suggests that lifelong supplementation of the food chain with vitamin D is thought to be contributing to the current epidemics of obesity and chronic disease.[52]

Sunlight benefits the heart

Heart disease

In Chapter Three we spoke of 'paradoxes' – examples of populations who apparently had 'unhealthy' lifestyles but did not suffer from the heart disease 'healthy eating' dictocrats would predict. While I suggested that it was evidence that their high-fat diet was actually protective, there may also be another reason: if one looks at disease patterns across the world, it is clear that there is a lot less cardiovascular disease at the Equator than there is in higher latitudes. The evidence is persuasive that this is because of the amount of sunlight.

Anyone who has travelled in Italy will know that most Italians love the sun. As a consequence, most Italians have healthy vitamin D levels in summer,[53] and the death rate from cardiovascular disease is relatively low. An Italian proverb states: 'Where the sun does not go, the doctor does.'

In France the numbers of deaths from heart disease are much lower in the south and west than in the north and east. Dr Marie Chapuy found that vitamin D levels in the blood of healthy adults in France followed a similar regional trend: mean blood levels in the sunnier and drier south and west were more than double those in the colder, wetter north.[54]

The Northern Ireland paradox also fits this paradigm.[55] Belfast has four times the numbers of heart deaths compared with Toulouse, despite having similar heart disease 'risk factors'. But Belfast is at 54°N and has 257 rainy days per year. Toulouse is 11° closer to the Equator and has only 74 rainy days per year.

Similar effects are seen in other 'paradoxical' countries. You will remember that despite its 'protective' consumption of polyunsaturated fats, Israel has a high death rate from heart disease.[56] But despite Israel being a sunny country, Jews, particularly orthodox ones, cover up in the sun and suffer from vitamin D deficiency.[57,58] The same is true of Moslems: average vitamin D levels among healthy adults in Lebanon are dangerously low.[59]

To compound this, 'healthy' mono- and polyunsaturated fats reduce the bioavailability of vitamin D;[60] saturated fats do not.

In Greece, there were quite remarkably large differences in blood cholesterol levels in both men and women at different altitudes when they were tested in 1979 in spite of similar diets.[61] Those who lived at high altitude, where the atmosphere is thinner, had much higher levels of vitamin D than those living at sea level.

The effect of altitude tends to be forgotten, despite the fact that heart disease mortality in the US showed a striking inverse correlation with altitude nearly 30 years ago: American populations at the highest altitude had about half the heart disease of sea level populations.[62] Most long-lived populations in the world live at high altitude.[63]

Dr Robert Scragg, Associate Professor of Epidemiology at the University of Auckland, New Zealand, has repeatedly shown that vitamin D explains many of observations about heart disease. These include the facts that heart disease is higher at higher latitudes, lower altitudes, in the winter, in African Americans, in the elderly, the inactive, and in more obese patients who are less likely to wear less in public.[64]

At the same time, vascular smooth muscle proliferation, reduced vascular calcification, decreased parathormone levels, reduced C reactive protein (CRP) and other markers of inflammation, and decreased rennin, which are all predictive of heart disease, are improved by vitamin D.[65]

Cholesterol-lowering statins and vitamin D

The results of studies show very clearly and consistently that we are in the midst of an epidemic of vitamin D deficiency of immense proportions. Study after study of nursing home populations, of nursing mothers, of healthy male and female volunteers and of various children's groups have consistently documented that optimal levels of vitamin D are very rarely found. Now consider the impact of cholesterol-lowering drugs. Vitamin D is manufactured directly out of cholesterol. Cholesterol must be available in our bodies in amounts sufficient to allow conversion to vitamin D. Yet we dump cholesterol-lowering statins into the population indiscriminately in a misguided attempt to bring everyone's natural level of cholesterol down to some artificially low level.

Congestive heart failure (CHF) is more prevalent in those with very low levels of vitamin D.[66] Furthermore, *NT-proANP*, a protein which is a predictor of the severity of CHF, is also increased when vitamin D levels are low.

Hypertension, a strong predictor of heart disease, follows a similar pattern, being higher where UV light has a lower intensity and in people with darker skin or who don't get out into the sun.[67] In Central Asia, Stage 1 hypertension was detected in 18% of Uighurs living at low altitude, but in only 1% of Kirghizs who live at high altitude.[68]

Summary

The evidence, of which the above is but a small part, is overwhelming: all around the world, the sunnier the climate, and the higher the altitude, the more people uncover and go into the sun, the more vitamin D there is in their blood and the less heart disease there is.

Diabetes

Diabetes also fits the same patterns as heart diseases, being more common further from the Equator, at lower altitude, in people with dark skins, in the aged and the obese. Across the world, blood sugar and haemoglobin A1c (see Glossary) are higher in the winter.[69,70] Numbers of cases of both type-2 and type-1 diabetes are higher where vitamin D levels are lower.[71]

In the US, while diets don't change, blood sugar levels are significantly higher in winter than in summer.[72] That finding from 1982 was massively reinforced by a recent study involving 285,705 veterans.[73]

Why does flu break out as the nights draw in?

Have you ever wondered why we get flu in the winter, but not in the summer? Or why the common cold is called a 'cold'? The answer to both questions is the same: it's because we tend to get both diseases when there is little sunlight.

The flu virus is with us all year round. Yet, in spite of people crowding together in the streets, factories, offices, on buses, trains, airplanes, cruise ships, and in nursing homes and hospitals, an outbreak of flu in the summer months is so rare that it makes the news.[74] Influenza is a disease of winter.[75] Furthermore, flu epidemics happen at the same season at the same latitude around the world, both north and south of the Equator.[76] The reason for this is that we don't get as much sunshine in the winter as we do in summer.

If you think about it, it should be obvious that the flu and cold season is the same as the vitamin D deficiency season. Activated vitamin D, a steroid hormone, has profound effects on human immunity: it dramatically stimulates the expression of potent anti-microbial peptides, which exist in neutrophils, monocytes, natural killer cells, and in epithelial cells lining the respiratory tract where they play a major part in protecting the lung from infection; our body's innate immunity, especially the production of natural antibiotics called antimicrobial peptides, also goes up and down every year with our vitamin D levels. Volunteers inoculated with live attenuated influenza virus are more likely to develop fever in the winter; and vitamin D deficiency predisposes children to respiratory infections.[77]

Flu vaccines don't work

In Britain, every winter, the over-65s, diabetics and those with other serious diseases among us will also be exhorted to visit their local doctor for their seasonal flu jab, because the World Health Organization (WHO) has claimed that flu vaccinations 'reduce the risk of serious complications or of death by 70 to 85%' in these groups. That claim is based on just one study which turns out to be wrong. A review of *all* of the studies has discovered that the flu vaccine is ineffective. One of the problems is that flu viruses have a nasty habit of mutating such that the flu vaccine given this year will be made from last year's flu virus, and won't work against this year's virus.

A recent review in the British journal, *The Lancet*, concluded: 'In elderly individuals living in the community, [influenza] vaccines were not significantly effective against influenza, influenza-like illness, or pneumonia.'[78] The authors concluded that the overall effect of flu shots is 'modest' at best.

The Canadians experimented with a flu vaccination programme which was universally free to those vaccinated, although it cost Ontario taxpayers more than C$200 million. It began in 2000. A study published in 2006, after the experiment had been running for five years, suggested that it appeared to have done nothing to cut the spread of influenza.[79] Research by the University of Ottawa, published in the journal, *Vaccine*, concluded that, not only had the per-capita flu rates in the province not fallen since the programme had been introduced, but the numbers of flu cases in Ontario had actually gone up from an average 109 per month in 1990 to 160 per month in 2005. Dianne Groll, the University of Ottawa professor who led the study, said: 'there has been a lot of money spent. The program was designed to reduce the incidence of flu, and this hasn't yet happened.'

Another large combined study from Italy and the US found that flu vaccines offer no protection for the elderly. Researchers compared monthly death rates from 1970 to 2001, and found no change in the mortality rates of seniors, even though the over-65s had been specifically targeted for flu vaccines for nearly 20 years.[80]

The flu vaccine's ineffectiveness also extends to younger people. Another study found that two-thirds of adults below the age of 65 still had influenza later in the season, as did a group of children over six years of age.[81]

This is not news. Twenty years ago, Edwin Kilbourne, the grandfather of American influenza specialists, found that: 'The effect of current vaccination programs on morbidity is insignificant, and that on mortality marginal.'[82]

Multiple sclerosis (MS)

Lastly, a great deal of epidemiological and experimental evidence suggests that high levels of vitamin D may decrease the risk of multiple sclerosis. A study of blood samples from over seven million US military personnel, together with MS cases identified through Army and Navy physical disability databases for 1992 through 2004, found that the risk of MS increased significantly with decreasing levels of vitamin D.[83]

Rickets

Rickets has been a childhood scourge for centuries. Before the Industrial Revolution in England it was a disease of the affluent, because of their style of clothing and the fact that they spent most of their time indoors. Later, urbanization and atmospheric pollution caused city-dwelling poor children to be more commonly affected. Rickets was largely eradicated in the middle of the last century – at least in civilized countries. Today, however, rickets is on the rise across the world in both developing and developed countries.[84]

Exposure of children to sunlight on the roof of a hospital in New York City in 1921 demonstrated that a common factor, later called vitamin D, was essential for skeletal health.[85] After this, sunbathing was promoted as a form of preventive medicine, parents were encouraged to put their offspring out in the sun,[86] and the condition largely disappeared. Now all that has changed and rickets is returning.[87] Over the past decade, the majority of cases in developed countries have occurred in children with inadequate sun exposure because of dark skin, or because they remain fully clothed for religious or social reasons.[88,89] The condition is more prevalent in south Asian children with dark skins.[90] It is also rife amongst breast-fed Moslem children whose mothers wear all-enveloping clothes and eat vitamin D deficient vegan diets,[91] in their children who cover up for religious reasons,[92] and in breast-fed children of black African origin.[88]

Recent 'healthy', low-fat dietary advice, coupled with anti-sun recommendations, has led to the re-emergence of this once-conquered disease in white-skinned children as well. In a paper which documents an association between use of sunscreens and vitamin D deficiency rickets, Professor Stanley Zlotkin, of the Department of Paediatrics and of Nutritional Sciences, University of Toronto, asks whether infants and children are at an increased risk of vitamin D deficiency because of the increasing use of sunscreens.[93] He suggests that infants who don't eat enough vitamin D and whose skin is protected by potent sunscreens should receive a vitamin D supplement. The strength of the sun in the higher latitudes of Britain and North America also makes it essential that *all* dark-skinned, breast-fed infants and children in these countries get out in the sun in the middle of the day during the summer months as much as possible, and receive vitamin D supplementation in the winter.

This problem is a particular worry in girls as vitamin D deficiency during adolescence may lead to carpopedal spasms, diffuse limb pains, deformities of the lower limbs, and generalized weakness as well as contributing to osteomalacia and osteoporosis in later life.[94]

Osteomalacia

Osteomalacia is a disease of the elderly which is similar to rickets in children. A dietary survey of elderly patients with osteomalacia showed more than half had very low levels of vitamin D.[95] One woman on a low-fat diet had none at all. Elderly women who were housebound – which was most of them – got no sunshine. If they also adopt low-fat diets, risks of vitamin D deficiency are particularly high.

Postmenopausal hip fracture

In a series of tests conducted between January 1995 and June 1998, a group of American scientists tested vitamin D levels in postmenopausal women who had suffered a hip fracture.[96] Hip fractures at this age are usually attributed to osteoporosis. However, in these tests, only a quarter of the women tested had osteoporosis. What was significant was that the women who had broken hips had lower levels of vitamin D.

Death

If all the above weren't enough reason to get out in the sun more, research published as this book was going to press showed clearly that people of all ages with the lowest blood levels of vitamin D were about twice as likely to die from any cause during an eight-year period than those with the highest levels.[97] This trend was particularly noticeable with heart-related deaths, which were significantly higher in people with low vitamin D levels.

Conclusion

Sunshine is one of the best, most misunderstood health remedies out there. Sun exposure can help you fight off a whole host of diseases and offers protection against several types of cancer by as much as 60%. It also reduces your risk of death overall. And it costs nothing. Or is that the problem?

On the other hand, the US economic burden due to vitamin D insufficiency from inadequate exposure to solar UVB was estimated at $40 billion to $56 billion in 2004, whereas the economic burden for excess UV irradiance was estimated at $6 billion to $7 billion. These findings are probably on the low side, because of the additional benefits found recently, such as protection against infectious diseases.[98]

The sun has a long legacy of healing. Prehistoric tribes and entire civilizations have worshipped the sun for its healing properties for centuries. 'Heliotherapy', the use of sunlight to treat medical conditions, has been used for thousands of years. Both Hippocrates and Pythagoras wrote about the many benefits of sunlight to promote healing. One Greek city, well-known for its temples of healing sunlight, was called Heliopolis. Herodotus wrote that exposure to the sun is necessary to help people overcome failing health.

With a vast history and backed up by a huge raft of studies showing that many different aspects of our health benefit from sunlight and subsequent vitamin D production, surely it is obvious that current advice to get as little sunshine on your body as possible is positively irresponsible. This is particularly important in children whose health for life may be irreparably damaged by inappropriate 'slip-slap-slop', cover-up-and-stay-out-of-the-sun messages.

We are 'children of the sun'. We need the vitamin D that is really only available from exposure to sunshine, during the middle of the day, and *without* a sun block. This might increase – slightly – the risk of skin cancers if we eat a 'healthy' polyunsaturated diet. But, even with that possible increase, most skin cancers are relatively benign when compared with all the other conditions and cancers that lack of sun exposure may cause.

A closing thought

Some years ago, the vicar of a parish in south Devon, who was not in favour of a nearby naturist beach, wrote in his parish magazine: 'If God had meant us to walk around without clothes, we'd have been born naked.' Well, of course, He did and we are – and for a very good reason. The sun heals.

Chapter Twelve

Exercise care

Touted as a cure for obesity, heart disease and myriad other conditions, we are all told to exercise more. All that does is burn energy, necessitating increased consumption – of the wrong foods. While exercise may increase fitness, it seems to have little benefit for health. Types of exercise generally promoted can do harm.

> The number of heart attacks occurring among the joggers should dampen the enthusiasm for this type of unsupervised sport among the laymen.
>
> *Dr Broda Barnes*

Together with diet, exercise is touted as a cure for obesity, diabetes, hypertension and other associated conditions. But does this hypothesis stand up to objective scrutiny. Just how much benefit is there really to undertaking a strenuous exercise regime? And can you have too much?

If you watch animals in the wild you will see that on the whole, they take as little exercise as possible. The lion, for example, spends most of his day lying down or asleep, yet he doesn't get fat or diabetic. It is his wife, the lioness, who does the shopping. But she hunts only once every two or three days and even then expends as little energy as possible doing it. Similarly, grazing animals have a slow and steady lifestyle, moving quickly only when threatened by a predator. The same is true of modern hunter-gatherer human tribes. Any traditional Inuit, for example, is always prepared for maximum walking, but nobody does it for fun or for 'exercise'. In the wild, Nature protects the heart from stress.

Think about when our ancestors were hunter-gatherers. They had a good brain, but not a lot of speed. Did they chase their prey? It's not very likely: their prey could mostly run or fly faster than them. No, hunters either crept up on animals stealthily until they were close enough to throw something at them or they used snares.

Animals that run for a living have efficient built-in shock absorbers in their legs; we haven't: merely the arch of the foot. We simply aren't designed to run far on a regular basis; we are designed for stealth and for walking at a slow, deliberate pace which does not send shock waves up our lower limbs. It is not surprising, therefore, that our current love affair with exercise has resulted in a huge burden on the health services from injuries sustained while running and jogging with a 10% per year increased demand for orthopaedic hospital beds as a result.

Exercise for weight loss

The combination of exercise and thinness is a well-established stereotype. The overweight are frequently criticized for not taking up the more strenuous physical activities enjoyed by slimmer people. Drs Andrew Prentice and Susan Jebb of the Medical Research Council pointed out that between 1980 and 1991 calorie intake in Britain fell by some 20%, while the number of people who were overweight doubled.[1] As we seem to be heeding the current dietary advice to eat less, but are nevertheless getting fatter, Prentice and Jebb concluded that the overweight are lazy. But are they?

Most modern diets advocate the twin strategies of taking in less energy (calorie-counting) while at the same time using more (exercising). And so dieters are urged to take up some form of physical activity to burn up the calories.

But the overriding philosophy – that exercise is the only sure way to lose fat – has always ignored one important fact: it doesn't work! Every single study on exercise to date, regardless of the type of exercise (aerobic, anaerobic, resistance training, split routines and combo approaches), has shown that exercise almost always fails to alleviate obesity – whether or not it is combined with a low-calorie or low-fat diet. This should not be surprising: everyone knows that, if they do more work, they get hungrier more quickly and eat more food. And the food they eat will be the same carbohydrate-rich food – candy bars, fizzy drinks – that made them overweight in the first place. This form of 'weight loss' is the best way to gain weight.

Not surprisingly, the great body of research, carried out in the hope of demonstrating that exercise reduces weight in the obese, has been consistently unsuccessful. Here are the results of some of them:

1. In 1976 Dr Per Björntorp and colleagues at the University of Gothenburg, Sweden, studied normal and overweight subjects on a six-month course of physical training.[2] Although those at normal weight did lose weight, the overweight ones didn't.
2. Two years later Dr Martin Krotkiewski and colleagues conducted a

similar study.[3] They found that while mildly obese patients did tend to lose weight, severely obese patients actually put on weight. These findings were not confined to Scandinavia.

3. In 1989 a study at McGill University, Montreal, and the University of Toronto, also found that exercise was fattening.[4] This showed that insulin remained much higher in obese patients for more than an hour after exercising, meaning that their bodies were taking glucose out of their blood and storing it as glycogen and fat.

4. Studies published in the early 1990s found no causal relationship between low physical activity and obesity in either children or the elderly.[5,6]

5. In 2000 a review found that the often-prescribed three to five hours per week of moderate to vigorous exercise had little or no impact on weight.[7]

There will be those who talk of doing very heavy work for long periods and who have lost weight. I lost a lot of weight myself when I was building my own house. But the amount of exercise which can be realistically done by the average person is ineffective for significant weight loss. The caloric burn of aerobic exercise, especially at the intensities that most mortals can sustain, is low – perhaps 5 kilocalories per minute. That's a fairly insignificant 300 kilocalories per hour. So, even after exhausting exercise, you will probably use up less than 150 kilocalories.

Children are the latest targets in the 'war against obesity'. In 2006, the *British Medical Journal* online published a study of 545 children with an average age of four years who exercised for 30 minutes, three times a week. It was studying the effects of the exercise on the children's body weight.[8] And did the children lose weight? No: all that exercise made no difference.

Research published in the *American Journal of Clinical Nutrition* assessed the relative roles of calorie intake and calories burned with regard to body weight changes in children.[9] It found that calories consumed rather than calories burned accounted for 74% of variation in weight. This means that what is eaten is far more important than exercise done.

And I do mean *what* is eaten, rather than how much. Between 1977 and 1999, 20 studies considered types of foods to determine which were more satisfying and staved off subsequent hunger longest. Sixteen of the studies showed that the lower the Glycaemic Index (GI) of foods, the better they were in this respect.[10] Significantly, an increase in GI of 50% *reduced* the satisfaction it gave by 50%. The best and lowest-GI foods are foods such as meat, fish, eggs, cheese, butter, cream, nuts and leafy vegetables. The worst GI foods included most starchy carbs such as breakfast cereals, bread, pasta, and rice. Yet these are exactly the types of foods promoted for eating after exercise – 'to top up glycogen levels'. For this reason, the carb-laced snack quickly wolfed down at the end of a workout is all it takes to put back all the weight lost during it.

All this is borne out by the following case history which shows that there is no need for exercise to lose weight if you eat the right foods.

Case history

E. K. has multiple sclerosis. She was first diagnosed with MS when she was 19. That's now over 20 years ago. Almost all of that time she has spent in a wheel chair, getting no exercise at all. You won't be surprised to hear that over the years she put on a lot of weight. Eventually, she decided to adopt the low-carb diet I recommended – and it worked beyond her wildest dreams. She didn't weigh herself; she couldn't. But she did know what she measured. After less that a year on the low-carb, high-fat diet, she had gone down three bra sizes and, she told me, 'it is getting expensive!' Three years after starting the diet, she was down to a normal weight and size, and she has now maintained it for over four years.

The truth is that the current recommendation for 30 minutes of aerobic exercise three times a week as an effective way of losing weight is a bad joke, and the impact of aerobic exercise on various parameters of weight loss is severely overstated.[11] And contrary to popular belief, aerobic exercise does *not* raise metabolic rate after training. Probably the biggest benefit of aerobics is that it improves the muscles' ability to use fat for fuel, by increasing mitochondrial density and the activity and number of aerobic enzymes. But that is only of use if you use fat as an energy source rather than glucose from carbs.

Exercise and energy stores

Your body stores energy in two forms: glycogen, a form of starch to serve as a short-term supply of glucose, and body fat or 'adipose tissue', which is a store of fat. The aim is to lose the fat. This means you must change your diet to one that is low in carbs or it won't work.

If you eat a carb-based, low-fat diet as most dieters do, then your body will be geared to burn glucose. When you exercise, you will use up the glucose in your bloodstream and then mobilize the glycogen stored in your muscles and liver. When this is getting low, it will look for another, quick-fix, source of glucose. And it will convert protein from your muscles into glucose. It's a process called *gluconeogenesis*.

As you cannot keep on exercising for ever without stopping, as soon as you eat your next carb-rich meal, your glucose and glycogen stores will be replenished. You will then be right back where you started – but weaker. And as every gram of glycogen is stored with about 3 grams of water, you can put that weight back on very quickly. On top of this you probably won't have burned up any body fat – which was the whole point of the exercise in the first place!

This form of exercising for weight loss is costly, short term, potentially dangerous and self-defeating. If, when you exercise, you burn up less energy than the amount of easily accessible glycogen stored in the liver and muscles, you won't use up any of your body fat – and therefore won't lose any weight. If you use more energy than is immediately available, any weight lost is at a cost of stress on your body.

To lose weight, you must mobilize your *fat* stores. This means getting your body to burn fat and that, in turn, means making it change from using glucose to using fat. And the only way to do that is to deprive your body of glucose in the long term, so it has no choice but to use fat.

If you think about it, it really is quite logical. To lose weight, you merely have to change to a low-carb, high-fat diet. Or you can starve (which is what low-calorie dieting is).

Exercise and heart disease

It has been suggested that regular exercise will enlarge the arteries, thus lessening the likelihood of their becoming blocked and so reducing the risk of coronary heart disease. It was noted in the 1950s that bus drivers had a higher incidence of coronary heart disease than bus conductors and, as the drivers had a less energetic working life, this might be seen to support the argument. It was also noted, however, that dock labourers had higher rates of heart disease than building labourers. This tends to defeat the argument as the amounts of exercise associated with their jobs are not likely to differ significantly.[12]

The claim that exercise may help in heart disease arose from the fact that seasoned athletes develop increased cardiovascular capacity. But the view that exercise necessarily protects against heart disease, a strongly emotive factor in the increasing pressure to indulge in high-intensity exercise regardless of physical status, can be dangerous.

Exercise recommendations rarely make a distinction between moderate and extreme exercise; they give no warning that the latter can *cause* cardiovascular disease and arrythmias that lead to sudden cardiac death.

People who are healthy do more of it; those who are unwell do less of it. And they are usually instinctively correct.[13]

The studies disagree

The results of the major studies published so far have found for the most part that there is no convincing correlation between exercise (or the lack of it) and heart disease. For example, a four-year study of 16,882 executive grade civil servants aged 40 to 64 suggested that heavy work such as swimming or gardening might be beneficial if continued for over 15 minutes, but its results were inconclusive.[14] Even when accurate reporting of the effects of voluntary exercise on heart patients is examined, the benefits appear to be minimal.[15]

In the UK Heart Disease Project, a part of the WHO European Study, however, the results were conclusive – and different. The Project studied 18,210 men, again in the 'coronary' age group, from 24 factories across Europe. Half were given the conventional advice on exercise and being overweight, the other half being given no specific advice. The results of this study showed that instead of the expected benefits, the group which followed the advice on exercise had significantly *higher* rates of heart problems and deaths than that which did not.[16] These results confirmed others that had been published in the US a few years earlier.

Data from the United States indicated that richer people tended to adopt health innovations more readily than poorer people, and this was particularly evident in the cases of smoking and exercise. Michael Stern of the University of Texas Health Science Center cites a dramatic illustration of the lack of benefit. Some 10,000 people participated in the New York Marathon. Of those, 80% had college degrees and, of these, half held graduate degrees. Stern points out that: 'Since in our society, whites are generally of higher socio-economic status than either blacks or Mexican-Americans, one might have expected that they would experience the steepest CHD mortality declines . . . The data, however, indicate the reverse has been true.'

The statistics from the period show that while mortality in the US from CHD declined by over 20% between 1968 and 1976, it seems that exercise increased the death rate.[17]

There may be a very good reason for this. I was in Ciechocinek, Poland, in late 2005 visiting Dr Jan Kwaśniewski, whose dietary ideas are similar to mine. Amongst other things, we discussed exercise and I was introduced to a work that has probably never been seen by any western doctor: a book published in East Germany in 1957, during the Cold War. One chapter demonstrated that the more work limbs and muscles do, the more cholesterol is found in the walls of the arteries that supply them.[18] Or, to put it another way, work may well increase atherosclerosis, the very process that is believed to contribute most to a heart attack. In which case, if you believe in the cholesterol hypothesis, exercising muscles such as the heart that are already hard at work even more, could be considered a form of suicide.

There is an alternative hypothesis: that the cholesterol is in the artery walls as a protective substance, in which case we want to encourage it by taking more exercise and making the heart work harder. But if that increases atherosclerosis as this book suggests it will, doesn't that destroy the case for atherosclerosis being a cause of heart attacks?

Exercise to prevent diabetes?

We are also advised to exercise to prevent type-2 diabetes. Sir Steve Redgrave was such an ardent exerciser that he won gold medals for rowing in five consecutive Olympic Games. But that didn't stop him becoming a type-2 diabetic in his 30s.

Exercising faith

In June 1991 the British government published its initial *Health of the Nation* green paper. In it, exercise was promoted on the grounds that it prevented heart disease. Given that a major national effort was invested in promoting exercise on the grounds that it prevents heart disease, you might think it fair to ask for some evidence to substantiate this claim. So the *British Medical Journal* conducted a debate into the merits of the green paper and contested the assertion that exercise was helpful. This led to two contributors to the debate revealing the anti-scientific mentality of the health promotion lobby. In their support of 'the role of exercise', Drs Henry Dargie and S. Grant took on the exercise sceptics by writing:

> 'Some would argue that there is no conclusive evidence from controlled trials that regular exercise reduces the number of deaths from coronary heart disease or substantially prolongs life. To demand such proof is to miss the point about exercise, which is that it is valuable for numerous other health benefits it confers and as a catalyst in the adoption of a healthier lifestyle.'[19]

So it seems there is no evidence after all for the benefits of exercise in heart disease – merely 'numerous *other* health benefits.' No doubt to request evidence for these benefits would also be to miss the point, which is that the health promoters firmly believe that exercise is conducive to a healthier lifestyle. It seems it is faith rather than science that justifies exhortations to change public behaviour. And such faith may place a trusting public at greater danger, for exercise is not always beneficial.

The dangers of over-exercising

'Fitness' is a multi-billion-pound or dollar industry which promotes books, exercise machinery, weights, footwear, clothing, and expensive gyms and exercise clubs. If someone tells you that you need to exercise, you would be wise to question whether there is any commercial bias behind their advice.

Sport and exercise of the right kind can be rewarding both as a social outlet and in making you feel good; it may boost your self-esteem if you treat it as a form of group therapy; and it helps to keep muscles in trim and give your body a better shape. As such it has an important part to play, particularly as leisure time for many of us is increasing. But it can easily be overdone with potentially disastrous consequences.

In women, exercise exhaustive enough to cause weight loss can delay the onset of puberty, cause amenorrhoea (cessation of periods), abnormal menstrual cycles, abnormal sex hormone patterns and impaired reproductive function, and the early development of osteoporosis.[20-22] Male long-distance runners may suffer reductions in the male sex hormone, testosterone.[23] For anyone contemplating taking up the more strenuous forms of exercise, advice from the *American Heart Journal* is:

> 'Be tested and have an exercise programme devised after clinical trials and tests on the heart as, although regular exercise will lower the overall risk of cardiovascular disease, there is a statistically significant increase in the risk of sudden death.'[24]

There are real risks if those who are not seasoned athletes attempt to break through the pain barrier, or as Jane Fonda puts it, 'go for the burn'. The pain barrier is the body's signal that its limit of toleration has been reached. Disregarding it is foolhardy. While seasoned athletes with their increased oxygenating capacity may be able to prolong their muscular activity before the onset of pain, the average person cannot and should not attempt to emulate them. The risk to health and even life is unacceptably high. Over the past few years there have been reports of significant numbers of cases of sudden death in healthy young men out jogging or playing squash because they disregarded the pain barrier.

Most sudden deaths in sport are caused by cardiovascular conditions, although one regularly hears that the benefits of exercise in terms of CHD are 'well established' and may reduce the risk of such events. Victims are often perceived as very fit but it should be noted that: 'extreme forms of conditioning, including marathon running, do not prevent severe atherosclerosis or sudden death.'[25]

There have also been a huge number of cases of broken bones, dislocations, and damage to internal organs, muscles, tendons and ligaments. A study from Japan cited a 25% incidence of injury in those undertaking exhaustive exercise and these figures are confirmed in similar western studies. The increase of sports-related injuries has been such that, had they been caused by a bacterium, it would have been classed as a serious epidemic.

Exercise-induced allergies – asthma, itching and urticaria (nettle rash) – are also on the increase, as are cases of cardiovascular collapse and respiratory obstruction.[26] While some conditions may be minor annoyances, others are definitely life threatening. They typically affect teenagers and young adults.

In a study of 42 Swedish elite runners, 23 had asthma and 31 had asthma-like symptoms. The prevalence of asthma in elite athletes in Finland whose mean age was 22.9 was similar. Of 103 athletes, 16 had documented asthma and 24 more had allergies. All of those with asthma and 14 of those with allergies reported having symptoms like exercise-induced asthma. Twenty-three of the remaining 63 also reported having asthma-like symptoms occasionally. Thus over half of the runners in this study were affected.[27]

The usual trigger for an attack of asthma is running, but some patients have collapsed after only a brisk walk. It is not possible to predict an attack even among people with a history of such attacks while running. Even joggers, who have been running for many years without incident, frequently collapse. Jim Fixx, author of *The Complete Book of Running*, invented jogging and advocated it to prevent heart attack. It is ironic that Fixx, himself, died of a heart attack while out jogging. Current advice to joggers is: never jog alone.

In spite of the risks, or more probably because they are not made aware of them, many people adopt exercise programmes which involve sudden intensive exertion such as squash or aerobics.

The term aerobics means 'using oxygen' and it is claimed that aerobic exercise is beneficial because it increases the amount of oxygen in the body tissues. In fact, the demand for oxygen may increase to a point where it cannot be met, so that, far from increasing tissue oxygenation, aerobic exercise decreases it. Aerobic exercise has been demonstrated to cause a significant and continuous drop in blood pressure – a sign of cardiac fatigue.[28] This can happen in as little as five minutes – and most aerobic sessions last for an hour!

There is another consideration, particularly where the overweight are concerned: by definition, people who are overweight are already carrying around extra weight. That fact alone means that they must already use more energy than slim people. There is a limit to how much more exercise someone who is massively overweight can do.

Athletes reach altered states such as 'the runner's high'. It makes them feel better and is a form of reward for their effort. The lower potential of overweight people means that they will be denied this satisfaction even if they do lose some weight.

Too much of a good thing?

The reason we have the potential for short-term rapid movement is that we have evolved to be able to escape from danger and to survive in a wide range of dangerous and adverse circumstances. This ability is built into our bodies' emergency system: the 'fight or flight reflex'. Activated by the need to run away from danger or stay and fight, or as a result of strenuous exercise, this reflex causes a number of automatic responses which prepare the body to face the danger to come: the heartbeat is accelerated; minor blood vessels are constricted so that more blood is fed to the brain and muscles; the lungs take in more oxygen; the amount of cholesterol in the blood is increased; adrenaline is pumped into the bloodstream helping these changes, stopping or slowing the digestive process, and stimulating the conversion of glycogen into glucose which the body can use more easily for energy.

These changes, in the natural world, are designed to last for a short time: the time of the emergency, after which the body can return to normal. In the case of prolonged physical exertion, however, the body is forced to continue, setting in motion a series of changes called the *General Adaptation Syndrome*. A major and important change is the prolonged production of a group of adrenal hormones called *corticosteroids*. An excessive production of corticosteroids has been shown to produce heart disease,[29] hypertension and stomach ulcers,[30] and harm the body's ability to fight infectious diseases and cancer;[31] the depletion of the corticosteroids may also cause rheumatoid arthritis.[32]

Other evidence emerged in 2005 which suggested that exercising may actually shorten your life.[33] Dr Peter Axt and his daughter, Dr Michaela Axt-Gadermann, who are both reformed long-distance runners, argue that exercising increases the production of harmful free radicals – unstable oxygen molecules believed to speed up the ageing process. They say: 'If you lead a stressful life and exercise excessively, your body produces hormones which lead to high blood pressure and can damage your heart and arteries.'

The correct exercise for health

I hope by bringing together some of the information above that I haven't put you off exercising altogether. That was not my intention as there are numerous benefits to health and well-being from exercise – if it is approached in the right way. I wrote what I wrote because there are two aspects to exercise: one is health, which I have covered above; the other is fitness. 'Health' and 'fitness' are not synonymous. There is not a great deal of evidence that exercise plays much part in health – unless you eat an unhealthy, 'healthy' diet – but exercise of the right kind will keep you fit:

that is, supple, strong and with stamina.

For health generally all that is necessary is moderate exercise. To increase the capacity of your cardiovascular system (that is, to increase your fitness), you need to work harder. But either way, it's a good idea to avoid repetitive 'bouncing' types of exercise that shock the system. This means that walking, cycling and swimming are good, but running and jogging are not.

Conclusion

People with only 10 pounds or so to lose may be able to lose it with exercise. But anyone who claims that exercise is the key to solving weight problems in the chronically obese is simply not telling the complete truth about what research on the subject has shown.

To sum up, moderate exercise and sport do have a healthy social role. However, excessive exercise is unnatural and can be dangerous. And don't be misled by the hype – athletes are not known for their longevity.

Chapter Thirteen

Homo carnivorous

Having shown that the health regimes we are exhorted to undertake have little or no evidential support, that leaves the question of what constitutes a truly healthy diet for us as a species. This chapter looks at our evolutionary history to show that we really should eat a very different diet from that advocated today. It also looks at the basis for our 'love affair with fat'.

Nature has taken good care that theory should have little effect on practice.

Samuel Johnson

Although the diet dictocrats continue to insist that we must eat starchy diets with lots of bread and breakfast cereals, low in meat and animal fat, we now know that the basis for our so-called 'healthy' diet is, as a doctor friend of mine puts it, 'scientifically untenable garbage'. But that leaves us with the question of what constitutes a truly healthy diet; what should we eat to be truly healthy and avoid all the pain, misery and cost?

'You are what you eat.' Dr Magnus Pike coined the expression in his book, *Food for all the Family*, in 1980. We now hear the expression frequently. It may, or may not, be true of what we eat today but it is certainly true that we are what our ancestors ate. And what they ate then is also what we should eat today for in this way we will eat the diet we have evolved to eat. To be healthy, we must eat a diet that is natural to us as a species.

What we need to determine, therefore, is what that diet is.

Do wild animals, in their natural environment, require instruction or frequent bulletins from a Department of Health to guide them in their choice of food? The answer is: No! The grazing animals seek and eat plant food; the carnivorous animals hunt and devour the plant eaters. Nature really is not complicated. Wild animals are perfect examples of optimum nutrition resulting from their respective correctly balanced diets. And that applies equally to humans. When did a primitive tribesman consult a calorie chart before deciding what and how much he should eat? They eat what comes naturally to them, in the quantities they want, and whenever they like.

We 'civilized' people forget that we, too, were also in this situation for millions of years before we began to acquire the assets of civilization. It is certain that Nature gave us a similar innate wisdom to choose foods best suited for us. So long as they remained nutritionally ignorant and uninformed our ancestors did a pretty creditable job of selecting their diet. If they hadn't, we wouldn't be here today.

Many claims are set forth stating what the 'natural' diet of humans is or should be. They vary widely from carnivore to vegetarian, fruitarian – even breatharians who believe it is possible to live just by breathing, without eating anything at all. To decide which is correct we must look at human diets from pre-history, and at cross-cultural dietary comparisons of primitive and modern societies. It is also useful to consider the diets of mankind's nearest relatives, the primates.

Primates

Apart from *Homo sapiens* (us), there are 192 other species of primate alive today. Many believe that we are the only one that is carnivorous; that all of the others are vegetarian. Some suggest, because of our similarities, we too are really a vegetarian species. But many studies have revealed that all the other primates are actually omnivorous. Never having been persuaded by the arguments of vegetarians, in addition to fruits, nuts, seeds, leaves and flowers, our primate cousins eat birds' eggs, insects, spiders, small animals and even other primates.[1-3]

Until Jane Goodall published her research in the 1960s,[4] it was assumed that chimpanzees ate only plant foods. But Goodall discovered that they kill and eat monkeys, baby baboons, and other small animals. Dian Fossey and Richard Perry also showed that gibbons, orangutans, and baboons kill and eat small animals regularly.[5,6] The most primitive primate of all, the tree shrew, is entirely carnivorous. These studies have led to primates being reclassified as omnivores.

An example of false assumptions involved the National Zoo in Washington. They attempted to breed the Amazon Golden Marmoset monkey in captivity, but failed – until animal protein was added to the monkeys' diet.[7] It had been wrongly assumed that marmosets were complete vegetarians, but we now know that they must have animal protein in order to be fertile.

Homo carnivorous

So, if every other primate eats meat, why not us? There is no reason at all. Indeed, the evidence is overwhelming that we took meat eating to the extreme, by eating little or nothing else for most of our existence. And we know that many human cultures still do today.

Archaeological and climate records tell us clearly what prehistoric Man ate: a diet of meat and fat, supplemented at certain times of the year, when available, with berries, nuts and leaves. It could not have been otherwise for, over at least the last two and a half million years, our ancestors lived, evolved and adapted during a long series of Ice Ages. The last Ice Age began to end a mere 9,000 years ago. But it didn't end everywhere at the same time. As the Earth warmed up, the ice cleared from the equatorial regions towards the poles over a period of 5,000 or 6,000 years. It was only after this that agriculture started to be practised. In evolutionary terms, that was yesterday.

The significance of this is that, if you are like me – a blond-haired, blue-eyed individual – whose evolutionary ancestry is in northern Europe, your genes, which are essentially the same as those of your early ancestors and control every function of your body, were developed during a long period of weather patterns that are not unlike those of present-day Greenland.

Even if your ancestry is in southern Europe, south-east Asia or Africa, your genes will be very much the same. And therein lies the problem, for your genes are concerned only with the foods that they have been programmed over millions of years to recognize as 'food'. They care nothing for what we place in our mouths today: they simply won't recognize many of them as 'food'. If they are fed properly these genes will do their job of keeping us healthy, but give these genes nutrients that are unfamiliar or in the wrong ratios, and they malfunction.

According to Dr S. Boyd Eaton, one of the foremost authorities on palaeolithic (pre-agriculture) diets, the foods we eat today are quite unlike anything our genetic makeup has prepared us for. Eaton makes the point that 99% of our genetic heritage dates from before our biological ancestors evolved into modern *Homo sapiens* about 40,000 years ago, and that 99.99% of our genes were formed before the development of agriculture. The less we eat like our ancestors, the more susceptible we will be to coronary heart disease, cancer, diabetes, and many other 'diseases of civilization.'[8] Yet, over the last 20 years our diet has changed out of all recognition.

Our natural diet

Books written by nutritionists and dieticians today tend to be contradictory, often reflecting current fads. As they cannot all be right, how are we to determine what is the diet to which we are best adapted?

The answer lies in our past, but not the immediate past. The way we live now is based on advanced agriculture and the domestication of plants and animals, recent innovations to which we cannot yet have become adapted. To determine what foods are likely to make up the diet we are best adapted to as a species, we must look further back.

We can trace human evolution from remains and artifacts of early hominids found in Africa and other parts of the world dated as long as 4 million years ago; we have fossilized bone records both of our hominid ancestors and of animals; we have stone tools and implements that must have been used for killing and cutting flesh or for grinding plants; we even have hominid faeces. These findings have led to a great deal of speculation about our diet. Are we a carnivorous, omnivorous or herbivorous species?

We call our ancestors, and the various modern primitive tribes, 'hunter/ gatherers'. In the world today, some tribes live exclusively on meat and fish; others live on fruit, nuts and roots, although meat is also highly prized; still more live without eating anything derived from animal sources. It is obvious, therefore, that as a species we can survive on a wide variety of foods. But which, if any, is the optimal diet that we have evolved to eat?

In our hunt for an answer, the first evidence to consider lies in the fossil sites of Africa, widely accepted as our birthplace. Here, where hominid remains are found, so also are animal bones – sometimes in their thousands.[9] If those hominids were not meat-eaters, why is that? Second, although many modern hunting tribes do eat plants, they have fire. There were very few plant foods with sufficient calorific value that our prehistoric ancestors could have digested without fire. There were fruits, of course, but there is not one prehistoric site in all Africa that indicates forests extensive enough to have supplied sufficient fruit to meet the needs of its inhabitants. There is also agreement that our ancestors did not dwell in the forests of Africa but on the savannah – that is, vast plains of grass. Yet grass is of no use whatsoever to our digestive system.

The walls of all plant cells are made of cellulose, a form of dietary fibre which is indigestible. There is no enzyme in the human digestive system that will break it down. With no means of breaking down raw plant cell walls, the nutrients inside those cells cannot be digested. Passing unaffected straight through the gut, they would be ejected as waste.

Neither is it likely that the seeds of the savannah grasses could have supplied early humans with the energy they required. Seeds are naturally indigestible, designed to pass through an animal's body, to be defecated and take root elsewhere surrounded in rich faecal fertilizer. There are two means whereby seeds can be made digestible: cooking and grinding.

Seeds could have been pounded to break down the plant cell walls, but no archaeologist has ever found a Stone Age tool suited to this task. If seeds had been ground down by chewing, fossilized teeth would show much more wear than they do; also, many seeds would have escaped and, passing through the body undigested, ended up in faeces. Fossilized hominid faeces, known as coprolites, have been studied in detail and almost none contain any plant material. And grass seeds are so much smaller than the cultivated grains of today, that gathering them would not have been profitable.

European Neanderthal coprolites dating from around 50,000 years ago, before fire was used, contain no plant material.[10] It was not until the Cro-Magnon colonization of Europe, some 35,000 years ago, that hearths became universal and plants could be cooked to break down the cell walls. But even then the evidence suggests that fires were used merely for warmth rather than cooking. At that time, Europe was in the grip of a succession of ice ages; times of long, cold winters and short, cool summers. Our Eurasian ancestors cannot have been plant eaters then – for most of the year there weren't any plants. They ate meat or died. And they ate that meat raw.

If you want to get ahead, get a brain

The evidence that we could not be a vegetarian species was already over-whelming when, in 1972, the publication of two independent investigations confirmed this.[11,12] They concerned fats. These studies showed that without the correct fats in the diet – fats that come only from animal sources – our brains could not have developed as they did.

About half our brain and nervous system is composed of complicated, long-chain, fatty acids. These are also used in the walls of our blood vessels. These fatty acids do not occur in plants. This is where plant-eating herbivores come in. Over the year, the herbivores convert the simple fatty acids found in grasses and seeds into intermediate, more complicated forms. By eating the herbivores we can convert their stores of these fatty acids into the ones we need.

About 2.5 million years ago, as the world grew colder and food plants became scarcer, animal foods began to occupy an increasingly prominent place in our ancestors' menus. Smaller molar size, less robust facial muscles and alterations in incisor shape from that time all suggest a greater emphasis on foods such as meat that require less grinding and more tearing.

An increasing proportion of meat in the diet would obviously have provided more animal protein, a factor perhaps related to the increase in stature which accompanied the transition from *Australopithecines* through *Homo habilis* to *Homo erectus*.[13] But greater availability of animal fat was probably a more important dietary alteration. Crude stone tools allowed early humans to break bones and allowed them access to brain and marrow fats from a broad range of animals. These and other carcass fats were probably as prized by early hominids as they are by modern human hunter-gatherers.[14] Not only did more animal fat in the diet mean considerably more energy; it was also a source of ready-made, long-chain, polyunsaturated fatty acids, including omega-6 arachidonic acid (AA), omega-3 docosatetraenoic acid (DTA) and omega-3 docosahexaenoic acid (DHA). These three fatty acids together make up over 90% of the fatty acids found in the brain matter of all mammalian species.[15]

Our brain is considerably larger than that of any ape. Looking back at the fossil records from early hominids to modern man, we see a remarkable increase in brain size from 375-550 millilitres at the time of *Australopithecus*, to 500-800 millilitres in *Homo habilis*, 775-1,225 millilitres in *Homo erectus*, and 1,350 millilitres in modern humans. While there is still speculation about *why* this should have happened, this increase in brain size could not have happened without an increased intake of preformed long-chain fatty acids which are an essential component in the formation of brain tissue.[16] It would never have occurred if our ancestors had not eaten meat – with its fat. Human breast milk contains the fatty acids needed for large brain development, cow's milk does not. It is no coincidence that, in relative terms, our brain is some 50 times the size of a cow's.

Where does the energy for our brain come from?

Around 20% of all the energy we use, is used by our brain. This is in contrast to the great apes whose brains use only about 8%. This makes our brains very expensive in energy terms. It means that our energy use compared with our body size should be considerably higher than that of other animals. Yet it isn't. This presents something of a puzzle: where do we humans get the extra energy to spend on our large brains? Researchers W. R. Leonard and M. L. Robertson conclude that the evolution of brain size implied changes in diet quality during hominid evolution. 'The shift to a more calorically dense diet', they said, 'was probably needed in order to substantially increase the amount of metabolic energy being used by the hominid brain. Thus, while nutritional factors alone are not sufficient to explain the evolution of our large brains, it seems clear that certain dietary changes were necessary for substantial brain evolution to take place.'[17] This confirms the Crawfords' work.[11]

We have a carnivore gut

There is another aspect to consider. Two scientists, L. C. Aiello and P. Wheeler, measured the sizes of brains and other body organs against organ size relative to body size predictions.[18] What they found was that the larger-than-expected size of the human brain was compensated for by a s*maller-than-expected* gut size. Measuring the other energy-expensive organs in the body – heart, kidneys, liver, and gastrointestinal tract – as these use the most energy after the brain, and comparing those of a 65-kilogram non-human primate with the organ sizes of an average 65-kilogram human, they found dramatic differences between the expected and actual sizes of the human brain, and gut: 'the splanchnic [abdominal/gut] organs were approximately 900 grams less than expected.' Almost all of this shortfall was due to our gut being only about 60% of that expected for a similar-sized primate.

Not only is our gut smaller than predicted compared with other primates, it is also configured very differently. Our small intestine is the major organ used to digest food and extract its nutrients for absorption into our bodies. Not surprisingly, it is more than 50% of the total volume of our gut. Our colon is used mainly to extract and so conserve water. For this reason, it represents only around 20% of our gut's volume. In contrast, the ratios in other primates are exactly the opposite. The small intestines of orangs and chimpanzees, which play a minor role in digestion, are around 25% of gut volume, and their colons, where bacteria are used to ferment plant fibre and where most digestion takes place, are around 53% by volume.[19]

This is not the only measurement that matters. So far I have compared our gut to that of our primate cousins who eat mostly plant food. If we also compare our gut to that of the great carnivores, we find that our gut is actually very much like theirs. The comparisons are done with respect to body weight as body weight is closely related to the metabolic energy requirements of an animal. This ratio, known as Kleiber's law, expresses the relationship between body mass (weight) and the body's metabolic energy requirements. The size of any organ that is directly concerned with metabolic turnover should comply with Kleiber's law. If we measure the size of these and they are in accordance with Kleiber's law, each part's gastrointestinal (GI) quotient should be 1.00. A GI greater than 1.00 means the organ is larger than expected, and GI less than 1.00 indicates a size smaller than expected.

In the gut, it is the surface area of various parts of the digestive tract which determines their relative absorptive ability. A test of major areas of the human digestive tract gave the following results:[20]

Stomach quotient	= 0.31
Small intestine quotient	= 0.76
Caecum quotient	= 0.16
Colon quotient	= 0.58

These values are all considerably less than 1.00. This is particularly obvious in the case of the caecum, a part of the gut between the small and large intestines which is present in all mammals, but with differing sizes depending on the mammal's natural food supply. Herbivores have a large caecum, hosting a large number of bacteria, which aid in the enzymatic breakdown of plant materials such as cellulose. Exclusive carnivores, whose diets contain little or no plant material, have a much smaller caecum, often partially or wholly replaced by the vermiform appendix. In humans, this is the case. Putting all this together we can come to only one conclusion: for the absorption of sufficient energy and nutrients for the body to function properly, food *must* be very energy and nutrient dense. Fat meat is the *only* universal class of food that falls into this category, thus there can be no doubt that humans fall into the carnivore class.

Brain quotient

Our gut is not the only part of our bodies to be analyzed in this way. It is in our brain size and high intelligence that we humans are unique. Relative to our body size, our brains are truly enormous. If we measure our brain quotient in the same way as we did for the gut, we can get some idea of just how big it really is.

In order to measure *encephalization* as it is called, statistical models were developed which compared brain size and body size in a wide range of species. This allowed an accurate estimation of the brain size for a given species based on its body mass. This is important because it allows the quantitative study and comparison of brain sizes between different species by automatically adjusting for body size. For example, elephants, which are plant eaters, and whales whether herbivores or carnivores, have larger brains than we do – but they also have much larger bodies. In this exercise it was noticed that the brain sizes of these animals also followed Kleiber's law.

When this test was conducted on humans, it put humans right at the very top of the primate scale. Our Encephalization Quotient was an outstanding 28.8.

With a brain so out of proportion to the rest of our bodies, it's not surprising that it uses such a large proportion of our total energy. As brain size and energy use are so high, and our gut size so small, the amount of energy available to the brain is dependent not only on how the body's total energy budget is allocated between the brain and other energy-intensive organs and systems, but on the ability of our gut to extract sufficient energy from our food. This confirms that the kind of diet we should eat must have the high nutrient density found in meat and animal fat.

Our brains are now getting smaller

With such a small gut with which to absorb all the nutrients and energy our bodies need, a modern low-calorie, low-fat, fibre-rich, plant-based diet is woefully inadequate as an energy source for our energy-hungry system to function at peak efficiency. That lack has begun to show.

Since the advent of agriculture, our brains have actually decreased in size. A recently updated and rigorous analysis of changes in human brain size found that our ancestors' brain size reached its peak with the first anatomically modern humans of approximately 90,000 years ago. That then remained fairly constant for a further 60,000 years.[21] Over the next 20,000 years there was a slight decline in brain size of about 3%. Since the advent of agriculture about 10,000 years ago, however, that decline has quickened significantly: now our brains are some 8% smaller.

This suggests some kind of recent historical deficiency in some aspect of overall human nutrition. The most obvious and far-reaching dietary change during the last 10,000 years is, of course, the enormous drop in consumption of high-energy, fat-rich foods of animal origin which formed probably over 90% of the diet, to as little as 10% today, coupled with a large rise in less energy-dense grain consumption.[22] This pattern still persists; it is even advocated today: it is the basis of our so-called 'healthy' diet.

Vitamin B$_{12}$

If you need any more convincing that we must be a meat-eating species, there is one other essential nutrient that is not found in any plant food but only in foods of animal origin. That nutrient is vitamin B$_{12}$.

The most important deficiency for anyone not eating foods from animal sources is that of vitamin B$_{12}$. By definition vitamin B$_{12}$ is essential to human life. It is essential for the synthesis of nucleic acids, the maintenance of the myelin sheath (the insulation around nerves which, when damaged, causes multiple sclerosis); indeed, its presence or deficiency affects nearly all body tissues, particularly those with rapidly dividing cells. Without vitamin B$_{12}$ we suffer from pernicious anaemia which is deadly, and degeneration of the nervous system.

Vitamin B$_{12}$ is unique among vitamins in that while it is found universally in foods of animal origin, where it is derived ultimately from bacteria, there is no active vitamin B$_{12}$ in anything which grows out of the ground. Where trace amounts of vitamin B$_{12}$ are found on plants it is there only fortuitously in bacterial contamination of the soil. And even that is lost if plants are washed thoroughly before eating them.

Bacteria in the human colon make prodigious amounts of vitamin B$_{12}$. Unfortunately, this is useless as it is not absorbed through the colon wall. Dr Sheila Callender tells of treating vegans with severe vitamin B$_{12}$ deficiency by making water extracts of their stools which she fed to them, thus effecting a cure.[23] An Iranian vegan sect unwittingly also makes use of this fact. Investigators could not understand how members of this sect remained healthy, until their investigations showed that they grew their vegetables in human manure – and then ate the vegetables without being too fussy about washing them first.[24]

To enable vegans to survive, vitamin B$_{12}$ is added artificially to breakfast cereals and may be bought in pill form. This is hardly a natural way to get food and it can be self-defeating. Unlike most other vitamins, vitamin B$_{12}$ occurs as a number of analogues, only one of which, *cyanocobalamin*, is active for humans. In collecting human stools for analysis, Dr Victor Herbert found that of each 100 micrograms of vitamin

B_{12} extracted, only 5 micrograms was of the cyanocobalamin analogue.[25] Thus even in this most prodigious source of the vitamin, 95% was composed of analogues which were useless.

Several fermented products such as tempeh, a soybean product, and spirulinas, used by strict vegans as a source of vitamin B_{12}, either do not contain significant amounts of the vitamin or contain analogues which are not active for humans.[26] Over half of the adults from a macrobiotic community tested in New England had low concentrations of vitamin B_{12}. Children were short in stature and low in weight. The community relied on sea vegetables for the vitamin.

This reliance on vegetables sources gives a false sense of security and could actually bring on the symptoms of vitamin B_{12} deficiency more quickly.

The amount of vitamin B_{12} we need is tiny: about 1 microgram per day. Eating more results in a reserve being built up in the body. When a person becomes a vegan, those stores are depleted – but only gradually. Thus it can be several years before the onset of symptoms. In England a carefully conducted study carried out on vegans showed that they all developed vitamin B_{12} deficiency eventually.[27]

There is one other, hidden danger. A largely vegetable-based diet provides large quantities of folic acid, which works in conjunction with vitamin B_{12}. The two need to be balanced, as excess folic acid can disguise the vitamin's deficiency. In such a case, irreparable damage to nerves and the spinal cord can take place such that, by the time symptoms become apparent, death is inevitable.

What matters as far as humans are concerned is that foods of animal origin are the only reliable food sources for vitamin B_{12}. This provides further evidence that such foods must have featured in our diet for a very long time.

Vitamin C

On the other side of the vitamin coin is vitamin C, believed by many to be available only in plants. This would argue for our being omnivores rather than carnivores – if it were true. Vitamin C is found in all animals. It is particularly high in adrenal glands. Canadian Indians, when they killed an animal, shared the adrenals amongst the family, where they were eaten raw.

The Inuit are renowned for eating little or no foods from plant sources, yet they don't get scurvy, the disease caused by vitamin C deficiency. The reason is that their wholly animal diet provided them with plenty of vitamin C. Seal liver, for example, contains 18-35 milligrams per 100 grams, narwhal skin has 18 milligrams, Beluga whale skin has 35 milligrams and its blubber has 5 milligrams. Cod roe has the highest content at 44 milligrams per 100 grams. Unfortunately for us in western society, apart from cod roe, these products aren't usually available in the supermarket, but you may be relieved to know that beef or lamb's liver has three times as much vitamin C as apples or pears, even after cooking. And all other meats also contain small amounts. Our total requirement for vitamin C is actually very low – unless we eat cereals, which don't contain any.

Agriculture and the first diet revolution

It was not until the last Ice Age came to an end that there was sufficient surplus food for some to be stored and some previously nomadic tribes were able to develop stable settlements. The cultivation of wild grass seeds began. Cooking solved the problem of their indigestibility.

This development caused a dramatic change in human lifestyle. The capacity to store controlled quantities of higher-energy starches meant populations could grow. And as numbers grew, it became more difficult to maintain food supplies through hunting alone. Thus our ancestors' basic diet changed from a high-protein, high-fat diet to one containing more starchy carbohydrates.

There is no evidence of nutritional diseases before the invention of agriculture. After it, there is. Cereals that became the modern staples, together with root crops which began to be cultivated, are all relatively deficient in protein, vitamins and several minerals, notably iron and calcium. Additionally, all cereals contain anti-nutrients. As a consequence, the coming of agriculture gave rise to nutritional diseases such as rickets, pellagra, dental caries, beri-beri, obesity, allergies and cancers: the so-called 'diseases of civilization'.

The Industrial Revolution and the second diet revolution

About 200 years ago the Industrial Revolution heralded a second dietary revolution which had two powerful but opposite effects on our health. Industrialized countries with their increased wealth no longer had to rely on home-produced, seasonally dependent foods. They could import what they wanted and could look forward to going through life without ever being hungry.

However, there were adverse effects. Many of the imported foods were unnatural to those eating them. New fruits tasted nice and, as a consequence, people changed from eating what they needed, to eating what they liked. But unaided by previous experience for such foods, the human autonomic nervous system had never learned when to stop. For example, you will find that you can eat sweets all day, but try eating butter with a spoon, and your body will soon let you know when it has had enough.

As time went by, science made possible the production of synthetic foods that had the appearance, texture and taste of the real thing, but with few of the proteins, fats and vitamins. Sugar became easy and cheap to produce, leading to a 30-fold increase in its consumption. The Industrial Revolution, therefore, was something of a double-edged sword: on the one hand it gave people a wider range of food than had ever before been possible; on the other it gave them diabetes, peptic ulcers, heart disease and a whole host of other new medical conditions. In the late 20th century the pace at which our diet became increasingly unnatural quickened – and so did the numbers of people getting these diseases.

Our love affair with fat

Despite these dramatic changes, our preference for meat, and fat meat in particular, continued. This is evidenced in written records over the last several thousand years. While I do not regard the Bible to be a scientific work, it does tell us what the peoples of the Middle East believed 2,000 to 3,000 years ago and what they liked to eat.

The first indication that fat was prized comes in Genesis, with the story of Cain and Abel and the account of the first recorded offering to Jehovah.

> 'And Abel was a keeper of sheep, but Cain was a tiller of the ground.
> And in process of time it came to pass, that Cain brought of the fruit of the ground an offering unto the Lord.
> And Abel, he also brought of the firstlings of his flock and of the fat thereof. And the Lord had respect unto Abel and to his offering.
> But unto Cain and to his offering he had not respect.'

This story tells us two things. Firstly, it represents the preferences of the Hebrew people themselves when they were living in the region of Babylon and Egypt: meat and fat were regarded as far superior to vegetables. Secondly, the inclusion of the words 'and of the fat thereof' means that Abel didn't only bring meat but also more fat separately as an added, superior, gift.

Further on in Genesis 45:17-18 we learn by inference that both Jews and Egyptians thought well of a high-fat diet:

> 'And Pharaoh said unto Joseph . . . "Take your father and your households, and come unto me; and I will give you the good of the land of Egypt, and ye shall eat the fat of the land".'

And from Isaiah 25:6:

> 'And in this mountain shall the Lord of hosts make unto all people a feast of fat things . . . of fat things full of marrow.'

From other passages of the Old Testament we know that the Israelites were thinking of fat mutton, or of mutton fat, when they spoke of 'the fat of the land'. The Bible tells us that mutton fat was considered the most delicious portion of any meat, and the tail and adjacent part the most exquisite morsel in the whole body. Biblical sheep were the Fat-Tailed variety, still found in

Syria and Palestine today.

The New Testament also has similar references, and we learn that beef fat was also held in high esteem: when the prodigal son returned home, his father didn't welcome him with an ordinary calf, he 'slew a fatted calf'. When Christianity spread northward, the Biblical phrase 'to live on the fat of the land' was readily understood across Europe.

Across the Mediterranean from the Holy lands, the Greeks too liked their meat fat and believed that their heroes preferred it so. You won't find a kind word about lean meat in the poems of Homer; but they are larded with praise of fat meats. Take the case of Agamemnon, who 'slew a fat bull of five years to most mighty Kronion' (*The Iliad*, Book II). In Book IX:

> 'Patroklos . . . cast down a great fleshing block in the firelight, and laid thereon a sheep's back, and a fat goat's, and a great hog's chine rich with fat.'

We find the same in the religious and profane classics of northern European peoples, preserved in the Scandinavian Eddas and Sagas. One Icelandic poem reads: 'There [in paradise] the feast will be set with clear wine, fat and marrow.'[28] That's bone marrow, by the way, not the vegetable kind.

The Norwegian explorer and scientist, Dr Carl Lumholtz (1851-1922), reported that the same was true in the southern hemisphere. When he was with the tropical forest-dwelling Aborigines of northern Australia, Lumholtz tells how they lived mainly on animal food, and never ate anything from a plant source if flesh was available. Lumholtz also noted that the Aborigines ate their meals like children will – the best things first. That was always meat, and the fatter the meat the better.

Sir Hubert Wilkins (1888-1958), Australia's most famous explorer, conducted a two-year expedition for the British Museum in northern Australia.[29] Wilkins confirmed Lumholtz's findings, and added certain observations along the same line: the Aborigines were cannibals, and the missionaries were having some difficulty breaking them of this habit. Wilkins noted that when a thin man died, all that was needed was a stern word from the missionaries, but when a fat man was buried, the missionaries had to stand watch over the grave. Even after some months the Aborigines would dig up fat corpses.

The earliest Indo-European scriptures – the Vedas Upanishads from around 2000 BC – also contain some very interesting observations regarding food. Meat, both wild and domestic, was highly prized despite the fact that agriculture was also practised. References to clashes between tribes in protecting the forest where wild game was available are many. And some of the old medical manuals were sophisticated enough to give us insights into the problem of tooth decay in the early days of agriculture. Royalty of the period, with abundant access to sweet and acidic fruit, had famous toothaches. Medicine men with narcotic pain killers were in high demand.

And it is no secret that the Lapps and Saami of northern Scandinavia, the peoples of Siberia, the Inuit of Greenland and the Canadian north, live entirely on animals and fish, even today. As do many peoples in the tropics: the Maasai, Samburu, Marsh Arabs, Berbers and so on. The Inuit today in their natural habitat do not eat vegetable matter. They live instead wholly on seal meat, caribou and fish; and they are among the healthiest people on earth. Only when they start eating the starch and sugar brought by Europeans does their health decline.

Similarly, up until the end of the 19th century, the North American Plains Indians lived almost exclusively on the meat of the buffalo, either fresh or made into pemmican (see Chapter Four).

There are others like them who live long, healthy lives on a diet which would cause today's western nutritionist to shudder. The Argentinean gauchos of European extraction are nearest to the Inuit as they too are almost exclusively meat eaters. After the gauchos, Australians ate more meat and fatter meat than any other people of European descent. Argentinean and Australian life-expectancy has traditionally been longer than in the industrialized nations of the northern hemisphere – although as Australians assume our way of eating, their health is declining.

The British also used to like fat. In English speech, fat food was called 'rich' food. This was the highest praise. In 19th-century Britain, the most esteemed part of the diet was fat. Describing good meat, Mrs Beeton said: 'Beef of the best quality is of a deep red colour; and when the animal has approached maturity, and has been well fed, the lean is intermixed with fat, giving it the mottled appearance which is so much esteemed.'[30] If meat didn't have much fat, that was a sign of poor quality. To my mind, it still is. And, of course, dietary recommendations shaped by Boyd Orr's work advised a high-fat diet until well into the second half of the 20th century.

Summary

This evidence tells us that fat has played a major part in the diet of peoples of every inhabited continent across the globe from the Arctic to the Equator and from primitive to civilized for the whole of our existence as a species.

But with the advent of 'healthy eating' all that seems to have been forgotten. Changing so radically from our accustomed high-fat diet to one unnaturally low in fats, not only have we lost the benefits from the fats we used to eat, we have replaced them with a source of energy for which we are genetically ill prepared – carbohydrates (starches and sugars). And carbohydrates, as we saw in earlier chapters, are very far from healthy.

The polyunsaturated margarines and cooking oils we now eat are also very different from those of our evolutionary background.

Are modern dietary studies out of context?

There is a tendency among most conventional scientists and nutritionists today to rely heavily, even exclusively, on modern clinical studies in discussing the health effects of modern diets without consideration of our history or our physiology. This is unfortunate and, quite frankly, narrow-minded, as it not only restricts study to unnatural and possibly irrelevant dietary matters, it ignores other important scientific information currently available from the fields of evolution, palaeontology and anthropology. Even though some formal dietary studies are ecological [epidemiological] and are based on the collection of large amounts of data, these studies require follow up clinical studies to confirm hypotheses suggested by the ecological data. So, one ends up right back with clinical studies.

Clinical dietary studies today are also always conducted with the assumption that current dietary recommendations are healthy. When participants eat a 'healthy' diet and then add or subtract foods to test the effects of such changes, there is an inevitable bias. In effect, the studies are conducted out of context. Food 'X' might be healthier than food 'Y' in an unhealthy background situation, but it is entirely possible that, in a more natural setting, food 'Y might be the healthier. It is also entirely possible that while a foodstuff may bring about an improvement to an otherwise unhealthy diet, what is really needed is a complete change of diet. We have to realize that if we don't get the context right, the answers we get may have no validity.

What we should be looking at is what we are genetically programmed to eat. When we look in that direction, we find that genetically we are still late palaeolithic, pre-agricultural hunter-gatherers.[31] Because of our genetic similarity, the diet of palaeolithic times is highly relevant today. Consequently, anthropological studies of real peoples in real situations, such as those conducted by Weston A. Price, Vilhjalmur Stefansson, and many others during the last two centuries are far more important and relevant to our understanding of foods and their effect on us than contrived studies conducted in unnatural surroundings with diets that are biased by 'politically correct' nutrition.

As a species, we have eaten animal fats and tropical oils – all of which have a significant amount of saturated fatty acids – for the whole of our existence. Until the 20th century, during which time coronary heart disease was extremely rare, such fats were the *only* ones we ate. With that background, you can understand, I trust, that the dietary advice we are given today is wholly alien to us. And that is why so many serious, chronic, degenerative diseases have skyrocketed since we embraced the nutritionists' recommendations.

Chapter Fourteen

The metabolic syndrome and the glycaemic index

Since we began to eat 'healthy' carbohydrate-rich foods, a constellation of serious degenerative diseases has emerged. Scientists have defined something they call the 'metabolic syndrome', or 'syndrome X'. This chapter looks at the causes and symptoms of the metabolic syndrome and of insulin resistance, and at the development and limited usefulness of the Glycaemic Index (GI).

> There is increasing evidence to indicate that the type of diet recommended in the USDA's food pyramid is discordant with the type of diet humans evolved with over eons of evolutionary experience.
>
> *Professor Loren Cordain*

Some scientists have recognized that as carbohydrate-rich foods increased in western populations, a wide range of diseases seemed to appear together. Professor Gerald Reaven at Stanford University School of Medicine coined the term, 'Syndrome X', to describe a constellation of markers that indicated a predisposition to these conditions. The definition and treatment are a matter of debate and there is no general agreement on a precise definition of the syndrome, but it encompasses *hypertriglyceridaemia* (high blood fats), *hyperinsulinaemia* (high blood insulin), *hyperglycaemia* (high blood glucose), *hypertension* (high blood pressure), low HDL, small, dense LDL molecules, and elevated uric acid. These factors appear to increase the risk of heart disease, obesity, type-2 diabetes and the other conditions discussed in this book. As there are two syndrome Xs, this one is now usually called the 'metabolic syndrome'. It is a condition that is caused entirely by incorrect diet.

And there is now considerable evidence that these are precisely the symptoms that respond to reduction in dietary carbohydrate and unnatural oils.

From glucose to fat as an energy source

The sole purpose of carbohydrate in the diet is to provide us with energy. With a low-carb diet, this can be replaced with protein from which glucose can also be made, or it can be replaced with fat. But the fuel that our body cells use for energy is neither of these; it is a chemical called *adenosine triphosphate* (ATP) which can be made from a variety of basic ingredients. A typical human cell may contain nearly one billion molecules of ATP at any one time, and those may be used and re-supplied every three minutes.[1] This huge demand for ATP, and our evolutionary history, result in our bodies needing several different pathways for its manufacture.

Oxygen and mitochondria

Living organisms have two means of producing the energy they need to live. The first is fermentation, a primitive process that doesn't require the presence of oxygen. This is the way that *anaerobic* (without oxygen) bacteria break down glucose to produce energy. Our body cells can use this method, but for most cells there is better method.

The second – *aerobic* (using oxygen) – method began after the Earth began to cool down and its atmosphere became rich in oxygen. After this event, a new type of cell – a *eukaryotic* cell – evolved to use it. Today all organisms more complex than bacteria use this property and all animal life requires oxygen to function. Oxygen's usefulness lies in its chemical ability to remove electrons from other molecules. When we breathe in, our lungs extract the oxygen in air and pass it to the bloodstream for transport through the body. In our bodies, it is our body cells' *mitochondria* – little power plants that produce most of the energy our bodies need – that use this oxygen. The process, called 'respiration', takes the basic fuel source and oxidizes it to produce ATP. The numbers of mitochondria in cells vary, but as much as half of a cell's volume can be mitochondria. The important point as far as diet is concerned is that mitochondria are primarily designed to use fats.

Which source of base material is best?

The question now, in this era of dietary plenty, is: which source of basic materials is healthiest? There are three possible choices our bodies can make:

- **Glucose**, which comes mainly from carbohydrates, although protein

can also be utilized by the body if necessary;
- **Fats,** both from the diet and from stored body fats;
- **Ketone bodies**, which are derived from the metabolism of fats.

These are explained elsewhere in this book.

Not all cells in our bodies use the same fuel

- Cells that can employ fatty acids are those that contain many mito-chondria: heart muscle cells, for example. These cells can make energy from fatty acids, glucose and ketone bodies, but given a choice, they much prefer to use fats.
- Cells that cannot use fats must use glucose and/or ketone bodies, and will shift to preferentially use more ketones which are derived from fats. These cells also contain some mitochondria.
- But we also have some cells that contain few or no mitochondria. Examples with few mitochondria are white blood cells, testes and inner parts of the kidneys; cells which contain no mitochondria are red blood cells, and cells that make up the retina, lens and cornea in the eyes. These are entirely dependent on glucose and must still be sustained by glucose.

This means that when we limit carb intake, the same energy sources must be used, but a greater amount of energy must be derived from fatty acids and ketones derived from fatty acids, and less energy from glucose.

Insulin resistance

We have about five litres of blood travelling around our bodies at any given moment. And in these five litres we have only about five grams of glucose (20 kilocalories) to supply the energy for all the body's processes that need it. Too much glucose is harmful to our health: it makes our blood thicker and more difficult for our hearts to pump round; it gets incorporated in red blood cells making their job of conveying oxygen around more difficult; and it also tends to clog up the tiny capillaries which can ultimately lead to the complete shut-off of blood to parts of the body, with disastrous results.

Our bodies recognize the dangers of too high a glucose level and have evolved a system to confine the level within safe limits. Glucose is metered in the brain by the hypothalamus. When blood sugar levels get too high, the hypothalamus stimulates the pancreas to produce insulin. Insulin helps the body utilize the blood sugar, glucose, by binding with receptors on cells like a key would fit into a lock. This stimulates glucose uptake from the blood into body tissues. Once the insulin key has unlocked the door, the glucose can pass from the blood into the cell. Inside the cell, glucose is either used for energy or stored for future use in the form of a starch called glycogen in liver or muscle cells, or as fat in the body's fat cells (*adipocytes*). This latter process is the way we put on weight.

But being overweight is only one consequence of eating a carbohydrate-rich diet. There comes a point where cells get fed up with continually taking in glucose they can't use. It then takes more and more insulin to achieve the same reduction of blood glucose. Insulin resistance occurs when the normal amount of insulin secreted by the pancreas is not able to unlock the doors to cells, and tissues have a diminished ability to respond to the action of insulin. To compensate for this and to maintain normal glucose levels, the pancreas secretes more insulin. Insulin-resistant persons normally have high blood insulin levels (*hyperinsulinaemia*). Many people who are insulin resistant produce large enough quantities of insulin to maintain near normal blood glucose levels. If you continue to eat the 'healthy' recommended diet for long enough, your pancreas will be continually producing insulin and, as well as having high levels of blood glucose, you will also have high levels of insulin. And that isn't healthy either. In about one-third of the people with insulin resistance, when the body cells resist or do not respond even to high levels of insulin, glucose builds up in the blood resulting in chronic high blood glucose levels. This is the progression to type-2 diabetes (see Chapter 20).

Sequence of events

You may be told that being overweight causes insulin resistance but insulin resistance has been shown to exist in a significant proportion of the normal weight population.[2] It really is a 'chicken and egg' situation because increases in body weight and insulin resistance occur at the same time. In simple lay terms the sequence of events is this:

- You eat small amounts of carbs and use the resultant glucose up. No problem.
- Then you start to eat a little more – 'five portions of fruit', et cetera.
- Now you start to get higher levels of glucose for which the body has no immediate use, and these trigger higher levels of insulin to reduce them.
- This starts the process of fat deposition and you start to put on weight.
- So you go on a low-fat, carb-based diet. This continues the cycle, increasing levels of glucose and insulin in the blood.
- Eventually, your body cells, both muscle cells and adipocytes, get to the point where they really don't want to know. Muscle cells refuse to take more glucose; fat cells release a hormone, *resistin*, and they too lose some of their insulin receptors. At this stage you are insulin resistant.

- As the excess glucose now has nowhere to go, this leads to uncontrolled increases in blood glucose and the onset of type-2 diabetes. And, of course, associated complications.

So, put bluntly, you become insulin resistant by the over-use of insulin.

There are three ways to decrease the blood glucose level and, thus, fat storage: you can exercise – but to accomplish the reduction in glucose needed you would need to run some three marathons a week, as a short run or aerobics class is quite useless; you can starve, which is what low-calorie dieting is; or you can keep your carbohydrate intake to less than 100 grams per day and make sure you aren't hungry by eating more fats. It's your choice.

But back to insulin resistance.

In 1976, Drs Kahn and Flier described two syndromes of severe insulin resistance, and research at the time began to focus on the newly described insulin receptor as the cause of insulin resistance.[3] Further studies, however, showed that the insulin receptor is usually not the cause of insulin resistance.[4]

Diseases of insulin resistance, particularly diabetes, occur with greater frequency in populations that have recently changed dietary habits from hunter-gatherer to western cereal grain-based regimes, compared with those having long histories of such diets. This is why obesity and diabetes are so much more common among peoples of African and Asian origin. It has been suggested that insulin resistance in hunter-gatherer populations may be an asset, as it would facilitate consumption of high-animal-based diets. The down-side of this is that when high-carbohydrate, grain-based diets replace traditional hunter-gatherer diets, insulin resistance becomes a liability and promotes type-2 diabetes.[5]

Several recent studies have measured insulin levels in various populations.[6] These noted higher insulin levels in people with high blood pressure and other vascular disease. For this reason, insulin resistance is now also considered a risk factor for heart disease. These studies have added a great deal of confusion to the field because many individuals with insulin resistance do not have diabetes, though that is where they are heading.

People who are insulin resistant typically have an imbalance in their blood fats (lipids): they have an increased level of *triglycerides*, a type of fat which increases the risk of heart attacks and decreases the level of HDL.

Insulin resistance is now a common condition. There is an enormous amount of evidence that the various facets of the metabolic syndrome are involved to a substantial degree in the cause and clinical course of the major diseases of western civilisation.[7] Emerging evidence suggests that the range and variety of diseases and abnormalities associated with insulin resistance may extend far beyond the common maladies that are frequently found in patients. Apart from those already mentioned above, such diverse abnormalities and illnesses as acne, myopia, reduced age of puberty and a trend for increased growth are all linked to insulin resistance by interactions with hormones.

What are the symptoms of insulin resistance?

There is only one easily recognized, outward physical sign of insulin resistance: that is the type of obesity known as 'apple shape' obesity – excess fat around the waist and upper half of the body. Other than that, a glucose tolerance test, during which insulin and blood glucose are measured, can help determine if someone is insulin resistant.

Insulin resistance is characterized by:

1. Resistance to insulin-mediated glucose uptake
2. Fat cells releasing a hormone *resistin* that causes insulin resistance
3. Glucose intolerance
4. High blood insulin levels
5. Increased levels of low-density lipoproteins (LDL)
6. Decreased high-density lipoprotein cholesterol (HDL)
7. High blood pressure
8. Excess weight and obesity, particularly around the waist and upper part of the body.

Why are so many people insulin resistant, and some more so than others?

Many millions of years ago, our primate ancestors ate a plant-based diet. The brain and reproductive tissues evolved a specific requirement for glucose as a source of fuel. But the Ice Ages which dominated the last two-and-a-half million years of human evolution changed all that. With little or no plant material around for much of the year, the diet must have changed to one much lower in carbohydrate and high in proteins and fat. This meant less glucose available directly from carbohydrates. Certain metabolic adaptations would have been necessary to accommodate the lower glucose intake. Studies in both humans and experimental animals indicate that the adaptation that took place is what we now call insulin resistance.

As the new low-carbohydrate, carnivorous diet would have disadvantaged reproduction in insulin-sensitive individuals, it would have positively selected for individuals with insulin resistance. Natural selection would therefore result in a high proportion of people with genetically-determined insulin resistance.

Many ethnic populations, such as the American Pima Indians, did not adopt agriculture until approximately 2,000 years ago.[8] Other populations, like the Inuit[9] and Australian Aborigines, continued to maintain a hunter-gatherer lifestyle until recently. Even the traditional carbohydrate foods of these and other ethnic populations have been shown to be low on the glycaemic index (see page 219), producing relatively small increases in blood glucose and insulin.[10]

The introduction of food processing which raised the quantity and quality of dietary carbohydrates, reversed the dietary evolution of the last two million years. That this is the cause of modern diseases appears to be the only theory that explains why the prevalence of these diseases is lower in those populations that developed agriculture earlier.[5]

The current high-glycaemic-index 'western' nutrition, with large amounts of sugar, high-fructose corn syrup, refined cereals, potatoes, and white rice, is, therefore, a new phenomenon which stresses the beta cells of the pancreas much more than previous carbohydrate-rich diets, and represents a chronic challenge. It is easy to imagine that this massive chronic stimulus may cause the beta cells of the pancreas to malfunction and overproduce, resulting in high blood insulin levels after meals, especially in genetically predisposed subjects.

Fats and insulin resistance

But there is another dietary change which also seems to play a part: we are eating the wrong types of dietary fat.

Fats are used in the construction of cell membranes. The traditional food oils, eaten until processed vegetable margarines began to come onto the market, produce cell membranes which allow for the easy transport of sugars and nutrients into cells. The new, engineered oils produce *stiff, sticky* cell membranes that restrict the normal absorption of sugars and nutrients.

Insulin resistance has puzzled many scientists. As the body has a vast store of *preadipocytes* to turn into fat cells to store excess glucose as fat, why do cells need to become resistant?

The reason is in the way that glucose enters body cells. Insulin is used to 'unlock' doorways in cell membranes that allow in the nutrients that cells need. These include glucose. To do this, insulin interacts with receptors on the cells' membranes. When insulin binds to a cell membrane receptor, it initiates a complex cascade of biochemical reactions inside the cell. These cause glucose transporters known as GLUT4 molecules to travel through the cell membrane. While in the membrane, they migrate to special areas of the membrane called *caveolae areas*.[11] There, by another series of biochemical reactions, they identify and hook up with glucose molecules and transport them into the interior of the cell by a process called *endocytosis*. Inside the cell, the glucose is then used as fuel by the mitochondria to produce energy to power the cells. In this way GLUT4 transporters lower glucose in the bloodstream by taking it out of the bloodstream into body cells.

Many of the molecules involved in these glucose- and insulin-mediated pathways are fatty acids. A healthy body cell membrane contains a variety of fatty acids including *cis*-type, omega-3 unsaturated fatty acids.[12] These make the membrane relatively fluid and slippery. When these *cis*-fatty acids are unavailable because of our diet, *trans*-fatty acids are substituted. These substitutions make the cellular membrane stiffer and stickier. And this, in turn, inhibits the transport of glucose from the bloodstream into cells.[13]

In this way, the mobility of the GLUT4 transporters is inhibited; the interior biochemistry of the cell is changed; glucose and other nutrients are not transported into cells; and insulin resistance develops.

Population studies support the hypotheses

Epidemiological studies support these hypotheses. High blood insulin levels are a common characteristic of several ethnic groups with a high prevalence of diabetes: Native Americans,[14] Mexican Americans[15] and Pacific Islanders.[16] The reason these populations develop high insulin levels after meals seems due to a limited genetic adaptation to high-carbohydrate, unnatural-fat nutrition, because they have been subjected to such a diet for a relatively short period of time.

When these populations, as well as Australian Aborigines,[17] urbanize and are exposed to high glycaemic-index nutrition, they develop hyper-insulinaemia and very high rates of type-2 diabetes. In Pima Indians, Nauruans and Mexican Americans, type-2 diabetes and obesity have reached epidemic proportions. Inuit, once thought to be resistant, are now also developing diabetes in increasing numbers.

Southern Europeans may have a relatively low incidence of diabetes compared with other populations because they were among the first to adopt agriculture, and their diet has been high in carbohydrate for several thousand years. Thus their beta cells have been exposed to high-carbohydrate nutrition for longer than any other group and are consequently better adapted to such a diet. But even amongst them, the dramatic increase in consumption of high-glycaemic-index food during the last quarter of the 20th century, in part as a result of low-fat, high-carbohydrate 'healthy' diets, together with a progressive increase in sugar consumption, which is now up to around 70 kilograms (150 lb) per head per year in most western countries,[18] has stressed the beta cells of even better adapted persons beyond limits. This explains the current epidemic of obesity and of the metabolic syndrome in western societies.

Genetic factors of obesity can also be explained by this hypothesis. The fact that obesity runs in families[19] may be due to a genetically determined higher susceptibility of the beta cells to foods that stimulate insulin production, or it may be because mothers teach their daughters to eat the same way that they do. Either way, these traits are passed on to the next generation.

The importance of insulin resistance is that it is accompanied by a progressive deterioration of the small capillaries supplying blood to many tissues, including the skeletal muscles that provide most of the body's insulin-mediated glucose disposal. These changes in the blood vessels and circulation may cause a decline in muscle blood flow and increase the severity of the metabolic disorder.[20]

Fruit and the metabolic syndrome

Fruit seems so natural and wholesome. How could it be anything but perfectly healthy? The problem arises in our ability to have fruit every day of the year, which is unnatural. Most fruit is all carbohydrate in the form of the fruit sugar, fructose, with only a trace of protein and no fat. In this sense, fruit is nothing more than nature's candy, and fructose has been shown to cause insulin resistance.

Scientists at the University of Florida noticed that the increase in obesity and the metabolic syndrome over the past two decades coincided with a marked increase in total fructose intake.[21] Unlike other sugars, the fruit sugar, fructose, causes serum uric acid levels to rise rapidly. This reduces levels of nitric oxide, which is a key mediator of insulin action, increasing blood flow to skeletal muscle and enhancing glucose uptake. As animals deficient in nitric oxide develop insulin resistance and other features of the metabolic syndrome, and changes in mean uric acid levels correlate with the increasing prevalence of metabolic syndrome in the US and developing countries, it seems likely that the epidemic of the metabolic syndrome is at least partly due to increased fructose intakes.

What should be done?

By 1999, it was quite clear that insulin resistance was caused primarily by dietary carbohydrates but the world's population being what it was, we could not do without them. It is also exacerbated by unnatural vegetable oils, endorsed by food manufacturers because they 'lowered cholesterol'. The medical profession and nutritionists had been telling people to eat lots of carbs, but diabetics in particular were having great difficulty eating what they were told and managing their disease successfully. Something had to be done. Professor Jennie Brand-Miller and colleagues at the Human Nutrition Unit, Sydney University, Australia, measured the amount that blood glucose rose after a wide range of meals containing carbohydrates in an attempt to come up with a way to differentiate carbs that might be 'bad' and carbs that might be 'good'. The resultant list, which now contains some 750 foods, is called the glycaemic index (GI). Today, 'GI diets' dominate popular diet book lists (my book, *Eat Fat, Get Thin!*, published in 2000, was one of the first). It's an idea that really 'took off' in the early 21st century as nutritionists and dieticians saw it as evidence supporting their advices. Unfortunately, it looks like it's making things worse.

GI blues

In March 2005, I was reading the latest copy of a popular woman's magazine which had a whole 10 pages devoted to the GI diet. It was billed on the cover as 'the healthiest low-carb plan around.' And it got it completely wrong!

The authors correctly stated that GI – the glycaemic index – is a measure of how much carbs raise blood glucose levels. But then, in lists of high-GI, medium-GI and low-GI foods they listed fatty foods as high-GI, when fats have a GI of zero – as low GI as you can get; 'omega-3 eggs' were listed as low-GI and 'eggs' as medium-GI, when both types of egg also have a GI of nothing. Low-fat cottage cheese was listed as low-GI, light cream cheese as medium-GI and full-fat cheese as high-GI when, yet again, their GIs are all nothing. In fact because fats, meat, fish, cheese and eggs don't raise blood glucose at all, they don't have a GI – or they have a GI of 0, depending how you look at it. And lastly, diet fizzy drinks were listed as both low-GI and high-GI depending on whether they contained caffeine – despite the fact that caffeine plays no part whatsoever in the GI tables. It looked like a classic case of ignorance trying to cash in on the latest fad.

The magazine article gave a recommended reading list of six recently published GI diet books. If the article was based on information from these books, then those authors had all got it wrong as well.

What is GI?

The glycaemic index (GI) was originally designed as an aid for diabetics. It is a measurement of the amount by which foods that contain carbohydrates raise glucose and, thus, insulin levels in the blood. It is a simple scale based on glucose being given the number 100 and other foods measured in relation to glucose. The higher the number against a food, the more it raises insulin levels.

GI has provided new insights into the relationship between foods and chronic disease. But it should not be taken in isolation. While observational studies suggest that diets with a high glycaemic *load*, that is a food's carbohydrate content as well as its GI, is an important consideration, GI and carb content are both independently associated with increased risk of type-2 diabetes and cardiovascular disease.[22]

The height to which glucose levels rise after meals plays a direct part in the process leading to metabolic syndrome diseases. Both high-GI food and large amounts of carbohydrates, and particularly a combination of the two, significantly increase the risk of obesity,[23] hypertension,[24] cardiovascular disease,[25] and type-2 diabetes,[26] and all their complications.

To compile this index, scientists fed 50 grams of glucose to their test subjects and measured how much this raised their subjects' blood glucose. That became their reference point; they labelled it 100. Then they tested their subjects with other foods and measured blood glucose response relative to the initial reference. If, for example, one of those foods raised their test subjects' blood glucose level to 50% of the reference, then it had a glycaemic index of 50, and so on. So far, so good.

But glucose is a bit too sweet for many people. Those being tested didn't like drinking 50 grams of the stuff and so, later, white bread was substituted. White bread has a GI of about 70 compared with glucose. The people doing the eating preferred this but unfortunately it generated another index in which bread was rated at 100.

There were now two GIs: one based on glucose = 100; the other based on white bread = 100. This started the confusion as both indexes came into general use – and many publications failed to say which one they were using.

How useful is GI?

In a nutshell, not very.

A GI of 70 or more is classed arbitrarily as 'high'; 56-69 is 'medium'; 55 and under is regarded as 'low.' But that doesn't tell us much because:

- One grain of sugar has a GI of 64; and a kilogram of sugar is also 64. So how much sugar can you eat? There is no way to tell. But as bread's GI is around 70, you can obviously eat more sugar than bread – or can you?

- In the example above I quoted the GI of sugar as 64 because that is the usually accepted figure. But 64 is really only the average of several tests which have been wildly different with the GI of sugar ranging between a low of 58,[27] and a high of 110.[28]

- We are frequently told to eat wholemeal bread in preference to white bread, with words like: 'Complex carbohydrates that come from whole grains, like whole-wheat flour, brown rice, whole oatmeal and other whole grains, take longer to process in the bloodstream, so insulin levels in the blood tend to be much steadier. These kinds of healthy carbohydrates are what the body needs for energy.' It's a myth. The difference between the GIs of white bread and wholemeal bread is only 2: white bread is 71 (on average); wholemeal is 69. A difference of only 2% is hardly earth-shattering. And those values are averages of several measurements in different countries. The only wholemeal bread made in the UK which is listed in the official International GI lists has a GI of 74 – which is higher than white bread!

- Then there is wholemeal flour. This is anything between 52 and 72 in Canada, 78 in Australia and is as high as 87 in Kenya. Again flour hasn't been tested in the UK so we don't know what the GI of wholemeal flour is here. But from the other data, it could be anything between low-GI and very high-GI.

- Another anomaly is that lower-GI doesn't necessarily mean lower glucose levels. A recent study compared blood glucose responses to either cornflakes or a bran cereal, both of which contained 50 grams of carbohydrate.[29] As the fibre-rich bran cereal had a GI less than half of the cornflakes' GI, you might expect the bran to have been beneficial. But you would be wrong: there was no significant difference between the two. What actually happened was that although the cornflakes raised glucose more initially, 20 minutes after the meal the bran had raised insulin levels almost twice as much as had the cornflakes. This removed glucose from the blood more quickly. Thus the lower GI of bran was not because it had a lower effect on raising glucose, but because it caused an earlier and bigger release of insulin. So, if you are insulin deficient, lower-GI foods such as bran might not be such a good idea.

- Another problem is that samples of the same food, made by the same manufacturer but in a different plant, can have widely differing GIs. Take Kellogg's All-Bran, for example: this has a GI of 30 in Australia, 38 in the US and 51 in Canada. I have no idea what the GI of Kellogg's All-Bran is in Britain – and neither has anyone else as it hasn't been tested.

- Then again the way a food is cooked or processed also makes a difference to its final GI, according to a trial conducted at the Department of Dietetics, Queen Elizabeth Hospital in Hong Kong.[30] So the GI of a food prepared by you may well have a different GI if it is prepared by someone else.

- And there are other strange anomalies. For example, you might think that foods containing sugar would have a higher GI than the same food made without sugar. But 'Banana cake, made with sugar' has a GI of 47, while 'Banana cake, made without sugar' is 55.

- And there is a last problem as far as diabetics are concerned. The GI of fructose (fruit sugar) is 22, very much lower than sucrose (table sugar) at 64. For this reason, diabetics are recommended to use fructose as a sweetener in preference to sugar. Yet fructose is far more damaging to a diabetic's health than sucrose (see Chapter 20). There is also no reason to suspect that it doesn't have a similarly harmful effect in non-diabetics.
- The same was true of other conditions. For example, carbohydrates are the major cause of cataracts. A study looking at the problem found that the glycaemic index of a carb was quite irrelevant. The only thing that mattered was the total amount of carbs eaten.[31]

Glycaemic load

Once the glycaemic index had been established, it was thought that it would make selecting carb-containing foods easier. As you can see from the above, it didn't. But even if the anomalies above didn't exist, there was still another problem because increase in blood glucose levels is dependent not just on GI, but also on the amount of the food you eat. And so yet another scale was created which tried to take this into consideration. That scale is the glycaemic load, or GL.

The GL table produces a scale by multiplying the amount of a food in grams by its GI. Although this gives a more realistic estimate of a food's glucose-raising potential, the GL is still of limited use, if only because it can be quite complicated to use. And it still takes no account of the effects of other ingredients a particular food is eaten with, such as thicker butter spread on bread.

That the GI and GL are of little use was shown in a five-year test at the University of South Carolina Arnold School of Public Health, the National Institute of Diabetes, Digestive, and Kidney Diseases, Bethesda, Maryland, US and the German Institute of Human Nutrition, Potsdam-Rehbruecke, Germany.[32] Starting in 1994-6 and following 1,255 adults for five years, the researchers evaluated GI and GL of foods eaten in relation to blood glucose levels measured before meals and two hours afterwards. When the dietary information was analysed researchers found no association between glycaemic index levels and blood sugar levels. They concluded that: 'present results call into question the utility of GI and GL to reflect glycaemic response to food adequately, when used in the context of usual diet.'

To sum up, the glycaemic index is a very weak tool which is over-simplified, over-hyped and over-sold. While it may have some limited use in a clinical setting, it is really of very little practical help to the general public; and the glycaemic load figures are far too complicated.

But even if these were more useful, they really have little practical value because what matters as far as your body is concerned is not the GI of a carbohydrate, but the total amount you eat: 100 grams of carbohydrate is 100 grams of carbohydrate whatever its GI may be.

Fruit may be as bad

Earlier I mentioned fructose, the type of sugar found in fruit. Because fructose does not stimulate insulin secretion from the pancreas, foods such as fruit that contain fructose produce smaller insulin surges than do glucose-containing carbohydrates such as bread and pasta. So, on the face of it, it looks as if fruit may be healthier. But there is a snag. Our bodies produce a hormone called *leptin* which controls weight gain: the more leptin produced, the less weight is put on. The production of leptin is regulated by insulin responses to meals. Thus fructose, by reducing insulin, also reduces circulating leptin concentrations. Dr Sharon Elliot and colleagues at the universities of California and Pennsylvania, say that the combined effects of insulin and lowered leptin in individuals who eat diets that are high in dietary fructose could increase the likelihood of weight gain and associated conditions.[33] In addition, they point out that fructose, compared with glucose, is preferentially metabolized to fat in the liver. In animal studies fructose consumption has been shown to induce insulin resistance, impair glucose tolerance and raise blood levels of insulin and triglycerides, as well as raising blood pressure, although the figures are not so clear in humans. Nevertheless, there are human data that suggest that eating more fructose may be detrimental in terms of increased fat storage and body weight and the illnesses associated with the metabolic syndrome.

We mustn't forget insulin

By now it must be obvious that both the glycaemic index and glycaemic load tables have little value. But there is one more aspect to factor in. Because insulin promotes the storage of excess blood glucose as body fat, a diet with a low GI or GL should make weight loss faster and easier – in theory at least. Nutritionists believed that a greater glycaemic response meant a greater insulin response. However, while the glucose/insulin link holds true with some foods, it doesn't hold true for all of them: protein reduces glucose – but increases insulin.

Over the years, there has been considerable uncertainty about the effects of protein intake on blood glucose levels. Recently a well-conducted study of people with type-2 diabetes showed clearly that protein improves overall glucose control.[34] In this study, protein intake was doubled while carbs were reduced proportionally. It produced impressive results by reducing 24-hour blood glucose by a massive 38%. There were also significant decreases in glycosylated haemoglobin and triglycerides after just five weeks. This was all to the good. However, the addition of 50 grams of beef had one drawback: it caused a prompt three-fold rise in blood insulin levels. Insulin was still at a maximum after two-and-a-half hours, and it did not return to a fasting value until more than six hours after the meal.

Two studies considered the effect of adding fats to carbs.[35,36] In both, the result was a significant flattening of the glucose curves after meals but insulin responses were not so affected. In one study insulin rose slightly and in the other it stayed about the same. This is an important finding because adding fat to any carb lowers the overall GI.

These findings change the picture fundamentally. GI and GL are concerned only with measuring the amount of *glucose* which carbohydrate-containing foods put in the bloodstream, not insulin. But raised insulin levels are just as important as they contribute both to weight gain and to the inability to lose weight, as well as other serious conditions such as heart disease and cancer. Blood glucose may be important, but it is only half the problem.

The other half is the amount that blood insulin is raised. And so, the scientists at the University of Sydney who gave us the GI later developed an 'Insulin Score' based on 38 common foods.[37] For this, subjects were given meals which all contained the same amount of energy (240 kilo-calories). You will note some very unexpected results in Table 14.1.

These figures are not to be confused with the Glycaemic Index. Dr Susanne Holt, the lead researcher, said: 'In the insulin index study, we measured glycemic scores and insulin scores for 1000 kJ portions of foods. They are not GI values. In a healthy person that has fasted for more than 10-12 hours overnight, cheese and steak can cause a small rise in blood glucose in the second hour of our two-hour test periods due to gluconeogenesis.'

This complication is because of the ways that different foods affect both blood glucose and insulin levels.

Limitations

Unfortunately, while a great deal of work has been done on carbs, proteins and fats separately, as well as on carbs-plus-proteins and carbs-plus-fats, no-one yet seems to have thought of studying the effects of fats-plus-proteins despite this combination forming the bulk of our traditional diets and being the basis of the way of eating which is recommended here.

Table 14.1: Insulin and glucose scores of common foods (Compiled from data in Reference 37.)

Food	Insulin Score	Glucose Score
Peanuts	12	20
Beef (very lean)	21	51
Fish	28	59
All-Bran*	32	40
Oranges	39	60
Porridge (Oatmeal)*	40	60
Muesli*	40	60
Eggs (poached)	42	31
White pasta	46	40
Apples	50	59
Potato chips (McCain's prefried)	52	61
Cheese (mature cheddar)	55	45
Cake	56	82
Grain [rye] bread	60	56
Popcorn	62	54
Lentils	62	58
Yogurt (strawberry fruit)	62	115
Doughnuts	63	74
Special K*	66	70
Honeysmacks*	67	60
Brown pasta	68	40
Ice cream	70	89
Sustain*	71	66
French fries	71	74
Croissants	74	79
Grapes	74	82
Cookies	74	92
Cornflakes*	75	76
Bananas	79	81
Mars bar	79	112
Whole-meal bread	97	96
White bread (REFERENCE)	**100**	**100**
Brown rice	104	62
White rice	110	79
Baked beans	114	120
Crackers	118	87
Jellybeans	118	160
Potatoes	141	121

*All cereals were served with semi-skimmed milk

However, as fats alone do not have any appreciable effect on either blood glucose or insulin levels, and as protein has no effect on glucose and only a modest effect on insulin, I am confident that the protein-plus-fat combination we have evolved to eat will turn out to be entirely harmless.

And finally

It is very important that we do not see insulin resistance as the problem *per se*. This approach has led conventional medicine to attempt to suppress the resistance with drugs. But that is a mistaken approach. Insulin resistance is a symptom of the problem, not its cause. The best answer – the healthiest answer – is to take away the need for the cells to put up resistance in the first place by giving insulin less of a job to do. As *all* dietary carbohydrate, whether it is bread, pasta, breakfast cereals, sugar or fruit, and whatever its GI, ultimately reaches the blood as glucose, the best way to reduce the need for increased insulin is to reduce dietary carbohydrate. And we also need to reduce our intakes of the cheap, engineered dietary oils and margarines. These two elements of our modern diet are a recipe for disaster.

It is essential that we never lose sight of this fact for it is a fundamental fact upon which all else depends.

Chapter Fifteen

Unhealthy dogma means unhealthy food

Food manufacturers have jumped on the lucrative 'healthy' bandwagon, making foods that are increasingly lacking in important nutrients, such as the many 'low-fat' dairy products. These have been shown to increase the risk of some cancers. 'Improving' foods has not only made them more hazardous for us to eat; it has also compromised the health of food animals.

Nothing is more terrible than ignorance in action.

Johann Wolfgang von Goethe

Public health recommendations over the last 30 years have been to reduce fat intake to as little as 30% of calories to lower the incidence of coronary artery disease. In the face of such recommendations, the agricultural industry started shifting food composition toward lower proportions of saturated fatty acids and then of all fats in general. Fat contents of foods have been replaced principally with carbohydrates. The unfounded, but still entrenched, belief in a connection between dietary fat and heart disease has spawned an enormous processed-foods industry based on those beliefs. It doesn't help consumers that such foods are cheap to produce and profits are greater for their manufacturers.

Fifty years ago, grocery stores stocked only about 200 items, most of which were grown, produced and processed within a few miles of the store. Today, a supermarket can carry 50,000 food items or more, most of which are highly processed and refined, and are transported thousands of miles. Europeans and Asians are increasingly following trends in the US where the population spend over 90% of their food budget on such commodities. These foods contain high levels of refined sugars, high fructose corn syrup, white flour, refined polyunsaturated oils and trans-fatty acids, as well as *excitotoxins* such as monosodium glutamate and aspartame. We are warned against junk foods; these are the real junk-foods. The logical result of these nutrient-depleted foods is that we in industrialised nations now have to consume much more of them to sat-isfy our bodies' basic nutritional requirements. And that, in turn, means that we are forced to consume a greater number of calories in order to satisfy our bodies' basic nutrient needs. The Americans have an apt name for this diet: they call it 'SAD-CRAP': Standard American Diet – Cereals Refined And Processed.

Recently, such a diet has become recognized as contributing to the ris-ing numbers of cases of metabolic syndrome and obesity. Blood fat and cholesterol patterns which lead to the formation of atherosclerosis and heart attacks are also recognized as being caused by such changes. De-spite these findings, the same recommendations are still promoted vigorously. As a consequence, the world is moving toward more unitary dietary recommendations; and agricultural practices have been adopted to decrease saturated fatty acids to as low as agriculturally possible. This has changed the composition of animals we eat; what used to be fresh, wholesome food, no longer is.

There are many examples. Meat is so lean today that Mrs Beeton would regard it as being of very poor quality indeed. I normally buy meat straight from the farmer, but recently I tried some beef that I bought from a supermarket; it was dry, tasteless and tough. That doesn't make it unhealthy, necessarily, but other changes brought about by 'healthy' dogma do. For example, in the UK, there are some truly depraved, overly-draconian laws forbidding pigs (even organic-raised pigs) from being fed on anything but denatured pellets made from low-grade grains and soy. Of course, even the most brain-dead specialist in wildlife is aware that pigs in the wild, such as wild boar, are true omnivores, which feed on thousands of varied, different things such as earthworms, insects, dead animal carcasses, grains, plants, leaves and grasses, roots, fruits and flowers, and even the bark off trees. But it seems the agricultural authori-ties are deathly afraid of more natural diets for domesticated animals. The pig diet, high in omega-6-rich seed oils, changes the composition of their body fat so that it is less saturated; cattle, which should eat grass, are also fed a 'healthy' diet based on grains and soya. These are posi-tively dangerous.

There are so many such examples that I'll give just one in detail: milk.

Milk: from healthy to harmful

In the 1930s, Sir John Boyd-Orr recommended that we drink more milk to improve our health. He was talking of full-cream milk, of course; skimmed milk was fed to pigs. Since then, milk and dairy products have been heavily promoted for their health-giving properties. But, although cow's milk is still enthusiastically promoted as providing adults with 'essential' vitamins and minerals, after the Committee on the Medical Aspects of Food Policy (COMA) introduced us to 'healthy eating' in 1984, the dogma about fat causing heart disease has transformed milk from healthy, fresh whole milk to a product which is utterly denuded of most of its essential nutrients – the most important of which is the fat in its cream.

How milk is processed

When I was young, milk was collected from a local farm, cooled and then delivered to households by horse and cart. At the door, the milk was measured out with a half-pint ladle. The cream floated naturally to the top of the churn; the delivery man had to stir it to make sure that everyone benefited. My mother had young children, so our milkman was careful to ensure that we got a bit more cream by ladling the creamier milk off the top. The milk was no older than the previous evening's milking. We were healthy in those days.

Today, raw milk is collected from farms daily for delivery to dairies by tanker for storage and processing. To make it 'safe for drinking' the raw milk is then heat-treated at a variety of temperatures to kill any bacteria and increase its shelf life. The lowest temperature is used in *pasteurization*; the highest is UHT (ultra-high temperature). Most milk in UK is pasteurized.

After pasteurization, milk to be sold as liquid milk is separated from its cream in a centrifuge. With the cream separated from it in this way, we are left with skimmed milk. The cream is then blended back into the skimmed milk in measured amounts to produce whole milk – 3.3% fat although whole milk would be over 4% naturally – and semi-skimmed milk (1.7% fat). Excess cream is sold as cream or used to make butter.

During the blending process the fat globules in the cream are usually broken up and dispersed throughout the liquid milk to give the finished product a more uniform texture. This process, called *homogenization*, also prevents the cream from rising to the top. Whole milk in supermarkets is homogenized.

After the entire process has been completed, the milk is heat treated yet again and then cooled before being packaged and sold to retailers.

Other than the addition of the cream back into the milk, every step in this process makes the finished product less and less healthy for consumers.

Skimmed milk and prostate cancer

Around 1975, scientists noted an apparent strong correlation between milk intake and deaths from prostate cancer. Since then, there have been growing suspicions of a causal link between the two which two studies published in 2007 appeared to confirm. The first was the CLUE II study which involved nearly 4,000 men in Washington County, Maryland.[1] This study found that men who consumed five or more servings a week of dairy foods were more likely to suffer from prostate cancer than those who ate a serving of one or less. The second study involved over 29,000 Finnish men taking part in the Alpha-tocopherol, Beta-Carotene Cancer Prevention Study (ATBC Study) which ran for 17 years.[2] This also found that the more dairy consumed, the higher the risk of cancer.

The first thing to be blamed for such an association, as it always seems to be, was the saturated fat in the cream.[3] But mounting evidence suggests that the truth is quite different because *full-cream* milk does *not* increase prostate cancer risk, only skimmed milk does. It was the stripping of fat from the milk – to make it 'healthier' – which actually increased the risk.

The 11-year Physicians' Health Study, involving over 20,000 men, found that *all* the increased risk of prostate cancer associated with dairy intake was attributable entirely to skimmed milk.[4]

In 2005, the first National Health and Nutrition Examination Epidemiologic Follow-up Study (NHEFS), involving more than 3,600 men and 10 years of follow-up, arrived at a similar conclusion. They found that men with the highest intakes of dairy were more than twice as likely to develop prostate cancer as men with the lowest intakes. But the risk was higher *only* with low-fat milk – not with whole milk or any other dairy. In fact, whole milk actually seemed to protect against prostate cancer.[5] Similar results were found in other countries. A Norwegian study of more than 25,000 men,[6] and an analysis of milk drinking and diet in 41 countries,[7] found that prostate-cancer death rates were associated *only* with the drinking of low-fat or skimmed milk.

Low-fat milk increases women's cancers too

Women are presently encouraged to consume dairy products as a source of calcium to prevent osteoporosis. And, because of the fat scare and the fact that all the calcium is in the milk, not in the cream, the milk women are advised to drink is skimmed.

Studies have looked at dairy intake and rates of ovarian cancer and found an increased ovarian cancer risk with milk drinking. But just as in the case with prostate cancer in men, there is no increased risk with whole milk; only with low-fat milk and skimmed milk. The Iowa

Women's Health Study investigated the association of epithelial ovarian cancer with dietary ingredients in a study of 29,083 postmenopausal women.[8] They found that skimmed milk, but not whole milk, was significantly associated with an increased incidence of ovarian cancer.

An even larger study published six years later confirmed the Iowa results. In the Brigham and Women's Hospital Nurses' Health Study, in which more than 80,000 women participated, those who consumed just one or more servings of skimmed or low-fat milk products per day had a 32% higher risk of any type of ovarian cancer, and a 69% higher risk of the most widespread form – serous ovarian cancer – compared with women who had three or fewer servings monthly. Yet again, whole milk did not increase the risk.[9]

Why more cancers with low-fat dairy?

But why should low-fat milk have such an effect? One theory is that removing the fat from milk strips it of certain nutritional components that are vital to health. Fat is found in milk for a reason. It contains vitamins A and D, both of which are necessary for the uptake and use of the calcium and protein elements in milk. Without these vitamins, milk protein and calcium are more difficult to absorb and can even become toxic to the body.

Calcium, particularly in large amounts, seems to have a specific adverse effect: it suppresses the formation of *calcitrol*, the hormonal form of vitamin D. Because calcitrol has anti-cancer effects on prostate cells, scientists have postulated that a reduction in the amount of calcitrol in the circulation could increase the risk of prostate cancer.[10]

The CLA connection

Another possible explanation is that stripping the fat from milk also removes other important anti-cancer components such as conjugated linoleic acid (CLA). CLA was identified as a component of milk and dairy products over 20 years ago, and studies have shown it to be a powerful anti-cancer agent. In the laboratory, when human breast and colon cancer cells were bathed in high-CLA milk fat from cows raised on pastureland, the number of cancer cells was reduced by between 58% and 90%.[11,12]

And women who consumed four or more servings a day of high-fat dairy foods were half as likely to develop colorectal cancer as women who ate less than one serving a day. Low-fat dairy had no such protective effect.[13]

Low-fat milk and infertility

Low-fat milk doesn't just increase the risk of cancers. A study conducted at Harvard University Medical School monitored 18,555 American women aged 24 to 42 between 1991 and 1999 and found that the risk of *anovulatory infertility*, a form of infertility due to lack of egg release from the ovaries, was also increased in women who drank low-fat milks.[14] The women studied, who were pregnant or trying to become pregnant, did not have a history of infertility. Nevertheless, the study showed that women who ate two or more servings of low-fat dairy products such as skimmed milk or low-fat yoghurt a day, increased their risk of anovulatory infertility by more than 85% compared with women who ate less than one serving of low-fat dairy a week. And women who ate one or more servings per week of skimmed or low-fat milk had a significantly higher risk of anovulatory infertility compared with those who ate less than one serving per week. Adding a serving of whole milk per day reduced the risk of infertility by more than 50%.

The authors of this study suggested that there might be a substance, vital for healthy ovaries, that requires the presence of fat for it to be properly absorbed. This would explain the lower risk of infertility from high-fat dairy foods. It might also explain the results of the prostate cancer studies.

Low-fat milk and acne

As well as more serious conditions, scientists have also noted a connection between low-fat milk and acne. Data, again from the Nurses' Health Study, also showed that women who frequently consumed low-fat dairy such as reduced-fat milk, skimmed milk and cottage cheese as teenagers were more likely to suffer from severe acne at the time.[15]

As skimmed milk showed the strongest association, the researchers speculate that changes in milk composition during the fat-extraction process could aggravate acne. Altering the balance of the hormones in milk, for example, might be an explanation.

Low-fat milk and coronary heart disease

Ironically, coronary heart disease, the very disease against which all the work was aimed, also seems to be made worse by low-fat milk. In 1998, William Grant published a review of all the epidemiological evidence concerning diet and heart disease, and also carried out his own researches, examining heart disease and dietary habits in 32 countries.[16] He found a correlation between low-fat milk, as well as calcium and milk sugars, with heart disease in both sexes.

The review points out that non-fat milk, which contains substantial amounts of dairy protein, is very low in B vitamins. The body's attempts to metabolize all this protein in the absence of B vitamins contributes to the build-up of *homocysteine*, a known marker for heart disease.

Processed milk increases asthma and allergies

Considering the negative health effects linked to low-fat milk, should we all go back to drinking full-cream milk?

Sadly, it's not that simple. While whole milk is a healthier option than low-fat or skimmed milk, it is still subjected to processing that destroys some of its nutrients. Pasteurization typically involves heating milk for 30 seconds at 63°C, which destroys beneficial bacteria as well as all the important enzymes that aid milk digestion. Essential vitamins and proteins are also damaged or destroyed.

Homogenization, a process that passes milk through a fine filter, causes other problems by reducing the size of fat globules by a factor of 10 or more. When protein molecules become attached to these smaller fat globules, this piggy-backing allows the proteins to bypass digestion in the stomach, which may lead to their incomplete digestion and to their causing allergic reactions.

Allergies, asthma, hay fever and 'atopic sensitization' skin problems, which have been increasing apace in the last quarter century in children drinking shop-bought, processed milk, are rare in children drinking raw, whole, unprocessed 'farm milk'.[17] Researchers found that the timing of exposure to raw milk was critical. Those children exposed during the first year of life showed the greatest protective effect.

But we aren't allowed to buy raw milk. We're told this is because there is a risk of brucellosis. However, studies have shown that the risk of brucellosis is very low in small herds, increasing as herd size goes up.[18] The animals' nutrition almost certainly plays a part. Small herds on fertile pasture or appropriate feed, plus regular testing, clean barns and milking machines, stainless steel tanks and refrigerated trucks all make it entirely possible to get healthy, clean, certified raw milk to the public. Tests are widely available to detect brucellosis in cattle, goats and sheep, and modern science makes brucellosis-free herds easily possible.

It is the alternative – pasteurized, processed milk from large herds crowded into barns and given hormones and antibiotics – which causes allergy problems for an increasing number of people. How many customers does the dairy industry have to lose to putative 'milk allergies' before it sees the light and opts for quality rather than quantity – for thousands of prosperous small dairies delivering directly to the consumer as in my youth, rather than small numbers of huge herds, confined to barns and producing dirty milk that must have its vital elements destroyed by pasteurization and processing?

Rather than avoiding all dairy products altogether, a more sensible option would be to consume milk in its most natural state: raw, unprocessed and full-fat – if you can find it. I can't, so I drink only cream.

But what about calcium?

Milk is touted as a great natural source of calcium, and we are told to eat plenty of calcium to prevent osteoporosis, or thinning of the bones. Sadly, eating available dairy products can increase the rate at which calcium is lost from the body and so hasten calcium deficiency diseases.

A recent meta-analysis found that a low intake of milk was not associated with any important increase in fracture risk in either men or women.[19]

Bureaucracy costs

Organ meats are hugely nutritious, but supermarkets don't sell them. Looking to source organs from local farmers, I recently discovered how difficult it can be to get them, as many who used to sell them now refuse to sell any organ-meats. Some told me that the main reason was that they had to pay a minimum of £100 per hour to both EU and UK vets in order for their meats to pass inspection, so it wasn't worth their while having the organ-meats inspected as well. Others said that the vets insisted on throwing away the organ meats. Either way, it's a criminal waste.

Conclusion

Milk should be, and could be, an important food source. It would be a shame to give it up. But current dietary dogma and processing methods have ruined it as a healthy food at this time.

Low-fat milk, milk processing and the other dietary modifications to make animal fats 'healthier' are crimes against nature.

But they aren't the only ones. There are many examples – from genetic modification to hormone controls, to developing animals such as Belgian Blue cattle that have double muscles and are too big to be born other than by Caesarian section – which are unnatural, dangerous and expensive. And with only one aim: to produce leaner meat.

In our arrogant tinkering with natural foods to make them 'healthier', we have inadvertently created a health crisis not only for ourselves but for our farm animals.

How long will it be before we learn that whenever we attempt to 'improve' on Nature, we end up paying for it with our health?

And when food is already so expensive, why overload the system with exorbitant costs?

Chapter Sixteen

So what should we eat?

We have seen that the healthiest diet for us is one low in carbohydrates, but there is little agreement on what we should eat instead. This chapter looks at proteins, fats and carbohydrates, their uses in the body and the amounts we need to each. The overwhelming conclusion is we should eat real, fresh food and avoid what is processed and artificial.

> The modern diet is not providing enough vitamins. Malnourishment is going to make you more vulnerable to illnesses and less able to cope with them.
>
> *Dr Mike Stroud*

Our hunter-gatherer ancestors lived from one animal hunt, fishing expedition or egg-gathering foray to the next. There must have been times when food was scarce. That was our forebears' lives probably since the human species began. To tide them over these periods of famine, their bodies evolved the ability to store energy as fat. Indeed, for as long as *Homo sapiens* has existed, our bodies' *preferred* source of fuel has been its stored fat. That is precisely why our bodies store it in that way. If a low-carb, high-fat diet were really as unhealthy for humans as we are constantly told, we simply wouldn't be here now.

Those conditions existed for us 'civilized' people until only a relatively few generations ago, and many modern hunter-gatherers still live that way today. There really hasn't been enough time for any significant genetic changes in our digestive, biochemical and endocrine systems. Genetically, we are basically the same now as our distant ancestors. In other words, we should eat today what our palaeolithic ancestors of 10,000 years ago ate.

As it happens, that is precisely what research published since 1999 shows: that a return to a diet based on foods of animal origin, cutting down on concentrated and processed carbohydrate foods such as bread and sugars, prevents many chronic degenerative diseases if they have not yet occurred, and cures them – or at least minimizes the symptoms – if they have.

At the moment, we are not eating real food. We are mostly eating food-like substances. We need to change our diets. This seems to be difficult for many people who have become addicted to their sugar-laden, non-food diets. But it only takes about three weeks to acquire new eating habits and then these people will find that the nutrient-depleted junk food they have been used to really doesn't satisfy them any longer.

But what should we change to? The evidence from both early epidemiological research and the clinical studies over recent decades strongly suggests that we should eat more naturally and reduce our reliance on carbohydrate-rich foods. We should eat a low-carb diet.

The problem now seems to be how to determine what exactly constitutes a 'low-carb diet' as such diets are variously called not just 'low-carb', but also 'high-protein', or 'high-fat', or 'ketogenic', depending on which macronutrient the restricted carbs are replaced with and at what level carb intake is set. There doesn't seem to be any agreement on what a low-carbohydrate diet really should be as different scientists and diet book authors have different ideas, and 'healthy eating' propaganda still colours many writers' recommendations.

What foods perform which functions?

Our bodies need a variety of nutrients. These are nearly all obtained from the food we eat. Our food contains *macronutrients*: carbohydrates, proteins and fats, which we eat in large amounts; and *micronutrients*: vitamins, minerals and trace elements of which we need very little. For the sake of brevity, I propose not to discuss the micronutrients as they are all included automatically if we eat the correct diet. It is in the macronutrients – particularly the foods that supply us with energy – that things are muddled. To understand what you need to eat to be healthy, you first need some knowledge of what happens to food and how your body metabolizes and regulates energy.

Proteins

Proteins are essential to the body, providing the material from which body cells are made and repaired. Proteins are composed of chains of amino acids. There are hundreds of these in Nature. Our bodies use around 20, which can be arranged in an almost infinite number of ways. Amino acids are usually split into two groups: *essential* and *non-essential*. The essential amino acids are those that the body cannot make for itself and which must be present in food. There are eight of them (infants need a ninth, *histidine*). If a protein contains the eight essential amino acids, in the correct proportions, it is called a *complete protein*; if it does not, it is said to be an *incomplete protein*.

Complete proteins are found in meat, fish, eggs and dairy products. Animal proteins, which are complete, have a high biological value for man. As we are part of the animal kingdom and composed of similar material to other animals, we can use animal proteins with the minimum of waste.

Sources of *incomplete proteins* are cereals, nuts, seeds and legumes. Proportions of amino acids in any one of these types of vegetable foods differ markedly from those we need. For example, maize is deficient in *tryptophan*, wheat is low in *lysine* and legumes are low in *methionine*, and soya is deficient in both *methionine* and *tryptophan*, all of which are essential. Proteins from these vegetable sources are said to be 'of low biological value'. It is necessary, therefore, to combine several vegetable protein sources, fairly accurately, to ensure that the body receives the right amino acid mixture.

In practical terms, it is not too difficult to combine vegetables to meet our bodies' protein requirements. In these circumstances, the real advantage of meat over the vegetables is their associated nutrients: the B vitamins, vitamin D, iron, calcium and the more complex fatty acids.

Our bodies need proteins continually but cannot store them in any quantity. Therefore, you should eat proteins regularly on a daily basis, and at the same meal, in quantities proportional to your size. But they must be complete proteins: if only one of the essential amino acids is missing, the cell rebuilding process will abort.

Daily protein requirements

Our bodies need complete proteins every day, and with proteins come calories. The average woman needing about one gram of protein per kilogram lean body weight per day could realistically get her protein needs from the foods in Table 16.1.

Although I do not advocate a low-fat diet, I have deliberately made this

Table 16.1: Example of minimum daily protein requirements

	Protein (grams)	kilocalories
125 grams lean meat	30	250
1 egg	6	75
50 grams cottage cheese	12	185
570 ml (1 pint) semi-skimmed milk	19	275
2 slices bread	7	120
Total	**74**	**905**

example typical of the kinds of foods we are advised to eat to illustrate realistically the extent of the danger of malnutrition if you cut calories too much.

Our bodies also need a certain amount of fat: if only to supply the essential fatty acids needed for proper brain function, you must eat at least 15 grams of these per day. That adds another 135 kilocalories to the daily energy intake, but as the foods in the examples all contain these fats, the calories they contain have already been included. It should be clear, therefore, that a 1,000-kilocalorie diet must be composed almost exclusively of foods which are very high in protein and fats if you are to take in the minimum amount of these nutrients to be healthy. Thus the 1,000-kilocalorie, low-fat, carbohydrate-based diets conventionally used for weight loss are invariably dangerously deficient in protein.

The importance of fat

The science of nutrition is complex and, even today, little is known about the vital part that fat plays in our health and well-being. Nutrients interact: a deficiency of one can have a profound effect on the metabolism of others. Today, a lack of dietary fat probably causes a wider range of abnormalities than deficiencies of any other single nutrient.

Fat does much more than provide energy. Restriction of dietary fat causes a range of problems including dry skin and eczema, damage to ovaries in females, infertility in males, kidney damage, and weight gain through water retention in the body. When there is little or no fat in the gut, there is nothing to stimulate the production of bile, the gall-bladder is not emptied and the bile is held in reserve. This can lead to the formation of gallstones. If a fat-free diet is continued for a long time, the gall bladder – an important part of a healthy digestive system – may atrophy.

Malabsorption of the fat-soluble vitamins A, D, E and K has consequences for yet more nutrients. If vitamin D and fat are not present in the intestine, for example, calcium is not absorbed. For a woman, whose chance of suffering from osteoporosis and osteomalacia is high, this is an important consideration. Dieters are usually told to drink skimmed milk. This has the advantage, they are told, that it contains more calcium than full-cream milk. This is true, but skimmed milk does not contain fat. As a consequence, while some 50% of the calcium is absorbed from full-cream milk, only around 25% is absorbed from semi-skimmed milk and 5% from skimmed milk. This small absorption of calcium is reduced still further if the skimmed milk is eaten with a bran-laden breakfast cereal. Calcium-enriched milk sold in supermarkets may seem worth the extra expense but as it is invariably calcium-enriched *skimmed* milk, all that extra calcium is simply excreted without doing any good at all.

Fat is best

All body cells require a continuous supply of various fatty acids. If insufficient are supplied from food, the body tries to make them from sugar. This causes blood sugar levels to fall, you feel very hungry and eat more, generally of the wrong things – and compromise your health.

Fat also has a satiety value: it takes longer to digest and stops you feeling hungry. Eat a hundred calories less fat at a meal and you will probably feel hungry so quickly that you will eat three times as many calories – in the form of sugary or starchy foods, because they are convenient.

It seems that the gut's nutrient-measuring system works so well with fat that it is difficult, if not impossible, to eat too much of it. Try and you will make yourself sick. But for the same reason, eating fat stops you eating too much in total. If your body needs 10 grams of fat, your appetite will not be satisfied until you have consumed those 10 grams. If you eat those 10 grams as 25 grams (1 oz) of cheddar cheese, you will take in about 125 kilocalories. If you eat them as wholemeal bread thinly spread with a very low-fat spread, you will need to eat eight slices – a total of about 200 kilocalories.

One big difficulty these days is that, after two decades of 'healthy eating' dogma, it isn't easy to buy healthy food. This means that getting sufficient fats into your diet is made more difficult than it was half a century ago. So:

- Buy the fattest meat you can find.
- Don't cut the fat off meat.
- Don't remove the skin from chicken, duck, goose or turkey.
- Use duck or goose in preference to chicken and turkey. They are fatter birds, taste better and provide lots of lovely, tasty fat for cooking.
- Use full-cream milk in preference to semi-skimmed or skimmed, or better still, as most of the milk is water, why not just buy cream? It's cheaper in the long run. And you can get the calcium and protein better from cheese. The best cheeses for calcium are parmesan, Swiss cheeses and cheddar.
- Eat your fruit with cream if you wish, put butter rather than gravy on cooked vegetables, and an olive oil dressing on salads.

Carbohydrates

Many people think of carbohydrates as things like bread and sugar – and they are right. But they also think that fruit and vegetables are not 'carbohydrates', they are 'fruit and vegetables'. I even know of nutritionists and dieticians who make this distinction (which demonstrates their level of ignorance). The fact is that *all* sugars and *all* starches, from whatever source, are carbohydrates; fructose, the sugar found in fruit, is as much a carbohydrate as table sugar; the sugars and starches in vegetables are also carbohydrates. Dietary fibre is another carbohydrate, although, as we cannot digest and absorb it, we tend to ignore this. We shouldn't; soluble dietary fibre can provide up to 2 kilocalories per gram.[1] The point is that, as far as your body is concerned, *all* digestible carbohydrate ultimately puts glucose into your blood stream. Significantly, carbohydrates are found almost exclusively in foods of plant origin – the very foods that form the basis of a 'healthy' diet.

So, in a nutshell, there are three macronutrients in our diet: fats, proteins and carbohydrates. Only two are essential and carbohydrate isn't one of them. This means that the message from official bodies is telling us to base our meals on the only foods we have no biological need for, and the only foods that our bodies are not best equipped to deal with. Is it any wonder that things have gone very wrong since we started to eat this way?

Get the ratios right

When you have selected the right foods and stocked your larder, all you need to know is in what proportion these foods should be eaten. It is determined, like everything else, by our evolution and our body's needs. For the best of health and for weight maintenance, research has shown that you should try for the following ratios of the three macronutrients:

Carbs – 10-15% of calories
Protein – 15-25% of calories
Fat – 60-70% of calories

Carbs. The ideal figure for carbohydrates has been found to be about 50-75 grams, equivalent to about five slices of bread. That amount avoids the problems that can be caused by a too drastic change of energy source from glucose to fats during the few weeks after the changeover period. It is also the maximum amount that a diabetic should eat. After your body has become accustomed to not getting the level of carbs it had previously, you can eat more or less as you like.

Protein and fat. To maintain your body and provide it with the amino acids it needs for cell regeneration and repair, plus the enzymes that control almost all body functions, your consumption should be at least 1 to 1.5 grams of good quality protein for each kilogram of lean body weight per day. This means in practice eating some 50 to 100 grams of protein per day. You then need to ingest sufficient fat for its essential role in body maintenance as well as to supply the energy your body needs to function. As only some 23% of lean meat is protein, whereas fat is practically all fat, this equates to eating meat which is about four to six parts lean to one part fat.

Not everyone eats the same amount: a smaller person will eat less than a tall one and a child will eat a different amount from an adult. Thus laying down specific total amounts can be misleading. Taking all this into consideration, let me put it another way, and suggest that you eat as much as will satisfy you while aiming for the ratios above.

You should also include organ meats like liver and kidneys as these contain the widest range of the vitamins, minerals and trace elements your body needs. Liver, in particular, is a superb food. In 1951, Dr Benjamin Ershoff divided laboratory rats into three groups. The first ate a basic diet, fortified with 11 vitamins. The second ate the same diet, with vitamin B complex added. The third ate the original diet but, instead of vitamin B complex, received 10% of their rations as powdered liver.[2] After several weeks, the animals were placed one by one into a drum of cold water from which they could not climb out. They had to swim or sink. Rats in the first two groups managed to swim for just over 13 minutes on average before succumbing; however, the liver group managed much, much longer: three swam for 63, 83 and 87 minutes and the other nine rats were still swimming vigorously when the test ended two hours later. Something in the liver had prevented them becoming exhausted.

Eat fresh food

Apart from the ratios between the three macronutrients found in traditional healthy diets, there is one other consideration: the food we eat must be fresh. Whether food is of animal or plant origin, all healthy traditional diets are composed of fresh or frozen, but unprocessed, materials. This is most important. It's when we start fiddling with things in our inept way that the problems start.

Animal foods should also be cooked as little as possible.

Important characteristics of traditional diets

There are lots of differences between the dietary patterns that Dr Weston Price found in traditional, healthy peoples and ours.

- All primitive and traditional diets have a high food-enzyme content from raw dairy products, meat and fish; raw honey; tropical fruits; cold-pressed oils; wine and unpasteurized beer; and naturally preserved, lacto-fermented vegetables such as sauerkraut, fruits, beverages, meats and condiments.
- Seeds, grains and nuts are soaked, sprouted, fermented or naturally leavened in order to neutralize the naturally-occurring anti-nutrients in these foods: the phytic acid, enzyme inhibitors, tannins, and other toxins.

- All healthy populations also consume some sort of animal protein and fat: meat of land animals; fish and other seafood; water and land fowl; eggs; raw milk and milk products; reptiles; and insects. Unfortunately, our pasteurized milk is not as healthy as raw milk, and homogenized milk is even less healthy.
- Traditional diets also contain 10 times more vitamin A and vitamin D than the western diet of today. These vitamins are found only in animal fats – butter, lard, egg yolks, fish oils and foods with fat-rich cellular membranes like liver and other organ meats, fish eggs and shell fish.
- There are also at least four times the minerals and water soluble vitamins – vitamin C and B complex – than there are in our western diet.

The first thing to recognize is that over 90% of the products sold from supermarket shelves are unsuitable for human consumption. They are composed of denatured foods: newly created foods from which many of the nutrients necessary to sustain healthy life have been reduced or removed altogether. That is why 'ready meals', which are becoming increasingly common, are now seen as an important cause of malnutrition in the UK and other industrialized countries. Indeed, as the *Daily Mail* has pointed out, our reliance on a junk diet is causing famine symptoms of the kind found in poverty-stricken African countries.[3] The number of hospital patients with malnutrition rose by 44% in five years to almost 4,000 cases in 2006. But experts have warned this is the tip of the iceberg, estimating that up to 6%, or some 3.6 million people, are malnourished in the UK. Dr Alistair McKinlay, an Aberdeen University gastroenterologist and a leading authority on malnutrition, estimated that the problem remained unidentified in 75% of cases.[3] Treatment of malnutrition costs the NHS over £7.3 billion a year. Dr Mike Stroud of Southampton University said: 'The modern diet is not providing enough vitamins. Malnourishment is going to make you more vulnerable to illnesses and less able to cope with them.'[3]

Foods to avoid are: refined sugars, fructose or corn syrup; white flour; canned foods; pasteurized, homogenized, skimmed or low-fat milk; refined or hydrogenated vegetable oils; protein powders; artificial vitamins or additives such as colourings and preservatives. And, of course, processed foods that contain them.

Artificial and damaged foods

There is a great difference between the fresh foods you buy in butchers' and greengrocers' shops or farmers' markets and the pre-packaged, processed foods supermarkets are full of. With that in mind, there is a simple rule of thumb: when buying from supermarkets, buy from around the perimeter: meat, fish, poultry, eggs, dairy, and other fresh produce. The only things edible in the aisles are olive oil, spices and condiments.

It's no secret that processed foods are liberally laced with colourings and preservatives so that foods look more attractive and have a longer shelf life. They are also usually made from the cheapest materials available. But there are three other factors to consider.

One is that heating, which is the most used form of processing, tends to denature many foods. If you buy these foods and cook them at home, that means heating them twice, which harms them even more. Secondly, real flavours tend to be more expensive than artificial ones because the real flavours have to come from real food. So, if, for example, you buy strawberries and some plain full-cream yogurt and mix them, you have an entirely natural and healthy dessert. On the other hand, if you buy strawberry-flavoured yogurt, you are likely to end up with a very different product. In Britain it seems impossible to discover what these flavourings are made of – it's a trade secret. Fortunately for us, the US's Freedom of Information Act allows access to the information. Via that route we find that the widely used strawberry flavour, MF129, is made up of:

Grams

17.25	Corps Praline (trade name of Firmench and Co)
362.05	alcohol, 95%; agitate and heat until dissolved, then add:
530.00	propylene glycol
10.00	glacial acetic acid
30.25	aldehyde C_{16}
22.75	benzyl acetate
11.25	vanillin
4.25	methyl cinnamate
2.25	methyl anthranilate
0.20	methyl heptine carbonate
2.25	methyl salicylate
2.25	ionine, beta
2.25	aldehyde C_{14}
2.25	diacetyl
0.75	anethol

The third difference is that even fresh foods may not be fresh: pre-packed supermarket foods are far more likely to have been picked fresh several days or even weeks before you take them off the supermarket shelves. This inevitably means that some of their original nutrients will have deteriorated or been lost. This can have unfortunate effects. Take strokes, for example. Doctors have known for a long time that potassium, widely available in fresh fruits and vegetables, can be a major player in reducing blood pressure. Their advice has been to eat more potassium-rich foods, while reducing sodium intake. But while a cup of fresh peas may contain several hundred milligrams of potassium and almost no sodium at all, if you use canned peas instead, you may get exactly the opposite.

Additives in processed foods

Even though additives must be listed on product labels, those labels may still tell only half the story, because enzymes, catalysts and other chemicals used in the *processing* of the product do *not* have to be listed. These are used to tenderize meat, to clean milk contaminated with antibiotics, to make modified starches, and in the baking and brewing industries. Some enzymes are made from plant or animal tissue but most are made by microbial fermentation. Naturally the industry says that they are safe but there have been a number of reports of allergic reactions to them in industry workers.

In all, the EU sanctions 395 additives: 71 thickeners and emulsifiers, 64 colours, 54 preservatives, 54 antioxidants, 54 anti-caking agents and acidity regulators, 52 miscellaneous, 27 additional chemicals and 19 flavour enhancers. New studies have emerged over the past few years that call into question whether such food additives, approved for use in Europe, are as harmless as regulators and the food industry suggest.

Dr Vyvyan Howard, a toxicologist and Professor of Bio-imaging at the University of Ulster, questions the practice of approving additives for use that have been tested alone. In 2005, he led a Liverpool University study that showed that, when combined, some additives in crisps and fizzy drinks had seven times the effect they had singly. Professor Howard avoids eating anything with E-numbers because: 'No one really knows what this chemical cocktail could be doing, particularly in the early stages of development. This cocktail is far too complex.'

Sodium benzoate, mitochondria and cancer

On 27 May 2007 *The Independent on Sunday* reported a new health scare over evidence that soft drinks might cause serious cell damage.[4]

Professor Peter Piper, a Professor of Molecular Biology and Biotechnology, and an expert in ageing at Sheffield University, had been working for 10 years on sodium benzoate (E211), a preservative used for decades by the £74bn global carbonated drinks industry. The danger lay, he thought, in the ability of sodium benzoate to switch off vital parts of DNA in the mitochondria to the point that it might totally inactivate them.

Professor Piper's findings could have serious consequences for the hundreds of millions of people worldwide who consume fizzy drinks. They should also intensify the controversy about food additives, which have been linked to hyperactivity in children.

Professor Piper stated that: 'The mitochondria consume oxygen to give you energy and if you damage them – as happens in a number of diseased states – then the cell starts to malfunction very seriously. And there is a whole array of diseases that are now being tied to damage to this DNA – Parkinson's and quite a lot of neuro-degenerative diseases, but above all the whole process of ageing.'

This is bad enough, but it is potentially even more serious. Cells' mitochondria play a central role in the process of programmed cell death which goes on throughout our lives, a process called *apoptosis*. In cancer cells, this process is switched off. By shutting down their mitochondria, cancer cells prevent this cell death and do not die when they should. This effectively makes cancer cells immortal and confers resistance to radiation and chemotherapeutic agents. It is why cancers are so dangerous and so difficult to kill.

Drinks manufacturers point out that sodium benzoate has been approved for use by the UK's Food Standards Agency (FSA). The FSA said additives had been approved by the European Commission. A review of sodium benzoate by the World Health Organization in 2000 also concluded that it was safe, although it noted that the available science supporting its safety was 'limited'. Professor Piper, whose work has been funded by a government research council, said tests conducted by the US Food and Drug Administration were out of date.

Sodium benzoate is found in a very wide range of foods and drinks: bakery products, pizzas, marinated herring, yoghurt, cheese, low-fat spreads, blue cheese dressing, fruit products, jams, figs, nut paste, pickles and sauces (e.g. horseradish), salad cream, sweets, candied peel, glace fruit, gelatin, desserts, toppings and fillings, milk shake syrups and fruit ice-cream. Also beer, cider, wine, perry, ginger ale, ginger beer, shandy, tonic water, barley water, fruit squashes, colas (other than Coca Cola), glucose drinks, cherryade, sparkling canned drinks, soda stream concentrates and frozen fruit juices.

It is also frequently used to preserve other additives, flavourings, colourings, anti-foaming agents and artificial sweeteners. In this case it is not necessarily declared on the packaging.

Potential harm from food containers

Another aspect of pre-packaged food is possible harmful effects from the packaging itself. For example, bisphenol A is a chemical that forms the building blocks of polycarbonate plastics, used for food containers. Small amounts leach from the plastics and are now commonly found in people's bodies. Research at Case Western Reserve University, Cleveland, Ohio, has found that environmental doses of bisphenol A may cause abnormalities in egg cells in future generations.[5] This means the toxic effects may not be seen until fetuses become adults and try to have their own children. A similar effect was seen in the 1970s when the prescribed drug DES was given to pregnant women. Their daughters grew up to have ovary damage.

For these reasons, processed, pre-packaged foods – and these are by far the majority on supermarket shelves – should be regarded as a last resort. Organic foods, if you can afford the extra premium, should be healthier. But please understand that conventionally grown vegetables which are fresh are healthier than organic ones that are older and wilted.

Foods from a supermarket's delicatessen counter and the fresh vegetables and fruits may be healthy but, being picked unripe and after travelling for several days before you get them, those that are imported have significantly lower levels of essential micronutrients. Wherever possible, it is usually healthier to buy direct from the food producers: farmers and horticulturists, farmers' markets and specialist shops that sell local produce. You will also help 'save the planet' by buying this way: it's an enormous waste of fuel to transport food around the world.

Artificial sweeteners

There is some debate about the role of the artificial sweeteners. Saccharine and aspartame contain no calories so, on the face of it, they appear to be an ideal substitute for those people with a sweet tooth who cannot give up sugar. But there are three problems with them.

A great deal has been said in the media about artificial sweeteners hampering weight loss. The suggestion is that the pancreas may start to produce insulin for the purpose of reducing blood glucose levels before those levels are elevated, merely in response to a sweet stimulus. Thus eating a calorie-free sweetener can trigger the production of insulin. And as no glucose enters the bloodstream, glucose already there is removed for storage, blood levels are driven down and the result is hunger and increased food intake. Whether or not this first point is correct, the second problem is that eating foods containing artificial or any other kind of sweeteners maintains the taste for over-sweetened foods. It is much better to reduce your use of *all* sweeteners gradually until the natural sweetness of foods tastes right for you. The sweetness to aim for is the natural sweetness found in non-tropical fruit such as strawberries.

The third problem is that artificial sweeteners aren't safe to eat.

Aspartame, for example, although widely used, has the capacity to harm. Scientists in South Africa assessed the potential effects of aspartame's components, phenylalanine and aspartic acid, methanol, and its break-down product formaldehyde, on the brain.[6] In their review, the authors detail the ability of aspartame to disrupt the chemistry of the brain, including its potential to lower levels of key brain chemicals such as serotonin (which may adversely influence all sorts of things including mood, behaviour, sleep and appetite). They also note that it additionally has the potential to disrupt amino acid metabolism, nerve function and hormonal balance in the body. They go on to suggest that aspartame's ability to destroy nerve cells may mimic or even cause Alzheimer's disease.

Genetic modification and plant toxins

Plants are chemical factories. Unlike animals, which have the luxury of teeth and claws and legs to help them get out of a tight spot, plants spend their lives in one place. But they have no desire to be eaten, so Nature gave them an elaborate set of physical and chemical defences to ward off unwanted predators. Thorns are obvious, but under the surface there are thousands of chemicals which are noxious or toxic to bacteria, fungi, insects, herbivores and, crucially, to us humans.

For this reason most plant species in the world are not edible. Over millennia, the process of domestication gradually reduced the levels of these toxins so that today the plant foods we eat are far less toxic than their wild relatives. But that has resulted in our modern food plants being much more susceptible to disease. To help them, some plants are being genetically modified to make them more resistant to disease again. But that raises the question: could genetic engineering inadvertently elevate the levels of natural plant toxins or make them produce new ones which may be harmful to us? The answer seems to be: we don't know.

Genetic modification of animals

In June 2007 came another very worrying report in *Chemistry & Indus-try,* the magazine of the Society of Chemical Industry.[7] It reported that scientists in New Zealand had identified cows with a natural ability to produce skimmed milk and said that their genes could be used to breed herds of animals producing only skimmed milk. The cows were discov-ered when biotech company, ViaLactia, screened the range of milk compositions across the entire herd of 4 million New Zealand cattle. They had also identified a single cow, named Marge, capable of produc-ing milk with the unique characteristics required to make a butter that is spreadable straight from the fridge. Why? Kept properly, *not* in a fridge, butter is always spreadable. The only way to make butter 'spread straight from the fridge' is for it to contain a high proportion of cancer-causing vegetable oils.

New Zealand dairy firm, Fonterra, has already made milk products from Marge's milk.

These cows could completely revolutionize the dairy industry. Ed Komorowski, technical director at Dairy UK, says that the New Zealand approach could be used to breed cows that still produce full-fat milk but with only the 'good fats'. The problem with this is that the so-called 'good fats' depend entirely on who decides which fats are good. At present, many of the fats regarded as 'good' are not.

In the UK, only 25% of milk sold is full fat. Komorowski says that: 'In future if whole milk can be made to contain unsaturated fats – which are good for you – then it might mean that people change back to whole milk products. The big thing about dairy products is taste, so this would be a way of giving the benefits of taste without the disadvantage of saturated fats.' (What disadvantage?) He continues: 'If you can genetically produce milk without fat then that may turn out to be a very good solution to what might later be a big disposal issue.' Producing skimmed and semi-skimmed milk means there is a lot of fat left over.

This sort of meddling is worrying. Naturally produced food is healthy. It is only when 'experts' start to 'make it healthier' with their dogmatic ideas of what constitutes a healthy diet that it becomes dangerous to eat, as we saw in the last chapter. These days, perhaps as little as 1% or 2% of all foods found in supermarkets is actually suitable for human consumption. This new development is certain to reduce the availability of healthy food even further. And has any thought been given to calves which need the energy in cream to grow healthily?

I don't doubt that 'skimmed milk straight from the cow' will increase the burden of chronic degenerative disease in the countries which adopt this unnatural product. But it will make a lot of money for the company that produces it.

No special low-carb foods are needed

In 2001 I joined a low-carb forum on the internet in an attempt to help people starting one of the several different, recently published, low-carb dietary regimes aimed at weight loss. The most frequently asked question by far was: 'Where can I buy low-carb foods?' The answer, of course, is: at any supermarket, butcher's shop, dairy, grocer's or farmers' market, because it is not necessary to buy anything 'special' with this way of eating.

No pills, nutritional supplements, meal replacements or special diet foods are required. In fact, I believe they defeat the whole object of this way of life, which should be as natural as possible. You should not look for low-carb bars, which contain processed protein powders, artificial sweeteners and harmful trans-fats. You don't need protein smoothies – made with cheap ingredients because the manufacturer is looking for a hefty profit. These are not healthy – what is the point in swapping one disease for another?

All the foods you need, to provide your body with all the nutrients it needs, and you with the pleasure you need, can be found in the meat, cheese, dairy, fish, and fruit and vegetable departments of any supermarket. You may have to add butter and other fats as meat today is bred so lean as to be tough and tasteless. But even this is far healthier than the junk that is beginning to be sold for the 'low-carb' market. And don't be afraid of eggs: they have a nearly perfect balance of nutrients and are excellent dietary sources of protein, vitamins, minerals and trace elements.

Think about *why* you eat

Sugar, sweets and other highly processed, carbohydrate-rich modern foods – and they include 'healthy', whole grain foods – are all highly addictive. People who have been eating such foods for many years, will probably find that any dietary health programme based on animal foods is difficult to accept.

Apart from the addictive nature of carbs, the relative importance we assign to food in our lives influences our decisions about health. Some people 'live to eat'; others 'eat to live'. In other words, some people eat food as an entertainment, primarily a source of pleasure, while some regard food merely as fuel. Most of us fall somewhere in between these extremes, but these days, the majority are encouraged by advertising and propaganda towards the 'live to eat' category, which biases them towards pleasurable but harmful foods. However, the more you regard food primarily as a fuel, the easier it is to gravitate to foods that promote health. This does not mean that eating simple foods cannot also be pleasurable. In fact, the tastes of plain foods – fresh raw milk (if you can get it), unadorned meat or fish, raw or lightly cooked with butter and seasoned, perhaps, with spices, and fermented vegetables – become more pronounced and satisfying when you avoid sugars and starchy sweets, breads and other prepared foods; try steak tartare, for example. The instant and temporary allure of sweets and starches is far less satisfying than the satiating taste of animal fats. And strawberries are more enjoyable when their delicate taste isn't obliterated with sugar.

Summary

To sum up, we should endeavour as much as is possible to choose our nutrition from those foods that were eaten by the many traditional populations known to be supremely healthy, before the introduction of the 'displacing foods of modern commerce', as Dr Weston Price put it. This means getting back to basics and eating as simply as possible. Avoid processed foods like the plague, as they are a primary source of many problems. Eat fresh, ideally locally grown, foods and prepare them yourself in your home with tender loving care.

Relax while eating

There is one last point: it concerns not what you eat, but how you eat it. There is a great deal of work demonstrating that, when people are put under stress, they show massive spikes in levels of blood sugar, insulin, triglycerides and certain clotting factors. The important times to avoid stress are while eating and immediately after eating. This is when the damage otherwise is done.

A Japanese experiment found that if people were laughing when they ate then they had much lower spikes of blood sugar;[8] people given mental tests to do had much higher blood sugar levels. The most powerful direct evidence came from a study showing that people who were given stress hormones, mimicking the levels found after various types of physical assault, e.g. car crash or surgical operation, were found to have spikes of blood sugar and insulin four times as high as 'normal'.[9] The Mediterranean Diet may be so healthy merely because those who eat it don't eat working lunches, but relax and have siestas after meals.

Conclusion

The message really is quite simple. Eat real, fresh, unprocessed food, mainly from animal sources, and relax while you eat.

Chapter Seventeen

Why low-carb diets must be high-fat, not high-protein

If we reduce the carbohydrate content of our diet, we either go hungry or replace the carbs lost with something else. There is currently a great deal of debate about what this should be. This chapter explains why carbs should be replaced with fats – and which fats they should be.

Fat is the most valuable food known to Man.

Professor John Yudkin

We now have seen why we should eat a diet that is low in carbohydrates. But a plethora of books published in the last decade have been low-carb, high-protein, or low-carb, high-fat, or low-carb, high-'good' fats, or all sorts of other mixtures. In other words, the real confusion lies in what we should replace the carbohydrates with: should it be protein or fats? And if fats, what sort of fats?

This chapter, I hope, will answer the question and put any doubts out of your mind. In a nutshell, carbs should be replaced with fats, and those fats should be mainly from animal sources.

Which source of base material is best?
The question now, in this era of dietary plenty, is: which energy source is healthiest? There are three possible choices:

- **glucose**, which comes mainly from carbohydrates, although protein can also be utilized as a source of glucose by the body if necessary;
- **fats,** both from the diet and from stored body fats;
- **ketones** which are derived from the metabolism of fats.

Not all cells in our bodies use the same fuel.

- Cells that can employ fatty acids are those that contain many mito-chondria: heart muscle cells, for example. These cells can make energy from fatty acids, glucose, and ketones, but given a choice, they much prefer to use fats.
- Cells that cannot use fats must use glucose and/or ketones, and will shift preferentially to use ketones. These cells also contain mitochon-dria.
- But we also have some cells that contain few or no mitochondria. Ex-amples of cells containing few mitochondria are white blood cells, testes and inner parts of the kidneys; and cells which contain no mito-chondria are red blood cells, and the cells of the retina, lens and cornea in the eyes. These are entirely dependent on glucose and must still be sustained by glucose.

This means that when we limit carb intake, the same energy sources can be used, but a greater amount of energy must be derived from fatty acids and the ketones, and less from glucose.

Sources of glucose

To understand how a low-carb diet works, we need to look at how we eat. This process is one of eating, digestion, hunger and eating again. During our evolution, we must have experienced periods when food was in short supply and we starved. It is a pattern our bodies are adapted to, and they have developed mechanisms to cope with such circumstances.

Firstly, the human body must contain adequate levels of energy to sus-tain the essential body parts that rely on glucose. The brain and central nervous system may be a particular case as, although the brain represents only a small percentage of body weight, it uses up to as much as a quar-ter of all the resting energy used by the body.[1] Fortunately the brain can also use ketones. During fasting in humans, and when we are short of food, blood glucose levels are maintained by the breakdown of glycogen in liver and muscle and by the production of glucose primarily from the breakdown of muscle proteins in a process called *gluconeogenesis*, which literally means 'glucose new birth'.[2]

But it is not sensible to use lean muscle tissue in this way: it weakens us. We should get the glucose our bodies need from what we eat. Some of that will come from carbs, the rest from dietary proteins. Our bodies need a constant supply of protein to sustain a healthy structure. This re-quires a fairly minimal amount of protein: about 1 to 1.5 grams per kilogram of lean body weight per day is all that is necessary to preserve muscle mass.[3] Any protein over and above this amount can be used as a source of glucose.

Dietary proteins are converted to glucose with less than 50%

efficiency, so approximately 100 grams of protein can produce less than 50 grams of glucose via gluconeogenesis.[4] Body fats are stored as triglycerides, molecules that contain three fatty acids combined with glycerol. During prolonged fasting, the fatty acids are used directly as a fuel; the glycerol is stripped off, but not wasted. Two molecules of glycerol released in this way combine to form one molecule of glucose and may account for nearly 20% of gluconeogenesis.[5]

The case for getting energy from fat and ketones

When most people think of eating a low-carb diet, they tend to think of it as being a high-protein one. They should not. All traditional carnivorous diets, whether eaten by animals or humans, are more fat than protein in calorie terms, with a ratio of about 75-80% of calories from fat and 20-25% of calories from protein. This works out at one-and-a-half grams of fat for each gram of protein. Or to put it in another, more usable, way: it is a piece of meat that is between about three and six parts lean to one part fat; or a full fat cheese.

Similarly, the main fuel produced by a modern low-carb diet should also be fatty acids derived from dietary fat and body fat. In practice, free fatty acids are higher in the bloodstream on a low-carb diet compared with a conventional diet.[6,7]

Fats also produce an important secondary fuel called 'ketone bodies.' Ketones were first discovered in the urine of diabetic patients in the mid-19th century; for almost 50 years thereafter, they were thought to be abnormal and undesirable by-products of incomplete fat oxidation. In the early 20th century, however, they were recognized as an important substitute for glucose. During prolonged periods of starvation, fatty acids are made from the breakdown of stored triglycerides in body fat.[8] On a low-carb diet, the fatty acids are derived from dietary fat and from body fat. Free fatty acids are converted to ketones by the liver. They then provide energy to all cells with mitochondria. Within a cell, ketones are used to generate ATP (see Glossary). And where glucose needs the intervention of bacteria, ketones can be used directly.

Reduction of carbohydrate intake stimulates the synthesis of ketones from body fat.[9] This is one reason why reducing carbs is important. Another is that reducing carbohydrate and protein intake also leads to a lower insulin level in the blood. This, in turn, reduces the risks associated with insulin resistance and the metabolic syndrome.

Ketone formation, and a shift to using more fatty acids, also reduces the body's overall need for glucose. Even during high energy demand from exercise, a low-carb diet has what are called 'glucoprotective' effects: ketosis arising from a low-carb diet is capable of accommodating a wide range of metabolic demands to sustain body functions and health while not using, and thus sparing, protein from lean muscle tissue.[10] As the levels of ketones in the blood reaches about 8 mmol/L, some 75% of our bodies' glucose requirement can be replaced by ketones. This significantly reduces the conversion of tissue protein into glucose, resulting in a substantial reduction of muscle loss. This means that more glucose is available for glucose-dependent tissues.

As it happens, ketones are also the preferred energy source for highly active tissues such as the heart muscle.[11]

The case against getting energy from protein

We know, then, that dietary fats can produce all the energy the body needs, either directly as fatty acids or as ketones. But, as there is still some debate about the health implications of using fats, you might say: 'why not play safe and eat more protein?'

There is one simple reason why not. While the body can use protein as an energy source in an emergency, it is not at all healthy to use this method in the long term.

All carbs are made up of just three elements: carbon, hydrogen and oxygen; fats are also made of the same three elements. Proteins, however, also contain nitrogen and other elements. When proteins are used to provide energy, these must be disposed of in some way. This is not only wasteful, it can put a strain on the body, particularly on the liver and kidneys.

Protein also requires fat-soluble vitamin A for its metabolism. A diet too high in protein without adequate fat rapidly depletes vitamin A stores, leading to serious consequences such as heart arrhythmias, kidney problems, auto-immune disease and thyroid disorders. High-protein diets also cause what the medical profession calls a 'negative calcium balance', where more calcium is lost from the body than is taken in. This condition leads to bone loss and nervous system disorders.

Many human cultures survive on a purely animal product diet, but *only* if it is high in fat.[12,13] All primitive peoples avoid protein-rich, low-fat diets. They can lead to nausea in as little as three days, the development of starvation symptoms in seven to 10 days, severe debilitation in 12 days and possibly death in just a few weeks. A high-fat diet, with moderate protein, on the other hand, is completely healthy for a lifetime.

Perhaps one of the best documented studies is that of the Arctic explorer, Vilhjalmur Stefansson, and a colleague.[14] They ate an all animal meat diet for more than a year to see whether such a diet could be healthy. Everything was fine until they were asked to eat only lean meat.

Dr McClelland, the lead scientist, wrote:

> 'At our request [Stefansson] began eating lean meat only, although he had previously noted, in the North, that very lean meat sometimes produced digestive disturbances. On the third day nausea and diarrhea developed. When fat meat was added to the diet, a full recovery was made in two days.'

This was during a hospital-based clinical study; but Stefansson had already lived for 11 years on an all-meat diet with the Canadian Inuit. He and his team suffered no ill effects whatsoever – except when only lean meat was available. When they could not get fat, they found that they developed what they called 'rabbit hunger' within a couple of days and had to find fat to cure the condition. So don't be tempted to add protein powders to raise the protein content without adding calories at the same time. The result could well be a low-carb, low-fat diet which is unnaturally high in protein. And that is probably the unhealthiest diet of all.

If you think about it, nature stores excess energy in our bodies as fat, not as protein. It makes much more sense, therefore, to use what we are designed by nature to use: fat.

Traditional fats are better for weight loss

No matter how careful you are, it is always possible to eat too much and put a bit of weight on. However, scientists at the Faculty of Medicine, University of Geneva in Switzerland, found that the more saturated a fat was, the less likely it was to increase a person's weight. Similarly, they found that fats which were composed of shorter chain fatty acids were also less fattening.[15]

This is because the unsaturated fats are fully digested to give more calories per gram than saturated fats. As animal fats are a mixture of both saturated and unsaturated fatty acids, a more accurate figure for fats from warm-blooded animals such as cattle and sheep is not the usually accepted 9 kilocalories per gram, but about 7.5 kilocalories per gram.

For this reason, fish oils are the most fattening; vegetable oils and olive oil come next; less likely to be fattening are animal fats; and least fattening of all is cocoa butter. This is another good reason to eat traditional animal fats and tropical oils, and avoid modern processed vegetable oils.

Potential of benefit for other diseases

The traditional Inuit diet is practically a no-carb diet. On this diet, blood cholesterol levels have been found to be very high as have free fatty acids, but – and this in much more important – triglycerides were low.[16,17] Traditional Inuit are of great interest to research scientists because they have practically none of the diseases we suffer, including obesity, coronary heart disease and diabetes.[18,19] It is also notable that the Inuit diet described by Drs Vilhjalmur Stefansson and Hugh Sinclair in the 1950s is very similar in regard to percentages of fat and protein intake to the experimental low-carb diets used in recent obesity studies.[20,21]

Conclusion

Our bodies store energy in the form of fat. Fat is our bodies' preferred energy source. And in what form do our bodies store fat? They store it as a mixture of saturated, monounsaturated and polyunsaturated fatty acids – a mixture very similar to the fat of other animals.

Don't be afraid of replacing the carbs missing from your diet with fats. If you eat naturally-occurring fats which haven't been processed or 'modified' you can't go far wrong.

Chapter Eighteen

Prevention is better

Prevention is better than cure, but this means starting with a healthy baby. This chapter looks at how to prepare in advance for healthy children, including eating the right things before conception and through pregnancy. It also looks at what constitutes a truly healthy diet for children up to the age of about seven years.

Long-term planning is not about making long-term decisions. It is about understanding the future consequences of today's decisions.

Gary Ryan Blair

Most health books are usually concerned with helping those who have succumbed to diseases after the event – to undo the damage caused by previous faulty dietary practice. But it must be self-evident that it is far better not to court ill-health in the first place. And this relies on correct nutrition from the start – that is, from a child's conception, for our nutritional status at our beginning has a profound effect on our health throughout life.[1-3] During the time the unborn child is forming, he requires an adequate supply of the right nutrients. If these are not supplied in the right quantity and at the right time, a damaged baby is the inevitable result.

Many mothers – and other family members, too – can be worn down by having a perpetually sick child, with constant colds, sniffles and recurrent ear infections. These often result in the prescription of antibiotics and other drugs from their well-meaning doctor. Some children undergo sinus surgery or tubes placed in their ears because doctors treat these conditions as they were taught to. As most children seem to suffer such frequent infections, they are regarded by both parents and their doctors as normal.

But I see things very differently. Illness is not an inevitable consequence of childhood. If a child suffers one infection after another, I suspect inadequate diet and a weakened immune system. Nutritional excellence is far superior to drugs in both recovery and prevention.

In her book, *Let's Have Healthy Children*,[4] the world-renowned nutritionist, Adele Davies, tells how, when pregnant and nursing mothers ate a proper diet, not only did they have more normal pregnancies and easier labours, their babies were born with no congenital abnormalities. Davies also found that children of well-nourished mothers, who were themselves well-nourished, suffered no colic, were more intelligent and attentive, and less prone to hyperactivity, allergies, colds and other ailments. On the other hand, expectant mothers who were malnourished to the point where they had small babies could expect their offspring to be more trouble to them and to have considerable difficulties in childhood and later life.

Birth-weight depends on what and how much the expectant mother eats

A study of diet toward the end of the first three months of pregnancy and subsequent birth-weights found that mothers of premature or low birth-weight babies ate significantly fewer essential nutrients than mothers of larger babies. The missing or deficient nutrients causing premature births were salt, magnesium, phosphorus and iron; those associated with low birth-weight were thiamine (vitamin B_1), salt, iron and magnesium, niacin (vitamin B_3) and riboflavin (vitamin B_2). Yet these are all abundant in meat and other high-protein foods. It is not surprising that the worst cases were always found in children born to mothers who were either eating vegetarian diets or on slimming diets while they were pregnant.[5]

There is also a growing body of research that demonstrates that high levels of insulin in an overweight mother's bloodstream have a fattening effect on her unborn baby.[6] This is caused by leakage of insulin-antibody pairs across the placenta.

This book does not pretend to be the definitive book on paediatric diet and nutrition but if its principles are followed from before conception, many of the trials and tribulations of infancy and of health in later life, as well as obesity, can be avoided.

Before conception

Pregnancy, and a proper diet for it, should always be planned. You may not realise that you are pregnant until after you have missed a period. By that time, your fetus could have been developing for four to eight weeks. It is during these weeks that all your baby's internal organs, limbs and face begin to develop. Damage at this sensitive time through unsuitable diet, smoking or drugs contributes to many malformations such as cleft palate, malformed limbs, and defects to eyes, hearing, heart or brain.

Obesity makes delivery more difficult for the mother and increases the risks for her baby. Babies born to obese women are twice as likely to need intensive care. But, as rapid weight-loss dieting is very harmful during pregnancy, excess weight should be lost before conception. What you eat immediately before and during pregnancy will also affect the amount of fat your baby will carry through life.

Difficulty conceiving

Difficulty in conceiving is often the result of poor nutrition. As we saw in Chapter 15, women who keep to a low-fat diet when trying to conceive dramatically reduce their chances of pregnancy, through *anovulatory infertility*, a condition in which ovulation stops.

Eating foods that contain trans-fats can have a similar effect.[7] Trans-fats are found not only in margarines and cooking oils, but also in commercially produced cakes, biscuits and cookies.

A deficiency of iron is yet another cause of anovulatory infertility.[8] The best sources of iron are liver and red meat.

You will note that all the possible causes of anovulatory infertility are related to diets that are high in carbs and low in foods from animal sources.

Overweight women and those on low-calorie diets who seem unable to conceive will find that the unrestricted-calorie diet advocated here, high in meat, fish and dairy produce, with fresh vegetables and fruit, and free from refined sugar and starch may well help to solve their problem.[9,10]

If difficulty conceiving turns out to be related to the man's sperm, then a dose of sunshine may help. Studies have shown that vitamin D is important for women wanting to get pregnant, but recent research from Dartmouth-Hitchcock Medical Center, New Hampshire, has shown that topping up levels of the 'sunshine vitamin' could also be critical for men, as higher levels of vitamin D in the blood appear to improve the number and activity of sperm.[11]

Diet during pregnancy

During pregnancy you really are eating for two. A poor diet during pregnancy is a major cause of low birth-weight babies, who have a much increased risk of perinatal death and of other health problems throughout life, and a reduced life-expectancy overall.

The ideal diet during pregnancy is one that has a high nutrient density with foods such as meat, fish, milk, and full-fat dairy products, and fresh vegetables and a little fruit. Professor David Barker and colleagues at the University of Southampton found that: 'Mothers who had high carbohydrate intakes in early pregnancy had babies with lower placental and birth weights. Low maternal intakes of dairy and meat protein in late pregnancy were also associated with lower placental and birth weights' which 'could have long term consequences for the offspring's risk of cardiovascular disease.'[12] Professor Barker's group has provided over-whelming evidence that malnutrition at a very early age in Britain in the 20th century resulted in earlier and more severe adult chronic disease.

Mother's size while pregnant doesn't seem to matter. What matters is what a mother has eaten during pregnancy.

During pregnancy there is an inevitable weight gain. This should be about ½-1 kg (1-2 lbs) in the first ten weeks, 3-5 kg (6-10 lbs) by the 20th week with about ½ kg (1 lb) a week after that to the end of preg-nancy: a total weight gain of about 13 kg (28 lbs) over the nine months.

If weight gain is substantially greater or less than this you should try to determine why. Excessive weight gain is usually caused by excessive intake of 'convenience food'.

The milky way

The Jesuits say that if they have a child for his first seven years, they have him for life. Similarly the way children are fed during these first formative years determines their eating patterns throughout life. Dietary habits learned during childhood are usually retained throughout life. This is because our eating habits are all acquired. We base our various diets on what our mothers cooked when we were young; what our society, ethnic, and religious groups prefer; what is advertised in print and elec-tronic media; and what is available in the local grocery store. But we seem to have lost our native wisdom as, today, these are rarely the foods we evolved to eat. So set your child's dietary habits on the right path early, as trying to change them later is not easy.

The way to good nutrition for your infant should not be difficult. There is one product that alone will provide your baby with all the nutrients he requires for at least the first six months or more of his life. That product, consisting of all the proteins, fats, carbohydrates, vitamins, minerals and trace elements your growing infant needs, formulated in exactly the right proportions, available when required at exactly the right temperature and germ free, is mother's milk. Not only is it the right food for growth, it will protect your baby from allergies, gastric and bowel disturbances, and many other diseases.

Given free access to the breast, your baby should not overeat, taking only as much as he needs. One bonus for you as a nursing mother might be that you are less stressed by a colicky child. Both you and your baby should be emotionally bonded and gain pleasure from the experience. And, unlike most things today, this amazing product is free.

Breast-feeding for your baby's health

There is little doubt that breast is best when it comes to feeding new-borns, with many long-lasting benefits to health throughout life:

- Breast-feeding seems to provide the best protection against disease and allergy such as asthma, acute or prolonged diarrhoea, respiratory tract infections, otitis media, urinary tract infection and neonatal septi-caemia.[13]
- Babies who had been exclusively breast-fed for at least the first four months of life had only half the amount of wheezing of those who were wholly bottle-fed. Children who part breast and part bottle-fed were little better than those wholly bottle-fed.[14]
- Blood pressure was also much higher in children who had been bottle-fed.
- In a 1999 study, breast milk growth factor reduced skin problems in children.[15]
- Breast-feeding appears to reduce leukaemia risk. The effect was strongest in children who were breast-fed for more than six months.[16]
- Breast-feeding improves heart health. Professor Alan Lucas and colleagues at the Medical Research Council's Childhood Nutrition Centre in London, found that adolescents who had been breast-fed in infancy had healthier cholesterol levels than those who had been given formula milk.[17] This indicates higher vitamin C levels.
- In another 1999 study, breast-feeding gave babies a three-point advantage in IQ over bottle-fed babies.[18] All studies but one in this analysis were based on breast-fed and not just breast-milk-fed children.
- Breast-fed infants are generally slimmer than formula-fed infants at one year.[19] In a 1995 study, obesity was reduced by more than 40% in children breast-fed exclusively for at least six months; bottle-fed children were nearly twice as likely to be obese when compared with breast-fed children.[20] Not surprisingly, perhaps, 95% of obese people had not been breast-fed.

If breast-feeding were carried out for longer, protection was improved.

Breast-feeding has also been shown to prevent infant deaths. *The Guardian* reported that, in the Philippines, only 16% of children between four and five months old are now exclusively breast-fed.[21] This, one of the lowest rates on Earth, is 33% down on just 10 years ago. And every year, according to the WHO, some 16,000 Filipino children die as a result of 'inappropriate feeding practices'.

Much of the responsibility for the decline in breast-feeding lies with baby formula manufacturers, who spend over $100 million each year advertising breast-milk substitutes in the Philippines. That is more than half the annual budget of the Philippines' Department of Health. Some families now spend as much as a third of their income on these products.

In 2006, the Department of Health issued a new set of rules which prohibited advertising and promotion of infant formula for children up to two years old. However, after lobbying from the US embassy, the US regional trade representative, and the chief executive of the US Chamber of Commerce, a restraining order effectively prevented this rule from taking effect.

A senior government lawyer, Nestor Ballocillo, tried to contest this order. He and his son were shot dead while walking from their home in a case that remains unsolved.

Switching from bottle to breast could prevent 13% of all childhood deaths. That's more than any other measure.

Breast-feeding helps mother too

Breast-feeding makes motherhood much less of a traumatic experience as the breast-fed baby will suffer fewer illnesses, smile more at one end and be less messy at the other.

An infant consumes large amounts of energy in the first six to nine months of life, so Nature guarantees this supply of energy in women's hips and thighs and has locked it up during the non-lactating phase. But you can lose it by breast-feeding. Scientists at the University of California found that women who breast-fed for 12 months or more lost weight much more easily than those who breast-fed for less than three months or didn't breast feed at all.[22] Indeed, women who fed their babies a formula feed tended to gain weight. The researchers concluded that 'lactation enhances weight loss postpartum if breast-feeding continues for at least 6 [months].' Dr Carol Janney and colleagues at the University of Michigan confirmed that women who breast-fed exclusively for at least six months regained their original weight much more easily and quickly than those who bottle-fed or only partly breast-fed their babies.[23]

There is no doubt in my mind that a mother's best 'hip and thigh diet' is the one she feeds to her baby.

Breast-feed immediately

Success with breast-feeding depends on how soon and how much a baby sucks. The breast produces milk only on demand: if your baby doesn't suck, you won't produce any milk. Your baby should be put to your breast immediately after birth. Under one hour old, a baby is responsive and alert, and will suck easily. When a baby is born, his blood-sugar level is usually low. In Nature, the first food a baby gets from the breast is colostrum. It may look a thin watery fluid but it has a high protein content. This amazing food, for which there is no substitute, is the start that all babies should have.

Bottle-feeding is inferior to breast-feeding both in the quality of the milk and for the mother-baby bonding process. Cow's milk, designed for a calf that must double its weight in a few days, is not suitable for a baby human. Formula milks are nearer to human milk but looking round the pharmacy at baby milk formulas I note that, without exception, they are now all made with polyunsaturated vegetable oils. These are unhealthy.

Baby-led weaning

Once a baby has become a few months old the issue of weaning onto solids arises. And this has become confused, creating a hole which baby-food manufacturers have been quick to fill. The baby-food market is currently worth some £354 million and increasing, despite a declining birth rate. Manufacturers say that the purées they usually produce are what parents want, but this way of feeding is not ideal. The point of weaning is to make the transition from milk to ordinary family food. It is at this phase in a child's life that the most care must be taken, for the foods that a child is introduced to at this stage of its life will govern its choices of foods throughout its life.

Baby-led weaning (BLW) is the method I advocate. BLW gradually weans a baby from a milk diet onto solid foods. Significantly, it does this in a way that allows the baby to control his solid food intake by self-feeding from the very beginning of the weaning process. Babies often begin by picking up and licking food, before progressing to eating. Babies should be offered a range of foods to provide a balanced diet from about six months of age. This is the typical age to begin self-feeding, although some infants will make a grab for food earlier and some will wait until seven or eight months. The beauty of this process is that it is tailored to suit each particular baby and his personal development.

The six-month guideline is based on research indicating the internal digestive system matures over the period from four to six months. It seems reasonable to posit that the gut matures in tandem with the baby's external faculties to self-feed. After 30 years of observation of infants, Gill Rapley, pioneer of this way of feeding and Deputy Programme Director of Unicef Baby Friendly Initiative, was convinced that parents should offer a variety of finger foods and let infants regulate what and how much they eat. 'Babies that are allowed to pick what to eat and feed themselves seem to be better at hand-eye coordination, less choosy and keener to try new foods and join in with the family. I even think that there are links between eating disorders and the way most people wean,' she said. Rapley also noticed that it is at around six months of age that most babies reach out and grab things to put in their mouths. 'It seemed blindingly obvious to me,' she said, 'that this development was perfectly timed to allow them to feed themselves.'

Babies who are allowed to feed themselves tend to accept a wide range of food. This is probably because they have more than just the flavour of the food to focus on – they are experiencing texture, colour, size, and shape as well. In addition, giving babies food separately, or in a way which enables them to separate them for themselves, enables them to learn about a range of different flavours and textures. And allowing them to leave anything they appear not to like will encourage them to be prepared to try new things.

The opposite appears to be true for a baby who is spoon fed, especially if foods are presented as purées containing more than one flavour. In this situation the baby has no way of isolating any flavour he doesn't like and will tend to reject the whole meal. Since his parents can only guess which food is causing the problem, they risk more food rejection until they track it down. In the meantime, the baby learns not to trust food and the range of food will accept can become severely limited. This can lead to his overall nutrition being compromised. Offering food separately, but together on the same plate, allows the baby to make his own decisions about mixing flavours.

Breast-feeding should be continued in conjunction with weaning; and milk should always be offered before solids in the first 12 months.

Appetite is a conditioned attitude to foodstuffs. An infant brought up on a diet of ants' eggs and worms, knowing no other, will be quite happy to eat them – although he might get some strange looks from his school pals if he takes these for his midday lunch. Similarly, if a child is taught to like sweet things, that is what he will prefer. Once the appetite is programmed in infancy it's very difficult to change later.

Weaning should not be started before four months for the reasons stated earlier; indeed there are advantages in not starting to feed solids until six months as avoiding them until this age dramatically reduces allergies,[24] but it should be started by six months. Breast-feeding may continue simultaneously for two years or more.

It is important that you don't sweeten anything. Don't worry if these foods do not taste sweet enough to you; your baby doesn't know the difference. If he doesn't become used to sweetened foods, he will not develop a taste for them.

Don't wean to carbs

Traditionally, the first weaning food given is a milled cereal but, not only is there is no nutritional reason for this, it can be counter-productive.

Different enzymes are needed to digest and metabolize different foods. While the enzymes needed for protein and fat digestion are adequate, pancreatic amylase secretion, which is used to digest starches, is essentially absent at birth and remains low through the first years of life.[25]

When a baby is born, he has a store of iron that will last for several months, but it will gradually be depleted. It is safer, therefore, to begin weaning with egg yolk which is a really great baby weaning food.[26,27] There is only one caveat: don't overcook the egg or this may oxidize both the cholesterol and fatty acids in the yolk. Eggs should be soft boiled or fried sunny side up. This not only helps replenish iron stores; it also helps provide the right fatty acids for brain development.[27,28]

Avoid soy milk

After breast-feeding is reduced or finished, many parents, worried by media articles about the healthiness or otherwise of cow's milk, use soy milk and other soy products. But this is not a good choice. Iron and zinc deficiency are substantial problems in small children in both developed and developing nations. Optimizing mineral absorption is an important strategy in minimizing this problem. Work at the Department of Pediatrics, Baylor College of Medicine, Texas, has shown that soy products could be harmful. The authors found that while beef protein increased both iron and zinc absorption, soy proteins actually inhibited the absorption of these minerals.[29]

Children need more dietary fats [30]

The Local, an English language newspaper in Sweden, reported a study from Gothenburg University which showed: 'that one in five four-year-olds have a body mass index (BMI) that is considered too high, while 2% are obese.' Yet none of these children was consuming more calories than required for their energy needs. What was different was the *type* of food eaten. The children with a high BMI were not the ones who regularly ate fatty foods; on the contrary: 'higher BMI was associated with lower fat and higher sucrose intake.' The children with a high BMI were also deficient in essential nutrients, vitamin D, omega-3 fatty acids and iron. The study's summary says it all: 'A lower fat intake was associated with higher BMI . . . insulin and insulin resistance were associated with increased growth rate from birth to the age of 4 . . . Risk factors for the metabolic syndrome can be identified already in healthy 4-year olds, especially in girls.'

Don't be frightened of natural animal fats. Dietary fat and cholesterol are needed to insulate nerve cells and prevent short circuits between nerves and subsequent brain damage. There is concern that infant formula milks do not provide the necessary long-chain fatty acids necessary for proper brain development.[31] For proper growth and brain development children under the age of two years need fat and cholesterol every day – particularly if they are chubby. Never forget that nature has designed breast milk to be the perfect food for babies, and 55% of the energy in breast milk is in the form of fat – and that is an animal fat, not a vegetable oil.

All food should be nutritious. A child has a lot of growing to do and only a small stomach. He must have the building blocks for bone, teeth, muscle and brain in the form of protein, fats, vitamins and minerals. He also will use an inordinate amount of energy. The most concentrated energy source is the fat. Don't cut it off; your child needs it.

Proteins

A baby's body – muscles, skin, internal organs, hair, nails, brain – is also made of proteins. Only when complete proteins of excellent quality are given every day, can every cell function properly and grow normally. It is vitally important, therefore, that a baby's stomach is not filled with foods such as breakfast cereals, fizzy drinks, potato chips, and so on. A child's stomach just hasn't got room for all that junk and real food as well.

You can tell easily whether a baby has enough of the right proteins: strong, well-formed muscles hold the body erect automatically. If muscles have had insufficient protein they lose their elasticity and posture is poor. A mother who has to tell her child, 'Stand up straight', is actually admitting her own failure to provide the proper nourishment.

If you do find this happening, it is surprising how quickly faulty posture can be improved with a diet containing adequate protein.

Commercial baby foods

It is important that babies are introduced to high quality foods from the start. Jars of commercial baby food are best avoided for a number of reasons:

- Using commercial foods usually means that the child's first solids are very different from the foods you will want him to eat a few months later.
- Commercial baby foods are made to 'healthy eating principles' and, as you now know, these are not healthy.
- These foods also contain large quantities of sugary or starchy fillers. Even those with 'no added sugar' usually contain fruit syrups, other sugars and starch thickeners to make them appear more like solid food. These not only predispose to obesity but also damage emerging teeth.

- There is no requirement that baby foods which contain meat have either their meat content, the species from which it comes, or which parts of the animal is used, stated on the jar. A 'Turkey Dinner' I had tested contained only 5% meat.
- Baby foods are highly processed and, as a consequence, nutrients may be destroyed. To make up this shortfall, manufacturers add vitamins. There is considerable evidence that vitamin supplements are not as healthy as vitamins found in their natural state.
- Baby foods also tend to be stored for a considerable time before being eaten. Lacking freshness and nutritional quality, they are the infant equivalent of junk food.

It is almost inevitable, I suppose, that you will want to use commercial baby foods for convenience from time to time. In which case scrutinize the labels and reject any that contain ingredients that are not 'food' in the accepted sense, or that you wouldn't want to eat yourself.

Making baby foods

Making foods yourself for weaning is not difficult. A whole month's supply can easily be made in one go, divided up into ice-cube trays and frozen in the freezer or refrigerator's ice box to be thawed out as required.

Drinks

When your child is thirsty, it means that his body is becoming dehydrated and requires water. Avoid fizzy drinks. The 'pop rot' can start early and quite subtly. Many baby drinks are also little better than sugared water: a single beaker of blackcurrant drink can contain six to nine spoons of sugar. Avoid also low-calorie diet drinks.

The best drink of all is water. Tap water is preferable to bottled water: the bottled water industry is not as well regulated as the tap water companies and, for safety reasons, bottled water is not recommended by the medical profession for infants.[32] If you live in an area where the tap water is fluoridated, however, you should not give it to your child. Although fluoride is prescribed to combat dental decay, it is a powerful enzyme disruptor which has many serious, long-term, adverse effects.[33] All sources of fluoride should be avoided at all costs.

Teething

At the age of about six months your baby will be grasping things and taking them to his mouth to suck. Later he will begin teething. At this time it is usual to give baby something to chew.

The old-fashioned bone teething ring is probably the best for her. Your baby can also chew on celery sticks or slices of carrot, swede or any other hard vegetable. These should be cut into chunks large enough to prevent their being inadvertently swallowed. Rusks are bad news. Even the low-sugar ones tend to contain a considerable amount of sugar. The first effect is that newly emerging teeth are bathed in the food of teeth-rotting bacteria and, secondly, baby will develop a taste for sweet things.

Growing up

Because of continued growth, children beyond infancy remain susceptible to nutritional disorders. Nutritional deficiencies are uncommon in western societies and, as a result, physicians may be unfamiliar with their clinical features. But they do occur, largely as a result of 'health-food' alternatives to milk.[28]

After the age of three, there is not much difference between the optimal diet for a child and an adult. The main issue at this age is how to account for the child's tastes. Children often crave fat but unwitting parents often try to encourage a diet that excludes it. Children need fat for proper neurological development in the early years, healthy immune function in the school-age years, and for sexual development in the teenage years. If they are not provided with adequate good fats in the diet, they will end up like so many western children as carbohydrate cravers.

Beware of breakfast cereals

Breakfast cereals should have no place at all in a healthy diet, particularly those aimed at children. No breakfast cereal is healthy, but those aimed at children are by far the worst of all. In a study of 161 brands, sugar accounted for more than one-third of the weight of children's cereals.[34] This is on top of the starchy carbs. They are also protein deficient. I cannot stress strongly enough how harmful these pseudo-foods are.

It's never too late

If your child is already eating cereals, sugar and sweets, begin to reduce the amounts slowly so that it is not noticeable. With sugar, you may find that you can cut amounts in some recipes by half without a noticeable difference to the taste. If you need to change eating patterns, try not to make it seem a punishment. One client's 11-month-old daughter took to her healthier lifestyle very quickly. With some trepidation, her parents threw out all her 'high-carb rubbish' and changed her to a healthy, meat-based, eating regime. She loved the change: she quickly sampled and liked sausages and black pudding. If given buttered toast, her father told me she loves to lick the butter off and 'the bread goes on the floor!'

Conclusion

Health patterns for life are set in early childhood. Not only childhood diseases such as rickets and colds, but the likelihood of heart disease and cancers in adulthood are also determined at this time as are most of the other conditions in this book. Teach your child good nutritional practices in the first few years and you lay the foundation for a long and healthy life.

You will devote a great deal of time, money and effort into bringing up your children. Don't let it go to waste.

Part Two

New Diet, New Epidemics

Chapter Nineteen

'Healthy eating' is fattening

Since the introduction in the 1980s of 'healthy eating', with its emphasis on low-fat, carbohydrate-rich foods, the number of overweight and obese people has risen exponentially. This chapter demonstrates that this is not a coincidence but a prime example of cause and effect and looks at why conventional advice on weight loss is totally at variance with both real life studies and clinical trials.

Diets high in fat do not appear to be the primary cause of the high prevalence of excess body fat in our society, and reductions in fat will not be a solution.

Professor Walter Willett

Being overweight has affected a small proportion of the population for centuries but clinical obesity was relatively rare until the 20th century. It remained at a fairly stable low level until about 1980, and then numbers began to increase dramatically in most industrialized countries. By 1991 one in three adults was overweight in the US. That was an increase of 8% of the population over just one decade, despite the fact that Americans were spending a massive $33 billion a year on 'slimming', as well as taking more exercise, and eating fewer calories and less fat than they had done 10 years before. And it has been getting worse.[1]

By 1992 one in every 10 people in Britain was obese; a mere five years later that figure had almost doubled. There is now a pandemic of increasing weight across the industrialized world. And nothing seems to work.

It is so bad that for some time the medical profession has been talking about giving up the fight. The 10 September 1994 edition of the *British Medical Journal* published two papers about it. One expressed grave reservations about the effectiveness of present dietary treatments[2] while the other, wondering if intervention was worthwhile, asked: should we treat obesity?[3]

Although it is widely believed that obesity is caused by taking in more energy in food than is used up by exercise, there is little evidence to support this hypothesis. The reason for obesity is not just that we eat too much, but that we eat too much of the wrong foods.

The first fact that must be grasped is that 'healthy eating' is not the answer to being overweight and obesity – it is part of the cause.

How a 'healthy diet' fattens

The prevailing wisdom over the past several years has been that fat makes you fat, and that if you simply stop eating fat, you'll lose weight without even trying. A typical example is:

> 'Fats are a concentrated form of energy, providing 9 calories per gram, compared to 4 calories per gram for both carbohydrates and protein. That is why high fat diets can lead to weight gain much easier than lower fat diets: it's easy to eat foods packed with calories and not realize you have eaten too much.'

That may sound plausible but, I'm sorry, it's not true. Cutting fat out doesn't work – but you have probably discovered that for yourself. Professor Walter Willett, of Harvard University School of Medicine, confirmed what some of us have known for years when he found that: 'fat consumption within the range of 18-40% of energy appears to have little if any effect on body fatness.'[4] Professor Willett continued: 'Moreover . . . a substantial decline in the percentage of energy from fat consumed during the past two decades has corresponded with a massive increase in obesity.' This has become blindingly obvious. Could cutting fat be the cause of obesity? Professor Willett concluded: 'Diets high in fat do not appear to be the primary cause of the high prevalence of excess body fat in our society, and reductions in fat will not be a solution.'

And there is more to this.

As fat in the diet is a significant contributor to being satisfied with a meal, low-fat diets often leave dieters very hungry. Those who tell you that, to maintain a normal weight you must eat a low-fat diet, want you to live your life hungry most of the time. And you simply can't do it. Your body is not designed to operate in this way and it rebels. No other animal on this planet counts the percentage of fat calories (or any other calories) in its diet; there is no need for us to, either.

As diet gurus and nutritionists have recommended low-fat diets for weight loss for decades, you might expect that there are lots of studies to support them. There aren't. Most such studies show marginal improvements in weight at best, and some actually show significant weight gains. Let's look at a typical example: a two-year study of 171 women on a low-fat, weight loss diet.[5] After six months, the greatest weight loss any one of them had achieved was 7.5 lb (3.4 kg), which isn't exactly earth-shattering; and by the second year some of that weight had been regained. In studies like these, not everyone will lose (or gain) the same amount; the average figure is a 'plus or minus' amount, called the 'standard deviation'. The standard deviation in this study was more than twice the average weight loss. This tells us that many of the people in the study actually *gained weight* on the low-fat diet.

The fact is that not one clinical study has ever shown that low-fat diets result in long-term reversal of obesity, *whether it is combined with exercise or not.* Indeed, over the past 20 or more years, fat consumption has consistently gone down – and national incidences of obesity have gone up at precisely the same time. In the US from 1976-80 to 1988-91:

- Average fat intake fell 11%.
- Average calorie intake fell from 1,854 kcal to 1,785 kcal.
- Percentage of population consuming low-calorie products rose from 19% to 76%.
- Those who were overweight *increased* 31%.

This doesn't mean that the one necessarily caused the other; however, with no change in the proportion of people with a sedentary lifestyle, the authors of this study conclude that it is 'reduced fat and calorie intake and frequent use of low-calorie food products' that are responsible for the 'paradoxical increase in the prevalence of obesity'.[6] There is no reason to suppose the trends in the UK are any different. If you know of any scientific study that does support a low-fat diet as an effective weight-loss diet, please e-mail me. My address is in the Appendix.

It's *not* all about calories

The orthodox Golden Rule for treating overweight is: calories in minus calories out equals weight change. As you will see later, although this hypothesis is plausible and has what looks like umpteen good, solid, rigorous, clinical studies appearing to support it, it is actually quite wrong. However, if we assume it is correct, that brings up the first big problem. How do we answer the apparently simple question: 'how many calories are there in an item of food?'

Despite supermarkets' desire for uniformity, natural food products vary widely from item to item. Weight for weight, for example, an early season fruit may be much lower in sugar than one from the peak of the season.

And that is only the first problem. The second is even harder to answer. How much energy do you use when you do something? If you walk a mile you will use less energy than someone else who walks the same distance, but weighs more. If you do it more quickly your energy usage will differ from someone doing it slowly. So there's really no way you can calculate accurately how much energy you are actually using.

When is a calorie not a calorie?

The second Golden Rule of orthodoxy is: 'a calorie is a calorie', whatever its source. This means that if you eat X number of calories more than you use, you will put on Y amount of weight, wherever those calories come from. So why is it that, in trials, dieters on fat-based diets consistently lose much more weight than dieters on carb-based diets, even when both diets have exactly the same number of calories?

There is an emerging scientific consensus that weight control is a highly complex topic and the old ideas that overweight people are lazy gluttons are now realized to be as absurd and insulting as the overweight have always thought they were.

Fats don't cause weight gain, carbs do

Carbs are the only foods that increase body weight. I know this is heresy to the 'healthy eating' dictocrats, but why it should be is a mystery: as long as humans have been raising animals for food, we have always fattened them on carbs. This is how it works.

Carbohydrates – it doesn't matter whether these are sugar, jam, bread, pasta, breakfast cereals or fruit – are all exactly the same as far as your body is concerned: they are *all* ultimately converted to the blood sugar, glucose.

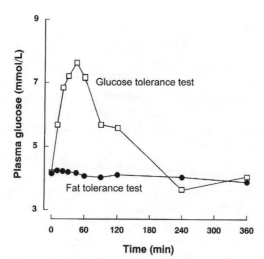

Figure 19.1: Blood glucose after 100 g of glucose or 40 g of fat

They are also digested quickly and raise blood glucose levels quickly, as can be seen in Figure 19.1. Our bodies regulate blood glucose and keep it within quite fine limits as high levels of glucose are harmful. If glucose rises too high, insulin is produced to take the excess glucose out of the bloodstream.

The glucose is converted first to a form of starch called *glycogen* which is stored in the liver and muscle cells but, as the body can store only a limited amount of glycogen in this way, all the other excess glucose is stored as body fat.

This is the process of putting on weight. And there is more. There is an inevitable time delay between cause and effect. You will notice in Figure 19.2 that when your blood glucose level is back down to a normal level of 6.0 mmol/L (108 mg/dL) after about 90 minutes, the insulin level in your bloodstream is still high and packing glucose away as fat in your fat cells. This drives glucose in your blood abnormally low (it's called *reactive hypoglycaemia*) and you soon feel hungry again. So you have a snack, usually of more carbohydrates and start the whole process over again. You're getting fatter but feeling hungry at the same time. During this, your blood sugar levels are fluctuating wildly – you are 'yo-yo dieting' by the hour. The answer is to eat *less* carbohydrate so that the blood sugar level does not fluctuate so violently, and eat *more* fat.

Because it takes a long time to digest, fat not only prevents those violent fluctuations in blood sugar levels, it also gives a feeling of satiety, which stops that feeling of hunger.

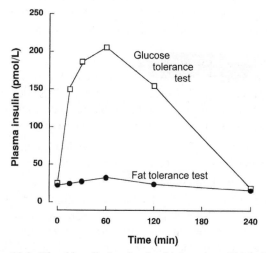

Figure 19.2: Blood insulin levels after high-carb and high-fat meals

The next problem is that insulin resistance, caused by the continual high levels of insulin in your bloodstream, impairs your insulin's ability to satisfy a satiety centre in your brain. This contributes to overeating, obesity and diabetes.[7]

This is the first crucial problem with the 'healthy eating' dogma. Eating the 'healthy' way, you can eat far more calories than your body needs as energy for the day, yet still feel hungry – and eat more. You enter a vicious cycle of continuous weight gain combined with hunger. Under such circumstances it is almost impossible not to overeat. Obesity is almost inevitable.[8]

Not surprisingly, a high insulin response to glucose has been shown to be a risk factor for long-term weight gain, and this effect is particularly so in people who are insulin-resistant.[9]

Note that, as the two graphs show, fat raises neither glucose levels nor insulin levels. This means that, despite what you have been told, dietary fat cannot make body fat. You may not realize it, but it has been known for half a century that excess fats aren't stored in the body. Any unused fat calories are excreted in urine and faeces.[10-12] Unless it is disguised in a carbohydrate-rich food, our bodies will not let us eat too much.[13]

Healthy eating inhibits weight loss

So far we have only considered half of the obesity problem. The other half is: having put weight on, you now need to lose it again. Here again 'healthy eating' hampers your efforts because eating a carbohydrate-based diet also stops you from losing weight.

If you are overweight, what is it that you actually want to lose? That's not as silly a question you might think. You don't want to lose weight – you can do that by having a leg amputated; what you really want to lose is fat, right?

The point is that, *to lose fat, your body must use that fat* as a fuel; there is no other way. And the only way your body will use its stored fat as a fuel is if you force it to. That means depriving it of its present supply of fuel – the blood sugar, glucose – so that it has no choice in the matter.

There are two ways to cut your body's glucose supply:

- you either starve – which is what low-calorie, low-fat dieting is, or
- you reduce the starches and sugars from which glucose is made and make it up with a source of a different fuel – fat.

The latter approach has two advantages over the traditional calorie-controlled approach: it means that you no longer have to go hungry and, by feeding your body on fats, it will stop trying to find glucose and change over naturally to using its own stored fat. This is by far the easiest way because:

'In the presence of dietary carbohydrate, the preferred fuel is glucose and the capacity to mobilize fat is limited. Factors that increase blood glucose during dieting may stimulate insulin release and all the metabolic sequelae of circulating insulin. Fatty acid synthesis is activated and lipolysis is profoundly inhibited by insulin even at very low concentrations of the hormone.' [14]

In other words, if you eat a carbohydrate-based, low-fat diet, you force your body into a fat-*making* mode, not a fat-*using* mode. Insulin's job is to get energy out of the bloodstream, not let more in. The study the extract above was taken from was published in 1992 but it merely confirmed what had been demonstrated decades before (but forgotten) when Dr Michael Somogyi showed clearly that 'carbohydrates . . . inhibit the burning of fats.' [15]

Control hormones

The hormones that control our bodies' responses to internal and external events were conditioned by our environment over the past couple of million years. These set in motion different combinations of hormonal responses. We have several hormones that raise levels of glucose in our bloodstream: adrenaline (epinephrine), glucagon, glucocorticoids (cortisol, cortisone, corticosterone) and growth hormone. But we have only one hormone – insulin – to bring glucose levels down. This strongly suggests that high glucose levels were not a problem in pre-historic times, meaning that we must have eaten a low-carb diet.

So, if you are overweight, is it your fault – or theirs?

Conventional nutritionists will invariably tell you, if you are overweight, it's your own fault: you are eating too much or not exercising enough – or both.

But are they right? In my experience, nobody wants to be overweight. Fat people are ridiculed, stared at, embarrassed to be seen in a bathing costume on the beach. In other words, if you are overweight you live a generally less happy life.

And it may not be your fault at all if you are doing what you are told by the 'diet police' because a lot of what you are told by them is nonsense.

A background of dietary nonsense

If you aren't convinced or are confused, let's look at current advice in more detail. This tells us all to base meals on starchy foods like bread, pasta, breakfast cereals, et cetera; 'eat five portions of fruit and vegetables a day'; and to cut down on sugary foods. Let me explain why I call this dietary nonsense:

'Cut down on . . . sugary foods'

This is one admonition that I don't disagree with. But I want to show you how it fits into a pattern of dietary nonsense.

The chemical name for table sugar is *sucrose*. Sucrose is a *disaccharide* (two sugars). Its chemical formula, $C_{12}H_{22}O_{11}$, means that it is made up of 12 atoms of carbon, 22 atoms of hydrogen and 11 atoms of oxygen. But our bodies will only accept *monosaccharides* (single sugars) from the gut. So the digestion breaks down (hydrolyzes) sucrose into glucose and fructose, both of which are monosaccharides whose formula is $C_6H_{12}O_6$. In this process one molecule of $C_{12}H_{22}O_{11}$ ends up as two molecules of $C_6H_{12}O_6$. But you may have noticed that sucrose has only 22 hydrogen and 11 oxygen atoms. To convert to glucose, it must gain two hydrogen atoms and one oxygen atom somehow. It does this by combining with water whose chemical formula is H_2O. The process is illustrated thus:

$$C_{12}H_{22}O_{11} + H_2O \rightarrow C_6H_{12}O_6 + C_6H_{12}O_6$$
1 sucrose + 1 water $\rightarrow$ 1 glucose +1 fructose

The addition of the water atoms to the sugar molecule increases the total energy content. In this way, 100 grams of sugar, which you would think contains 400 calories, ends up as 105 grams of glucose plus fructose, which is 420 calories.

'Base meals and snacks on starchy foods'

We are then told to base meals on starchy foods: bread, breakfast cereals, pasta, rice and root vegetables such as potatoes. Starch, which is made up of strings of thousands of sugar molecules fastened together, is called a 'complex carbohydrate' or *polysaccharide* (many sugars). The formula for each individual glucose molecule in starch is $C_6H_{10}O_5$ so, to make them into $C_6H_{12}O_6$, we again need two hydrogen atoms and one oxygen atom. In a similar way to the digestion of sugar, one molecule of water, H_2O, is combined with each of the starch molecules, thus:

$$C_6H_{10}O_5 + H_2O \rightarrow C_6H_{12}O_6$$

But as the atoms from the water now form a greater proportion of the total in this equation, 100 grams of starch actually becomes 111 grams of glucose or 444 calories. That's more than the sugar.

So if you are trying to lose weight by reducing your calorie intake, basing meals on starchy foods doesn't look like a very clever thing to do.

So what went wrong?

With all the evidence that it is carbs and not fats that are the cause of obesity, why is it that those in nutritional authority can't see it? The answer seems to lie in their implicit belief in the First Law of

Thermodynamics, otherwise known as the Law of Conservation of Energy. This states that energy cannot be created or destroyed, merely changed, and is the basis for the 'calorie is a calorie' argument.

Towards the end of the 19th century, based on the First Law, doctors devised a simple concept. They likened the body to a tank, into which energy is poured in the form of food. This, they said, was then either used up or stored. If you used up more than you poured in, you got thinner and if you poured in more than you used, you got fatter. The theory was easy to understand, made sense, obeyed the laws of physics, and for a while it seemed satisfactory. Doctors could now say, apparently with scientific backing, that fat people must either be eating too much or working too little.

By the start of the First World War doubts were creeping in. The treatment for diabetics at that time involved completely depriving them of carbohydrate. In this case, scientists found that the energy input/energy output sums simply did not add up.

By the early 1920s, interest in the theory had been renewed. It was found to be impossible to measure the total amount of water in a person at any one time; therefore, any discrepancy in the balance between energy input/output and excess weight was put down to water retention or loss. It was decades before this convenient theory was disproved.

In the 1950s, isotope techniques were developed which allowed more accurate measurement of body fat turnover. In addition, it was demonstrated that different foods could alter the amounts of body fat; and that body fat could also be affected by certain responsive glands – the adrenal, thyroid and pituitary glands – even when energy intake was constant. Now the faults began to emerge.

The flaws exposed

The calorie is a unit of heat. The way the energy content of a food is determined is by burning it in a device called a 'bomb calorimeter' and measuring the amount of heat it gives off. One gram of carbohydrate burnt in this way gives an energy value of 4.2 calories, or more correctly kilocalories (kcals, see Glossary). A gram of protein gives 5.25 kcals but one kilocalorie is deducted because a gram of protein does not oxidize readily. That gives a final figure for protein of 4.25 kcals. Burning a gram of fat in the bomb calorimeter gives 9.2 kcals.

These figures are then rounded to the nearest whole number – 4, 4 and 9 respectively – and are used in calorie charts to indicate the energy values of foodstuffs and, thus, to allow dieters to measure their food intake.

But there are two basic flaws in using these figures to determine the amounts of food we should eat.

The more obvious flaw in the argument is that our bodies do not burn foods in the same way that they are burned in a bomb calorimeter. Our digestive process is quite inefficient. The chemical process whereby blood sugar is oxidized to provide energy produces carbon dioxide. About half is exhaled as carbon dioxide in the breath; the other half is excreted in sweat, urine and faeces as energy-containing molecules, the energy values of which must be deducted from the original food intake. All of these vary.

The second and more important flaw in the argument is that the body does not use all its food to provide energy. The primary function of dietary proteins is body cell manufacture and repair; enzymes that control practically all body processes are also proteins. The amount of protein needed for these purposes is about one gram per kilogram of lean body weight. As meats contain approximately 23 grams of protein per 100 grams, a person weighing, say, 70 kilograms (155 lbs) needs to eat about 300 grams (11 oz) of meat, or its equivalent, every day just to supply his basic protein needs. Even eating this volume of lean chicken would provide some 465 kilocalories. These calories are not used to supply energy; they contribute nothing to the body's calorie needs and so must be deducted from the total.

Much of the fat we eat is also used to provide materials used by the body in processes other than the production of energy: the manufacture of bile acids, prostaglandins, prostacyclins, leukotrienes, thromboxanes, hormones and so on. These also contribute nothing to energy production and so all these must be deducted.

Thus trying to determine, from food intake and energy expenditure alone, how much excess energy your body will store as fat, without knowing all this other information, will give a completely wrong answer. These other factors cannot be measured; therefore, calorie-counting, which is the foundation of most modern slimming diets, is a waste of time.

And there is one more flaw. We are told by the 'experts' that 'a calorie is a calorie.' What they mean is that it is impossible for two diets containing exactly the same number of calories to lead to different weight losses. Yet, over the last century many dietary studies have found that isn't true: calorie for calorie, low-carb, high-fat diets are much better at reducing weight than the traditional low-fat diets. 'Experts' have heavily criticized these studies saying that the data must be wrong because that would violate the laws of thermodynamics.

They don't. It is important to realize that there is more than one law of thermodynamics. The narrow view that 'a calorie is a calorie' might comply with the First Law, but it violates the Second Law of

Thermodynamics. There is no doubt at all that low-carb, high-fat diets *do* have a metabolic advantage when it comes to weight loss, whatever the 'experts' say.[16] And this metabolic advantage complies fully with the Second Law of Thermodynamics.

The First Law is a *conservation* law. The Second Law is a *dissipation* law; it is this Second Law which governs the use of energy in chemical reactions within our bodies.

Let me use an analogy. The energy in the petrol that fuels your car makes the car go along, but it also produces heat through friction and noise, which is wasted energy. The Second Law is all about efficiency – how much of the energy we put in does useful work and how much is wasted. Although all of the energy in the petrol is accounted for and complies with the First Law, the actual moving of the car, if the waste products (heat and noise) are removed from the equation, does not. The Second Law was developed in this context.

The Second Law says that no machine is completely efficient. Some of the available energy is lost as heat or in the internal rearrangement of chemical compounds and other changes. And as different foods use different metabolic pathways, with different levels of efficiency, variations in efficiency must be expected. For this reason, the dogma that a 'calorie is a calorie' violates the Second Law of Thermodynamics as a matter of principle.

What the diet dictocrats fail to take into consideration when considering the laws of thermodynamics are the energy losses incurred in the different chemical changes within our bodies. When they are, neither law of thermodynamics is violated.

Normalization of controls

Our bodies have a control system that works extremely efficiently, without any conscious effort on our part, as long as it is allowed to. Appetite and hunger are natural and vital signals which are part of this system – and both must be satisfied. Therefore, any diet should follow a pattern that is normal and natural.

Modern low-calorie diets, whether they rely on a very restricted range of nutrient-poor foods such as raw vegetables or cabbage soup, or require a more subtle reduction of calorific intake, are abnormal and unnatural. They all encourage hunger but do not satisfy it. Neither, usually, do they satisfy the appetite.

The most important prerequisite of any diet, then, is to get your body's systems working normally again – and, crucially, reduce the production of insulin. That means cutting carbs and increasing fats.

Low-fat diets cause muscle loss

There is more to the question about which is the better way to lose weight than mere weight loss. I asked earlier what it was you wanted to lose, and suggested that it was fat. All weight loss diets will reduce your weight, but not all of them do it by reducing fat.

With all low-fat, calorie controlled diets, weight is lost from muscles. This is because, conditioned to using glucose as a fuel, and deprived of its necessary supply from carbs, the calorie-controlled dieter's body uses an alternative source to produce glucose: proteins from lean muscle tissue are cannibalized – and that weakens you.

So this is another area where low-carb diets win over the low-calorie ones: by changing the dieter's body to using fats, they preserve muscle mass and favour fat loss. This effect was ably demonstrated in the small study done by Dr Charlotte Young in the early 1970s.[17] Her overweight patients all consumed 1800 kilocalories per day and they all consumed 115 grams of protein per day. Only the fat and carb content was varied. Those eating the most fat (133 grams/day) and least carb (30 grams) lost more body fat and less muscle mass than those getting less fat (103 grams/day) and more carb (104 grams/day).

When we are talking of obesity, these findings are tremendously important. Muscles use more energy than fat. This means that, if muscle mass is lost, this lowers the rate at which your body uses energy. Weight loss that involves a significant loss of muscle mass is much more likely to result in rebound weight gain. That's another good reason to lower your intake of carbs, not fats.

Eat fat, get thin

If we are to overcome the obesity epidemic we *must* reject outright ideas that have been shown to be unproductive. That means abandoning starvation-type, calorie-controlled diets for something that has been shown to work: low-carb, high-fat diets.

Low-carb, high-fat diets are said by those with scant knowledge of the subject, to be a recent dietary fad with no long-term evidence in their support. Nothing could be further from the truth: they have actually been around for over 140 years. (And that is without counting anthropological studies of our ancestors or modern hunter-gatherer cultures who eat them.)

It is almost a century and a half since a Londoner, William Banting, wrote the first low-carb diet book entitled *Letter on Corpulence Addressed to the Public*. Banting had been plagued by obesity for over 30 years and suffered an increasing number of other complaints. The doctors of the day were no better at treating obesity than are today's nutritionists. Then Banting met a Dr William Harvey, FRCS. Harvey put Banting on a low-carb diet, and within a year all his ailments had 'passed into a matter of history'. Since then, inspired by Banting, many studies have shown over and over again that a low-carb, high-fat diet is the best way to lose weight and, more importantly, maintain that lower weight.

An early study was conducted at the Royal Infirmary, Edinburgh. Drs D. M. Lyon and D. M. Dunlop noticed that healthy adults maintained an almost constant body weight over long periods, in spite of considerable variations of physical activity and of food intake. They further noticed that those who regularly over-ate did not necessarily become overweight; neither did those who had a poor appetite necessarily become thin. During 1931 they conducted a controlled dietary trial using a large variety of diets, ranging from 800 to 2,700 calories.[18] So that comparisons would be more meaningful, all the patients were put initially on 1,000-kilocalorie slimming diets. On these, average losses were found to depend not on the calorie content of the diets but on the carbohydrate content. The average daily losses on the 1,000-kilocalorie diets were:

high-carbohydrate/low-fat diet   –   49 grams
high-carbohydrate/low-protein   –   122 grams
low-carbohydrate/high-protein   –   183 grams
low-carbohydrate/high-fat   –   205 grams

It was expected that on the 1,700 to 2,700-kilocalorie diets patients would not lose weight. In fact all but three did lose weight. Lyon and Dunlop, in their conclusions said:

'The most striking feature . . . is that the losses appear to be inversely proportionate to the carbohydrate content of the food. Where the carbohydrate intake is low the rate of loss in weight is greater and conversely.'

There have been many such trials and they still continue today: Published in the year 2000, a prospective study was conducted to evaluate the effect of a low-carb, high-protein/fat diet in achieving short-term weight loss.[19] Researchers at the Center for Health Services Research in Primary Care, Durham, North Carolina, reported data from a six-month study that included 51 individuals who were overweight, but otherwise healthy. The subjects received nutritional supplements and attended bi-weekly group meetings, where they received dietary counselling on consuming a low-carbohydrate, high-protein/fat diet. After six months, they had lost, on average, more than 10% of their weight and their total cholesterol had dropped by an average 10.5 mg/dl (0.27 mmol/L). Twenty subjects chose to continue the diet, and after 12 months, their mean weight loss was 10.9% and their total cholesterol had decreased by 14.1 mg/dl (0.37 mmol/L).

All these recommendations and evidence could have saved a great deal of grief, trauma and ill-health if two other doctors had been listened to in 1994. Professor Susan Wooley and Dr David Garner highlighted the professional's role in people's increasing weight, saying:[2]

> 'The failure of fat people to achieve a goal they seem to want – and to want above all else – must now be admitted for what it is: a failure not of those people but of the methods of treatment that are used.'

Blaming the overweight for their problem and telling them they are eating too much and must cut down, is simply not good enough. It is the dieticians' advice and the treatment offered that are wrong. Wooley and Garner concluded:

> 'We should stop offering ineffective treatments aimed at weight loss. Researchers who think they have invented a better mousetrap should test it in controlled research before setting out their bait for the entire population. Only by admitting that our treatments do not work – and showing that we mean it by refraining from offering them – can we begin to undo a century of recruiting fat people for failure.'

But there is a 'better mousetrap'. William Banting wrote of it nearly a century and a half ago.

Being overweight is healthier than being underweight

The 'weight loss industry' has created a popular belief that being overweight and obese leads inevitably to a premature death. This belief, nurtured with the backing of powerful marketing and political interests, lays the foundation for a money-making 'obesity' industry.

But, yet again, the truth is quite different. Being overweight is not as bad as you might think. Indeed, the healthiest weight is not the 'normal' BMI between 18.5 and 25; it is actually the 'overweight' BMI range of between 25 and 30. It seems that being thin is 25% more dangerous than being the government recommended 'healthy' weight.[20] Thinness is riskiest of all for those over age 60 and puts them at double the risk of 'normal' weight people. It's even riskier than being very obese (BMI over 35).

The Rancho Bernardo Study added to the evidence when it found that:

> 'In elderly adults without clinically recognized CHD, body weight and fat distribution do not predict coronary artery plaque burden. These results raise questions about the value of weight reduction diets for preventing heart disease in elderly survivors without clinical heart disease.'[21]

So, if you are happy with the weight you are, but are thinking you should lose weight for your health's sake, you may wish to reconsider.

The correct way to lose weight – and maintain it

The reason so many people are getting fatter now is because they are told to eat the very foods that are the most fattening: carbohydrates. That was recognized nearly half a century ago. In 1963 a team writing in the *Journal of the American Medical Association* said:

> 'It may be stated categorically that the storage of fat, and therefore the production and maintenance of obesity, cannot take place unless glucose is being metabolized. Since glucose cannot be used by most tissues without the presence of insulin, it also may be stated categorically that obesity is impossible in the absence of adequate tissue concentration of insulin . . . Thus an abundant supply of carbohydrate food exerts a powerful influence in directing the stream of glucose metabolism into lipogenesis, whereas a relatively low carbohydrate intake tends to minimize the storage of fat.'[22]

It's so obvious yet it is completely unknown to the conventional diet gurus of today. But until it is understood and acknowledged, things will only continue to get worse.

Low-fat, low-calorie diets (which are essentially the same thing as starving) generate a series of biochemical signals in your body that will take you out of balance, making it more difficult to access stored body fat for energy. People on restrictive diets get tired of feeling hungry and deprived. They go off their diets, put the weight back on, and then feel bad about themselves for not having enough willpower, discipline or motivation.

But you shouldn't need willpower – no other animal does; all you really need is the right information.

If you change what you eat to a more natural way of eating – a way of eating more like our pre-agricultural ancestors – you won't have to be concerned about how much you eat at all and be continually counting calories. Your body will do that for you, the way it is genetically programmed to do.

Chapter Twenty

Diabetes deceit

Because diabetics are more prone to heart disease, they too are advised to eat a low-fat, high-carbohydrate diet. But this is what caused their condition in the first place. This chapter looks at how conventional dietary treatment makes diabetes worse and suggests an alternative diet that both helps and prevents diabetes.

> They say: 'You really need a high level of proof to change the recommendations,' which is ironic because they never had a high level of proof to set them.
>
> *Professor Walter Willett*

People who are overweight often go on to develop type-2 diabetes. For this reason, obesity is generally blamed for the condition. In fact, the two conditions are caused by the same thing: a diet high in carbohydrates. Obesity only seems to come first because it is easier to spot. Everyone knows that type-2 diabetes is an epidemic caused by the modern lifestyle and diet – everyone, that is, except doctors, according to a new study in which researchers discovered that doctors took a very casual view of the disease, often failing to suggest even a change of diet.[1]

Not that the doctor would have much to say even if he was prepared to offer advice from the goodness of his heart. Medical schools devote little time to diabetes prevention, and so doctors tend to learn about the disease while observing other physicians who, by and large, had the same teachers.

Background

Every cell in the human body needs energy in order to function. One of the body's primary energy sources is glucose. Glucose from the digested food circulates in the blood as a ready energy source for any cells that need it. But too much glucose in the blood is harmful; it must be strictly controlled. Insulin, a hormone produced by the beta-cells in the pancreas, is the control: it helps to regulate blood sugar levels by taking any excess glucose out of the bloodstream and putting it into body cells, either to be used as fuel or to be stored as glycogen and fat. It does this by bonding to a receptor site on the outside of body cells and acting like a key to open a doorway into the cells through which glucose can enter.

When there is not enough insulin produced by the pancreas, or when the doorway no longer recognizes the insulin key, as in the case of insulin resistance, glucose stays in the blood rather than entering the cells. This causes blood glucose to rise to abnormally high levels, a condition called *hyperglycaemia*.

The body will attempt to combat this high level of glucose in the blood by drawing water out of the cells and into the bloodstream in an effort to dilute the sugar and excrete it in the urine. It is not unusual for people with undiagnosed diabetes to be constantly thirsty, to drink large quantities of water, and to urinate frequently as their bodies try to get rid of the extra glucose. At the same time, because glucose does not enter the cells that need it, the cells send hunger signals to the body which results in their owners eating more food.

This essentially is the condition called 'diabetes'.

Diabetes

The word 'diabetes' comes from a Greek word meaning a 'flowing through'. It refers to the increased amount of urine excreted in the disease, a phenomenon called *polyuria*. The commonest form is called *diabetes mellitus*, or 'sweet flowing through', because glucose appears in urine.

Diabetes mellitus is a chronic disorder of carbohydrate metabolism. It is not contagious; you can't catch it from someone who has it. Diabetes impairs the body's ability to use food properly such that blood sugars are not oxidized to produce energy. This is due to a malfunction of the hormone insulin which is produced in the beta cells of the pancreas.

People with diabetes fall into two broad groups:

- In type-1 diabetes, the pancreas produces little or no insulin.
- In type-2 diabetes, the pancreas does produce insulin but there is a reduction in the body's ability to use that insulin because of insulin resistance.

Type-1 diabetes

Type-1, characterized by a sudden onset, is generally believed to be inherited as it is more likely to occur in people who have close relatives with diabetes. However, this seems unlikely as type-1 diabetes is not found in the animal kingdom either in meat-eating or in plant-eating animals, where those animals live in their natural habitat. Neither does type-1 diabetes exist amongst human cultures whose diets are typically low in carbohydrates.[2] While not a single case of type-1 diabetes has been found among the meat- and fat-eating Inuit population of Alaska, there have been cases of the maturity onset, type-2 diabetes.[3] These appear to be the result of increasing carbohydrates introduced into the modern Inuit diet by 'civilization'.

As type-1 is wholly restricted to peoples of western industrialized civilization, it cannot have a genetic origin, although family dietary traits and lifestyle can play a major part in its appearance within families.

Another explanation is that type-1 is an auto-immune disease, and this is more likely. The question then is: what causes that auto-immune reaction? The answer seems to be a cereal-based 'healthy' diet:

- ***Maternal diet.*** If a pregnant woman eats too much carbohydrate, this will raise her insulin levels. It is not thought that insulin itself crosses the placenta from mother to unborn child. However, insulin antibodies do.[4] These increase glycogen and fat deposits resulting in an abnormally large baby. It may also predispose that baby to diabetes.

- ***Infant diet.*** The development of auto-immune type-1 diabetes involves complex interactions among several genes and environmental agents. Human type-1 diabetics show an unusually high frequency of wheat gluten-sensitivity. Gluten is closely linked with the auto-immune attack in the pancreas and is strongly associated with pancreatic islet inflammation and damage.[5] Thus early weaning to a diet which contains a gluten-containing cereal such as wheat, barley, rye or oats is likely to increase the risk of type-1 diabetes.[6] To avoid that risk, such foods should not be used before at least six months of age. And, even then they should be introduced slowly, if at all.

Type-2 diabetes

Much more common, over 90% of diabetics have type-2. Type-2 is also called maturity-onset or adult-onset diabetes as it generally affects people later in life. It is also called non-insulin-dependent diabetes mellitus (NIDDM), although this term is somewhat misleading as patients with type-2 are often prescribed insulin when conventional dietary and drug treatments fail.

In type-2 diabetes, the pancreas often produces high levels of insulin, but cells have become resistant to the insulin and it may not work as effectively.

Excessively high insulin levels in the blood (*hyperinsulinaemia*) exists in childhood in populations at high risk for type-2. Stimulated by a high-carb, high vegetable-fat diet, insulin resistance develops, accompanied by impaired glucose tolerance. The pressure from continual high-carbohydrate meals continues this process until blood glucose eventually makes the beta cells unable to secrete sufficient insulin to bring the levels down and you also have high glucose levels.[7]

Symptoms of type-2 diabetes can begin so gradually that people may not know that they have it. These include:

- High blood glucose level (*hyperglycaemia*)
- Glucose in urine (*glycosuria*)
- Frequent thirst
- Increased urination
- Fatigue, drowsiness
- Blurred vision
- Infections that will not heal quickly
- Sometimes nausea and vomiting
- Women may also complain of urinary tract infections or vaginal itching
- People with type-1 or type-2 diabetes are at higher risk of contracting respiratory, urinary tract and skin infections than people without diabetes.

In the same way that type-1 diabetes is not found in the wild animal kingdom or in primitive man, neither is type-2. That this form of the disease is a result of environmental and lifestyle factors is demonstrated when people migrate and adopt the eating habits of their new country. Populations who migrate to westernized countries with more sedentary lifestyles have greater risks of type-2 diabetes than their counterparts who remain in their native countries.[9] But it is not just the change in exercise patterns that causes the greater susceptibility to diabetes; populations undergoing westernization in the absence of migration – for example, Native Americans[9] and Western Samoans,[10] who remain in their own countries – have also experienced increases in both obesity and type-2 diabetes.

Gestational diabetes

Another form of diabetes, called gestational diabetes, can develop during pregnancy, usually during the second or third trimester and generally resolves after the baby has been delivered. The condition is usually treated by diet; however, insulin injections may be required. Women who have this form of diabetes are at increased risk for developing type-2 diabetes within five to 10 years.

The scale of the problem

Diabetes was once a very rare condition, but it has become so common since the advent of 'healthy eating' that it will soon touch most people's lives. According to Diabetes UK, there are currently 1.4 million diagnosed diabetics in the UK, with a further million undiagnosed. With 33,000 diabetic deaths in the UK every year – that's one death in every seven – diabetes is now reckoned to be the fourth leading cause of death after heart disease, cancer and doctors. Diabetics also account for 49,419,319 patient days in hospital, based on 1999/2000 figures.

Many people think of diabetes as a minor complaint. It isn't. People with diabetes are at greatly increased risk of coronary heart disease (CHD). For example, women aged 40-59 with diabetes are eight times more likely to die of CHD than women without diabetes.

A wide range of complications occurs among patients with diabetes. These are caused by damage to small blood vessels (microvascular complications) leading in turn to blindness (*retinopathy*), kidney failure (*nephropathy*) and nerve damage (*neuropathy*); and damage to the larger arteries (macrovascular complications) leading in turn to damage to the brain (stroke), the heart (CHD) or to the legs and feet (peripheral vascular disease). It can also lead to difficulties in pregnancy, infection, periodontal disease and many other conditions. So a diagnosis of diabetes should be taken very seriously even though, as will become clear later, its cure and prevention are easily accomplished.

The UK Prospective Diabetes Study (UKPDS) – a multi-centre trial on people with newly diagnosed type-2 diabetes – found that nearly half of those recruited to the trial had one or more complication.[11] About a quarter already had CHD. The US National Diabetes Data Group and the World Health Organization have established that much of type-2 diabetes is undiagnosed, that onset of type-2 occurs at least seven years before its diagnosis, and that significant ill health and premature deaths occur in subjects with undiagnosed diabetes. Table 20.1 lists the complications

Table 20.1: Prevalence of complications of diabetes amongst people with newly diagnosed diabetes, 1977/91, United Kingdom, in percentages [12]

Retinopathy	21%
Abnormal electro-cardiogram	18%
Myocardial infarction	2%
Angina	3%
Stroke/transient ischaemic attack	1%
Intermittent claudication	3%
Absent foot pulses/ischaemic feet	14%
Impaired reflexes/decreased sense of vibration	7%

already evident in people newly diagnosed with diabetes. Note that, as these are new cases, they are likely to be the healthiest. Diabetes is often not diagnosed until complications have occurred.

The Global Burden of Disease Project estimates that in established market economies such as the UK, 3% of years of life lost in disability are due to diabetes. This is only slightly less than the years of life lost in disability due to cancer at 4%.[13,14] What is more, diabetes is becoming epidemic in the UK, with the number of sufferers set to double in a decade.

To address this, the Government published the *National Service Framework for Diabetes: Delivery Strategy* in January 2003, outlining clinical targets for reducing the impact of diabetes:

- Improving blood glucose control as hyperglycaemia is the major contributor to diabetic complications.[15]
- Reducing cholesterol levels in people with diabetes.
- And, as most type-2 diabetics are overweight, a reduction in weight.

Diagnosis

If you are diagnosed as diabetic, you should take the diagnosis seriously, but don't think you are necessarily doomed to a shorter life full of ill-health. The good news is that there's plenty of evidence that with the right diet, you will have no symptoms and can live a normal life without ever having to resort to drugs.

The diagnosis of diabetes is based solely on numbers – the fasting level of glucose in the blood of 7 mmols/L (126 mg/dL) and glucose levels two hours after eating of 11 mmols/L (200 mg/dL) of glucose. Above those numbers you are diabetic, below them you are not. So, get your glucose levels down and, essentially, your diabetes is cured. And as glucose is raised almost entirely by dietary carbohydrates, a switch to a low-carb, high-fat diet is an instant cure for type-2 diabetes, although the underlying insulin resistance will still remain; and also greatly helps with type-1.

Conventional treatment worsens diabetes

When someone is diagnosed as diabetic, they are advised on diet and lifestyle ostensibly so that they can modify those risks and live a healthier life with their condition under control. However, greater patient 'knowledge' does not translate into a better outcome: diabetics do not get better; they almost invariably get worse. For this reason it is assumed by the 'experts' that the knowledge patients are given by their doctors is not being complied with.

However, dietary maltreatment of diabetes is endemic in our society. Patients *are* listening and complying but they are being given the wrong information by the medical profession. That this is so was highlighted in a study published in 2005 which revealed the ineptitude of diabetic advisors and the inadequacy of current treatment for diabetes.[16]

Doctors are poor teachers because they themselves are taught wrongly – by very large and wealthy corporations, including pharmaceutical companies, whose motives are not to improve people's health, but to maximize profit. The truth is being, well, 'doctored'.

And so drugs are still dispensed to type-2 diabetics to lower blood sugar, even though such drugs essentially force the beta cells of the pancreas to produce more and more insulin until such time that overstressed beta cells are worn out. At this point, the type-2 diabetic, who originally produced plenty of insulin, and whose problem was merely one of insulin resistance, now starts losing the ability to produce insulin and becomes insulin deficient (type-1) as well. This is a much more serious and problematic disorder – and it's entirely his doctor's fault.

In a similar way, type-1 diabetics, by being told to inject as much insulin as necessary to compensate for their wholly unsuitable – but recommended – diet, which is extremely high in foods that convert into sugar, ultimately acquire insulin resistance, and develop type-2 diabetes as well.

The diabetes authorities are well aware their policies are harmful. This is illustrated by the following text from the American Diabetes Association's website, which, under the heading 'THE DIABETES FOOD PYRAMID: STARCHES', reads: 'The message today: Eat more starches! It is healthiest for everyone to eat more whole grains, beans, and starchy vegetables such as peas, corn, potatoes and winter squash.' The ADA's website then admits that: 'Yes, foods with carbohydrate – starches, vegetables, fruits, and dairy products – will raise your blood glucose more quickly than meats and fats.' This, of course, is exactly what every diabetic should avoid doing at all costs. But the ADA say that these high-carbohydrate foods: 'are the healthiest' for diabetics. Are they serious? They warn patients: 'Your doctor may need to adjust your medications when you eat more carbohydrates.' I'll say he will – upwards!

It goes on: 'You may need to increase your activity level or try spacing carbohydrates throughout the day.' In other words, you have now got to find a way to minimize the harm that increased carbohydrate intake causes. Surely this advice borders on insanity.

Let's get some sanity back into diabetes treatment

It is a disgrace that diabetics of both types become worse by following current medical recommendations and treatment. This is a disease that is reversible, and in most cases curable by paying attention to decades of metabolic science.

Sanity for type-1

The medical profession generally regards type-1 diabetes as incurable. It is managed conventionally with a low-fat, carbohydrate-based diet. As such a diet inevitably puts large amounts of glucose in the bloodstream, daily insulin injections have to be administered to bring these high levels down to normal. This means walking a tightrope for life, as exactly the right amount of insulin must be given or it will either reduce glucose levels too much or not enough. But the human body rarely produces no insulin at all. At diagnosis of type-1 diabetes, some 5 to 15% of the pancreas's beta cells are usually still producing insulin. If these are relieved of the burden of continually reducing excessive levels of glucose, this helps to preserve beta cell function and they can often produce sufficient insulin for the variety of other metabolic processes that need it, without supplementation with injected insulin.

Until recently, the only hope of reversing the disease seemed to be replacement of beta cells by transplantation. However, in 2005, a team from the University of California in Los Angeles showed that most people with long-standing type-1 diabetes – in some cases as long as 60 years – still had detectable insulin-producing beta cells in their pancreas.[17] Regeneration of beta-cells may well be possible if they are not taxed by a high-carb intake. In which case type-1 diabetes may be reversible.

One of the mechanisms underlying this increased beta cell death involves glucose toxicity. Thus, merely reducing carbohydrate intake, particularly from fruit and cereals, may be all that is required to cure the condition, or at least reduce the symptoms of type-1 diabetes from a serious health hazard to a mere annoyance. And, even if it is still necessary to inject insulin, the amount needed can be reduced substantially.

This hypothesis that type-1 diabetics could live a normal life without having to inject insulin has the backing of evidence from a Polish doctor, Jan Kwaśniewski, who has successfully treated type-1 diabetics for over 30 years merely by reducing their carbohydrate intake to 'an amount dictated by the insulin-producing capacity of the sufferer', he told me. This amount, he says, typically equates to 1.5 grams of carbohydrate per kilogram body weight for a growing child and between 40 and 50 grams for an adult per day. With this regime, the main energy source is animal fat. On such a diet, his type-1 diabetic patients no longer needed to inject insulin.

Sanity for type-2

Lech Wałęsa, the leader of the Solidarity union in Poland, the man primarily responsible for the downfall of the Communist regime in that country, and its first president after the downfall, was an insulin-using, type-2 diabetic. He was treated by the best diabetic professors in Poland as well as an American doctor and a Japanese professor – and he was getting steadily worse. By the time he consulted Dr Kwaśniewski in 2002, Wałęsa had been on insulin for 10 years and was injecting 52 units a day. His condition was so serious that he also had to spend three days a month in hospital. After he adopted a new diet, however, all that changed. In 2005, Wałęsa no longer injected insulin or took drugs; he had no symptoms and was effectively no longer diabetic. The diet he changed to is the diet recommended in this book.

Type-2 diabetes is easily treated without the need for any drugs at all. It is also very easily prevented. All it needs is a reduction in carbohydrate consumption – particularly from cereal grains (bread, pasta, rice, breakfast cereals, et cetera) and fruit, replacing the energy lost with animal fats.

And as the last chapter demonstrated, such a diet is also the best to reduce obesity, so it kills both birds with the one stone.

Carbs alone raise blood glucose and insulin

All carbs are digested quickly. Within a very short time after a carb-rich 'healthy' meal the level of glucose in your bloodstream will rise rapidly.[18] We saw in Figure 19.1 of the last chapter that a high-carb meal increased blood glucose dramatically whereas a high-fat meal had practically no effect at all.

High blood glucose levels are harmful to the body and, as levels of glucose rise rapidly in the bloodstream, your pancreas produces a large amount of insulin to take the excess glucose out. This was shown clearly in Figure 19.2. A healthy insulin level is one below 40 pmol/L.

Not surprisingly, a 'healthy' carbohydrate-based diet, whether or not it is low-GI, gives by far the worst control of blood glucose and insulin levels. You will note that insulin levels after a carb-rich meal don't return to normal for some four hours.

Protein reduces glucose – but increases insulin

Current research confirms what has been known for many years: a high-protein diet lowers blood glucose levels after meals in people with type-2 diabetes and improves overall glucose control.[19] A study in which protein intake was doubled while carbs were reduced gave impressive results by reducing 24-hour blood glucose by a huge 40%. There were also significant decreases in glycosylated haemoglobin and triglycerides after just five weeks. This was all to the good. However, while the effect on

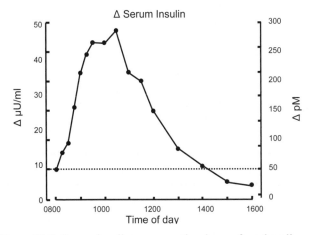

Figure 20.1: Serum insulin response: the change from baseline.

glucose was beneficial, the addition of 50 grams of beef caused a prompt three-fold rise in mean insulin levels. Figure 20.1 shows that this was still at a maximum after two-and-a-half hours, and it did not return to a fasting value until more than six hours after the meal. This effect may not be so beneficial.

Fat gives the best control

We are often told that eating fat increases glucose and insulin levels. Like most dietary advice today it is quite wrong: dietary fat has practically no effect on either glucose or insulin. This has been confirmed by many studies, some of which were discussed in the previous chapter, that have shown clearly that eating fat gives by far the best control over glucose and insulin levels.

To sum up: carbs raise both blood glucose and insulin; protein reduces glucose, but increases insulin; only fat gives good control over both. Not surprisingly, currently recommended, 'healthy' carbohydrate-based diets for diabetics look to be totally inappropriate.

High fibre carbs don't help . . .

Diabetics are told to eat high-fibre foods such as wholemeal bread as, having a 'lower glycaemic index', they don't raise insulin levels so quickly. But, like many other recommendations, it doesn't work very well in practice.[20] Wholemeal flour is only marginally better than white flour. The real answer is to cut out bread altogether.

... and fruit is not a healthy addition

Diabetics are also told to eat 'five portions of fruit and vegetables a day.' But fruit and vegetables contain the sugar, fructose.

The belief is that, while glucose raises blood levels and, consequently, insulin levels quickly, as fructose doesn't require insulin, it is healthier for diabetics. But again it isn't that simple. The aim of the dietary advice is to reduce the risk of complications. In this respect fructose does not seem to be a good choice because according to established evidence: 'Fructose glycosylates haemoglobin seven times faster than glucose.'[21] 'Glycosylates' means that it combines with protein. Haemoglobin is the protein in red blood cells that carries oxygen around the body. When haemoglobin is glycosylated in this way, this stops it from performing its function properly. Glycosylation also makes blood 'sticky'. This renders it more likely to clot, to stick to the artery walls and to block the small capillaries in the eyes, kidneys, brain and lower legs so that fresh, oxygenated blood cannot reach these parts. This is the cause of the damage to eyes, kidneys, nerves and peripheral blood vessels associated with diabetes.

This tendency to glycosylation is also important because glycosylation of proteins such as LDL and HDL particles increases the growth rate of atheroma, generally believed to cause heart disease.[22] Fructose also appears to increase total cholesterol primarily by raising LDL.[23]

It appears that LDL rises by more than 1% for every 2% increase in dietary fructose. Dr Swanson and colleagues at the Department of Medicine, School of Public Health, University of Minnesota, say: 'There is now reason to believe that dietary fructose will increase the risk of atherosclerosis.'[23] So one has to ask: why are diabetics told to eat so much fruit?

The uselessness of drug treatment

As a result of current advice, type-2 diabetics can expect to put on weight, and to have increasing levels of blood glucose and insulin. They will then be put on drugs which operate in several ways:

- Alpha glucosidase inhibitors (acarbose) inhibit absorption of glucose from the gut. (If you are going to stop the absorption of a food, why waste money on buying it in the first place?)
- Biguanides (metformin) force muscle cells to absorb more glucose. (Wouldn't it be better not to get too much glucose in the blood in the first place?)
- Sulphonylureas make the pancreas produce and release ever more insulin to combat the rising levels of glucose in the blood. (Again, wouldn't it be better not to get too much glucose in the blood in the first place?)

Eventually, they may be forced to inject insulin when their pancreas is finally worn out by this constant excessive production of insulin and gives up.

More recently added to the anti-diabetic drugs arsenal are the *PPAR-gamma agonists*, *Actos* and *Avandia*. These activate *PPAR-gamma receptors*, which are nuclear receptors designed to multiply fat cells. So, these drugs lower your blood sugar by increasing the number of fat cells faster to accommodate more fat. They don't fix the underlying problem – over-consumption of carbohydrates – they merely allow your body to reduce its blood glucose by storing more of it as fat. And once those fat cells become resistant to insulin you're back to where you started – only a lot fatter. So your drug doses are increased (again), and you end up in a never-ending vicious cycle of increasing weight and deteriorating health. It doesn't help that both drugs apparently significantly increase your risk of heart failure.[24]

The problems of high insulin

As we saw in the previous chapter, a carbohydrate-based meal causes a large and rapid rise in blood insulin. The insulin takes excess energy out of the bloodstream and stores it as fat. The result of this is weight gain. Insulin also inhibits use of energy from fat cells, which means that you won't lose any weight.

But insulin does much more harm than that. It:

- increases the risk of thrombosis (blood clots),
- increases arterial plaque formation (the 'furring up' of arteries leading to heart attacks and strokes),
- prevents plaque regression,
- stimulates connective tissue synthesis and also stimulates the production of insulin-like growth factor 1 (IGF-1).[25,26]
- raises systolic and diastolic blood pressure levels significantly both before and after meals.
- increases blood pressure by forcing the kidneys to retain sodium and by enhancing the flow of sodium and calcium into artery walls.

All of these factors increase the risk of both heart attack and stroke.

And it doesn't stop there: insulin is known to increase cancer risk, particularly prostate, endometrial and breast cancers,[27] and it makes cancers more likely to spread (metastasize).[28] It is also associated with polycystic ovarian syndrome (PCOS).[29] And insulin is suspected to be involved in gestational hypertension, pre-eclampsia[30] and osteoporosis.[28]

Diabetes and heart disease

The reasoning behind conventional dietary treatments is based on the fact that diabetics suffer higher rates of heart disease than non-diabetics. With this in mind, it didn't seem like a good idea to advise a high-fat diet. However, while diabetics suffer a rate of heart disease eight times as high as non-diabetics, they don't have cholesterol levels that are eight times as high. Going back to the days of relative sanity in diabetes treatment, Dr Elliot P. Joslin of Boston, Massachusetts, traced 97% of his diabetes cases over a 36-year period. He was aware of the believed importance of cholesterol in heart disease so he measured it against the amount of arteriosclerosis in his patients. He found that blood cholesterol values were not high in adults with arteriosclerosis. Neither were their cholesterol levels definitely correlated with any impending or existing arteriosclerotic process. In fact, he said: 'The group with the lowest average cholesterol is the group with the greatest arteriosclerosis.'[31]

That was in 1930. In 1995 it was again shown that a 'healthy' carb-based diet increased the risk of a heart attack in diabetics. Dr Y. D. Chen and colleagues say: 'In general, study has demonstrated that multiple risk factors for coronary heart disease are worsened for diabetics who consume the low-fat, high-carbohydrate diet so often recommended to reduce these risks.'[32] This was published in the medical journal, *Diabetes Care*, so the people who are still promoting such diets can hardly say they don't know.

Cholesterol-lowering drugs and nerve damage

One of the complications of diabetes is damage to nerves in the feet, legs and other extremities called *peripheral neuropathy*. Because of the increased heart disease risk, diabetics are also preferentially prescribed cholesterol-lowering statin drugs. However, a Danish study has reported that a small percentage of healthy people who took statin drugs were four to 14 times more likely to develop neuropathies than those who did not take statins.[33] To compound this, such neuropathies will almost invariably be attributed to diabetes. Physicians should be aware of this potential toxicity, monitor patients appropriately[34] and not give statins to diabetics.

Conclusion

A low-fat, high-carbohydrate diet plus regular exercise is the regime currently advised for diabetics. But it is self-evident that such a diet is less than satisfactory: carbohydrate-based diets raise blood glucose and insulin secretion after meals, thereby increasing the risk of CHD, high blood pressure, high blood cholesterol, obesity and even diabetes itself.

Over the past three decades, there has been a significant decrease in fat consumption and an increase in carbohydrate consumption. The current epidemics of diabetes and obesity are concurrent with this change in diet.

It is now clear that, from a public health point of view, an alternative dietary approach is needed. Carbohydrate restriction is a prima facie candidate for dietary control of diabetes. Evidence from randomized controlled trials over many years shows that such diets are not only safe and effective, but have other positive health benefits as well.

The objections continually raised in the scientific literature about low-carb, high-fat regimes have very little evidential basis. Type-2 diabetes is easily treated without any need to resort to drugs. It is also very easily prevented.

Type-1 diabetes is also better treated with such a low-carb, high-fat diet. In this case it is even possible that injected insulin may no longer be needed. But even if it is, lowering carb intake will certainly reduce insulin which, in turn, will make blood sugar levels easier to control.

In a nutshell, you should drastically reduce your carb consumption – particularly from grains, sugars and fruit – and increase your intake of fat and protein from animal sources. This will lower your carbohydrate load, slow your blood glucose rise and markedly improve glycaemic control.

This is not just a treatment regime for diabetes, it is a complete cure, at least for type-2. It is also preventative for anyone at high risk of diabetes and its many complications.

WARNING
If you are a type-1 diabetic injecting insulin, or a type-2 taking a drug that increases your pancreas's insulin production, then you MUST reduce the dose as you reduce your carb intake to compensate for the lower levels of glucose in your blood or you risk a hypo. The way to do this is to lower both carbs and insulin (or drug) simultaneously in small amounts over several weeks. Remember, if you only make small changes, you can only make small mistakes.

Chapter Twenty-One

Diseases of the heart and blood vessels

Most cardiovascular diseases are attributed to dietary fats and cholesterol. This chapter looks at alternative, evidence-based possibilities and finds the case for carbohydrates and consequent high blood insulin levels being to blame more persuasive.

All published efforts to help by drug or dietary reduction of blood cholesterol have uniformly failed.

Professor Sir John McMichael

By the time the establishment began its crusade aimed at preventing premature heart disease deaths in the 1980s, the number of such deaths had already fallen by 30% from their peak in the 1960s. Today, people are exercising like crazy, changing their diets, gulping supplements and taking expensive drugs to lower their cholesterol. Yet none of this is making a dent in heart attack statistics. Indeed, 'healthy' advice to increase fruit and starches in the diet and eat less fat appears to have had the opposite effect to that intended, and numbers of cases of cardiovascular diseases have risen since we took that advice on board.

Atherosclerosis

Atherosclerosis is what 'healthy eating' is aimed at preventing. It is a condition in which arteries become blocked or partially blocked, effectively reducing the interior diameter of the artery, thus restricting blood flow. The body then either increases blood pressure, or oxygen transport around the body is decreased. If the coronary arteries are involved, the heart muscle is starved of the oxygen it needs. That results in the chest pain called angina and, eventually, as arteries become completely blocked by either atherosclerosis or a blood clot, a heart attack.

Orthodox treatment for atherosclerosis includes bypass surgery in which the blocked coronary artery is removed and a piece of vein is grafted in to replace it. Another method is a 'stent', a metal lattice which is inserted into the partially blocked artery to hold it open. Neither treatment addresses the cause of the disease, nor does either do anything to help other arteries which may be affected. Both treatments are expensive, invasive and potentially life-threatening;[1] often their benefits do not last long and they have to be repeated. The few times they have been studied to assess their usefulness they have failed to demonstrate any improvement in the long-term survival.

In 1953 a brilliant Canadian physician, Dr G. C. Willis, made the crucial observation that atherosclerosis mainly occurs in the vessels near the heart. What was so special about them? Although wide and apparently strong, Willis thought it was their very proximity to the heart that was the problem. The sheer pumping force of the heart put those vessels under constant mechanical stress, thus weakening them. So, the deposition of fat, he suggested, was a means of artificially thickening the arteries to prevent damage.[2] It was a valid hypothesis. Thirty years later, Drs Michael Brown and Joseph Goldstein were awarded the 1985 Nobel Prize in Medicine for the discovery that atherosclerotic plaques are deposited in response to injury of the blood vessel wall.[3] Where arteries pass through bony channels in the skull or through the heart muscle, they never develop atherosclerosis. This suggests that the stiffening action of atherosclerosis is actually a protective measure.[4]

And atherosclerosis may not be so important as was thought. A report published in 2005 on autopsies of adults who had suffered sudden cardiac deaths found that the most common cause of heart deaths was not blockage of the coronary arteries, but arrhythmia.[5] As far as we know, arrhythmia is *not* caused by any dietary constituent, but by physical or mental stress.

Here is a curious fact which you can check with any veterinary surgeon. There are three basic types of animal when it comes to diet: herbivores which eat only plants, omnivores which eat both meat and plants, and carnivores, which eat only meat. While all three types can suffer a heart attack, the only animals in which atherosclerosis builds up are those that eat plants, whether they eat plants exclusively or together with meat. And this includes humans. This suggests that, contrary to popular wisdom, it is not something in meat that is the contributory factor, but something in plants.

Coronary heart disease

Coronary heart disease took off in the 1920s, but atherosclerosis of the coronary arteries, which the medical establishment teaches is the cause, doesn't happen overnight; it takes many years. So what factor introduced in the late 19th century could explain the later occurrence of the disease?

Dr Kilmer McCully, Chief of Pathology and Laboratory Medicine, Boston, told me that: 'The introduction of food processing with the Industrial Revolution in the 19th century and the use of chemical additives and other processes in the 20th century is the only satisfactory explanation for the dramatic changes in incidence of vascular disease in the 20th century.' The major dietary change brought about by such food processing was a marked reduction in the B group of vitamins in such processed foods. This leads to an increase in an amino acid called *homocysteine* in the blood. Numerous studies have shown an independent relationship between raised levels of homocysteine and cardiovascular diseases.[6] Starting at 10 μmol/L, there is a linear increase in cardiovascular risk as homocysteine levels rise.[7] The B vitamins, particularly B_{12} and folic acid, prevent this occurrence and, thus, prevent diseases affecting the blood system. There is strong evidence that we should ditch unreliable measurements of cholesterol (more on that below) and concentrate on increasing B vitamins while using homocysteine as a measuring tool.

Studies challenge the cholesterol theory

None of the many human intervention studies into the causes of heart disease conducted over the last half century looked solely at one aspect of diet – fat. They were all 'multiple interventions' which changed several dietary constituents, and included other factors such as exercise, cigarette smoking and so on. For this reason, ascribing any benefit to just one aspect is impossible.

In 1988, however, an opportunity presented itself when a trial was conducted on a group of people suffering multiple food allergies who had high cholesterol levels.[8] Because of their range of allergies, their diet was restricted to cut out sugar (sucrose), milk and all cereal grains. In this diet most of their calories came not just from fat, but from beef fat. We are told that beef fat is 'unhealthy' because it raises cholesterol levels, but that was not confirmed in this study. Instead of rising, the patients' total blood cholesterol levels *fell* by 27.5% from an average of 6.84 mmol/L (263 mg/dL) to an average of 4.9 mmol/L (189 mg/dL); their HDL increased from 21% of the total to 32%; and their triglyceride levels decreased from an average of 1.13 g/L to a more healthy average of 0.74 g/L. The authors say:

'These findings raise an interesting question: are elevated serum cholesterol levels caused in part not by eating animal fat (an extremely "old food"), but by some factor in grains, sucrose, or milk ("new foods") that interferes with cholesterol metabolism?'

After such a study, it should be no surprise that a survey conducted in South Carolina of adults with 'bad' dietary habits – the eating of red meat, animal fats, fried foods, butter, eggs, whole milk, bacon, sausage, cheese and the using of solid fats to cook vegetables – found their blood cholesterol levels were only marginally affected by their diet.[9]

We saw in Chapter Three that CHD is rare in Polynesians who eat a high saturated fat diet. It's the same in the US. Dr William Castelli, Director of the Framingham Study, wrote in 1992: 'In Framingham, Massachusetts, the more saturated fat one ate, the more cholesterol one ate, the more calories one ate, the lower people's serum cholesterol. . .'[10]

Because cholesterol is a major component in all animals' bodies, eggs have a very high cholesterol content. That is why we are still told to eat no more than three a week. Dr Uffe Ravnskov did his own test of this theory by eating a total of 59 eggs over nine days. Did his cholesterol level shoot up? No, it fell by more than 11% from 7.23 mmol/L to 6.39 mmol/L.[11]

However, a study of one isn't much of a study. In 2008 a bigger study was published.[12] This, tabled below, also showed that total cholesterol went *down* as more eggs were eaten.

Dr George V. Mann was involved with the Framingham Study and also conducted extensive studies of the Maasai, whose diet is very high in saturated fat but who do not suffer from CHD at all. He concluded that:

> 'The diet-heart hypothesis has been repeatedly shown to be wrong, and yet, for complicated reasons or pride, profit and prejudice, the hypothesis continues to be exploited by scientists, fund-raising enterprises, food companies and even governmental agencies. The public is being deceived by the greatest health scam of the century.'[13]

In 2002 the hearts of 11 adults aged under 35 years, who had died within an hour of the onset of cardiac symptoms, were examined for the type of underlying plaque complication and the time of onset of clot formation.

Table 21.1: Intake of eggs and blood cholesterol levels

Number of eggs eaten	<1 a week	1 a week	2-4 a week	5-6 a week	1 a day	2 or more a day
Number of participants	4527	6621	697	141	1473	264
Percentage with high cholesterol	14%	12%	11%	11%	11%	9%

'High cholesterol' was defined as over 240 mg/dL (6.25 mmol/l).

Only one of the 11 culprit lesions was rich in cholesterol.[14] Careful analysis of the available data, including randomized trials, indicates that, contrary to widespread opinion, cholesterol lowering is not a very effective way of reducing cardiac deaths or overall mortality in the general population.[15]

Plants may be a danger

Because cholesterol is found only in animal products, more and more people have turned away from meat and towards eating foods from plants. But *chole*-sterol is only one of a whole family of sterols. Cholesterol is found only in animals; the other sterols are found in plants. Dr J. Plat and colleagues at Maastricht University's Department of Human Biology in the Netherlands, say that these plant sterols may actually be more important in heart disease than cholesterol. Because plant sterols are structurally related to cholesterol, Plat and colleagues examined whether oxidized plant sterols (*oxyphytosterols*) could be identified in human blood and soy-based fat emulsions. They could. Approximately 1.4% of the plant sterol, sitosterol, in blood was oxidized. This may not seem very much, but it is 140 times as much as the 0.01% oxidatively modified cholesterol normally seen in human blood. The same was also found in two soy emulsions.[16] Latest research on both humans and animals suggests that 'functional foods' aimed at lowering cholesterol may actually increase the risk of a heart attack.[17]

If any sterols are to blame, plant sterols are much more likely candidates than *chole*sterol because the popular idea that animal products, specifically protein, cholesterol, and saturated fatty acids, somehow factor in causing atherosclerosis, stroke or heart disease is not supported by any available data, including from research in the field of lipid biochemistry.[11,13,18,19] On this point, it is interesting that Dr Ancel Keys, whose 1953 hypothesis began the fatty-diet-causes-heart-disease dogma did *not* recommend cutting down on animal fats. He recommended cutting vegetable oils.

Oxidized LDL

Where the problem with LDL lies is when fatty acids that are transported *with* LDL are attacked by oxygen and oxidized.[20] In 2004 a study was conducted with patients eating two different diets.[21] Both reduced total and saturated fat intakes and increased polyunsaturated fat intakes. Conventional wisdom says that these revised diets should be 'healthier'. In fact, what happened was that the levels of *oxidized* LDL in the bloodstream *rose* in both – by 27% and 19%. Another contributor to heart disease, lipoprotein (a), also rose by 7% and 9%.

Fatty acids come in a variety of lengths. As the chain length of a fatty acid increases, it acts more and more like an oil which will not mix with water or blood. Short- and medium-chain fatty acids will mix in blood; they exit the intestine bound to the protein, albumin, whereas long-chain fatty acids with more than 12 carbon atoms do not mix and must be transported in lipoprotein carriers. LDL is used to transport these long-chain fatty acids. This may be why, in a 10-year study of fats and the numbers of heart events, researchers found that only polyunsaturated fats significantly *increased* heart disease.[22]

There is also another anomaly. You may not be aware of it, but cholesterol levels are always measured in blood taken from a vein, yet nowhere in the medical literature is there a single case of cholesterol having caused obstruction of a vein; atherosclerosis only affects arteries. As blood moves far more slowly in veins than in arteries, wouldn't that make it be more inclined to leave cholesterol deposits – if the assumption that cholesterol was the cause were true?

Carbohydrates and cardiovascular diseases

Recent large epidemiological studies have contradicted the traditional diet-heart disease hypothesis by finding that fat intake has no association with heart disease, whereas carbohydrate intake does.[23]

In 2005 a study conducted at Johns Hopkins Bloomberg School of Public Health on diagnosed and undiagnosed diabetics showed clearly that high blood glucose levels were strongly associated with heart disease.[24] This points to 'healthy' carbs being the culprit – not saturated fats. It supports another strong indicator that carbohydrates are to blame from a study of coeliac patients at the University of Nottingham. Coeliacs mustn't eat cereal grains. Although rates of heart attack and stroke were similar, adults with coeliac disease had less hypertension compared with the general population.[25]

Healthy eating' increases heart disease . . .

Heart disease deaths peaked and started to decline in the mid-20th century in both the UK and in the US. However, the number of Americans who develop heart disease may no longer be declining, say researchers.[26] Analysis showed that the number of people with any signs of coronary artery disease which had been declining, levelled off around 1995 and started to increase. The team concluded that their findings suggested that 'declines in coronary disease prevalence have ended.'

Here are some quotes from trials of our so-called 'healthy' diet:

In diabetics. 'In general, study has demonstrated that multiple risk factors for coronary heart disease are worsened for diabetics who consume the low-fat, high-carbohydrate diet so often recommended to reduce these risks.'[27] This is because high levels of glucose in the blood over a long period of time 'glycosylate' haemoglobin (see Chapter 20). This glycosylation was found to increase the risk of a heart attack in both diabetics and non-diabetics in another Johns Hopkins study,[28] in which non-diabetics' risk was more than doubled.

In older women. 'Low-fat, high-carbohydrate diets [15% protein, 60% carbohydrate, 25% fat] increase the risk of heart disease in post-menopausal women.'[29]

In the elderly. We have known for a very long time that blood choles-terol levels tend to increase as we get older. Several studies from around the world show that the elderly with high cholesterol live longer than those with low cholesterol. An East German doctor, Max Bürger, dem-onstrated almost half a century ago that, as we age, cholesterol is lost from body tissues and neurons (brain cells).[30] These findings were pub-lished in Leipzig during the Communist era, so it is unlikely that any western clinician has ever seen, let alone read them. Putting these two facts together, is it not probable that the increases in blood cholesterol seen as we age are our bodies' way of replacing cholesterol lost from tissues and nerve cells?

This has huge implications in the context of 'healthy eating'. Advice today is aimed at lowering cholesterol levels in people of all ages, but these facts together suggest that drug or dietary regimes aimed at lower-ing cholesterol in people aged over 70 might shorten their lives.

In everyone. In 2000, scientists from Stanford University School of Medicine, California, compared the effects of a low-fat, high-carb diet with a high-fat, low-carb diet, on blood fats and cholesterol. They found that subjects on the high-carb diet had significantly higher blood triglyc-erides and significantly lower HDL. These effects are not desirable. The authors concluded:

> 'Given the atherogenic potential of these changes in lipoprotein metabo-lism, it seems appropriate to question the wisdom of recommending that all Americans should replace dietary saturated fat with [carbohydrate].'[31]

Similarly, while presenting two-year results of the Glucose Abnormalities in Patients with Myocardial Infarction (GAMI) study at the European Society of Cardiology Congress 2004,[32] Dr Lars of the Rydén Karolinska University Hospital, Solna, Sweden, said that abnormal glucose metabolism is common in acute heart attack patients. Even high-normal levels, below the diagnostic target for diabetes, increase the risk for mortality and cardiovascular disease. Forget cholesterol; the strongest predictor of a future heart attack was high blood glucose. The following year another study confirmed that when blood glucose levels were raised for significant lengths of time, the risk of a heart attack was greatly increased.[27] Long-term blood glucose levels are measured by the amount they glycosylate haemoglobin. The measurement is known as 'HbA1c' or 'haemoglobin A1c'. What this study showed was that, in diabetic adults, each 1% increase in HbA1c increased the risk of a heart attack by 14%. And in non-diabetics with a level of over 4.6%, each 1% increase in HbA1c increased the risk of a heart attack by a huge 136%. Long-term high glucose levels are, of course, only caused by eating a 'healthy' diet.

High-fat, low-carb diets reduce heart disease risk

By the end of the 20th century, low-carb diets were becoming increasingly popular and nutritionists kept insisting that they would increase cholesterol. In 2002, scientists at the University of Connecticut decided to test this claim with a very low-carbohydrate, high-fat diet on normal-weight men with normal cholesterol levels. The diet contained only 8% of calories from carbs, with 61% of their calories from fats.[33] With a diet in which nearly two-thirds of calories came from fat, you might expect – because that is what you have been led to believe – that cholesterol would rise. In fact, it did just the opposite: cholesterol actually fell by 29% and HDL went up by more than 11%. But this wasn't all: triglycerides, which are more harmful in terms of heart disease, fell by a whopping 33% and insulin fell by 34%.

That last study covered only six weeks. In the same year, doctors at the Division of General Internal Medicine, Duke University, conducted a similar six-month study.[34] Patients could eat as much meat, cheese, eggs, fish, butter and fat as they wanted, but their carb intake was restricted to no more than 25 grams a day. Over the period of the study, the participants lost an average of 9.7 kilograms (21.3 lbs), their cholesterol fell by 6.1%, there was an almost 40% drop in the level of triglycerides in their blood and their HDL increased by about 7%. In an interview for Reuters Health, the study's main author, Dr Eric Westman, said: 'We were somewhat surprised to find that patients' blood lipid profiles improved, even though there was much more fat in the diet. We had thought the fat in the diet would increase the cholesterol.'

Summary

Ever since 'healthy eating' was introduced in the 1980s, the establishment has tried to show that a diet high in animal-fat is harmful. Yet not a single trial has ever managed to do this. This might surprise you, but it should not as it was shown as long ago as 1968 that 'hyperlipidaemia [high blood fats] can be controlled by a diet which is low in *unsaturated* fat . . .'[35] (emphasis added). You see, the only fats that have *ever* been implicated in heart disease are polyunsaturated vegetable oils. Yet, perversely, we are told to eat more of them!

Early testing doesn't help

Doctors reckon that, to reduce heart disease, it is necessary to screen for the disease regularly so that it can be caught in its earliest stages and treated before it gets too bad. Unfortunately, the figures don't support the theory. Doctors in Canada and the US ordered more cardiac tests and procedures between 1993 and 2001 than ever before – yet there was no reduction in the number of heart attacks over the period. This is extremely worrying, they said, as all this testing is pushing the Canadian health insurance system to breaking point and heart care costs have doubled in the last decade.[36]

But early testing will never be of benefit if the follow-up care is based on a flawed premise. What the evidence shows is that it is carbs and polyunsaturated fatty acids that increase the heart attack risk. Yet those are exactly the foods that people thought to be at risk of a heart attack are told to eat. It's lunacy – and expensive lunacy, at that.

Congestive heart failure

It seems that high blood glucose levels may also be an important cause of another disease of the heart: congestive heart failure (CHF). United States researchers had found evidence to suggest that raised fasting blood glucose levels were a risk factor for CHF among elderly individuals, particularly those who had diabetes. CHF and diabetes are disorders that frequently coexist.

Despite this, there was uncertainty as to whether raised glucose levels act as a risk factor for CHF, as studies produced conflicting results. To investigate this further, Dr Joshua Barzilay and colleagues at Emory University School of Medicine, Atlanta, Georgia, studied patients, aged 65 years and above, for up to eight years.[37] They discovered that each one 'standard deviation' increase in fasting blood glucose *increased* the risk of CHF by 41%. Dr Barzilay and team suggested that raised glucose levels might affect CHF risk in several ways: the glucose might compromise artery linings and affect blood flow to the heart, or cause fibrosis and stiffness of the heart muscle itself.

Or is it low cholesterol?

'In patients with CHF, lower serum total cholesterol is independently associated with a worse prognosis.' Those were the conclusions of a study looking at the relationship between blood cholesterol levels and CHF.[38] The study found that for each *increase* of 1.0 mmol/L (38.5 mg/dL) in blood cholesterol: 'The chance of survival increased 25%.' The best predictor of *increased* death rate in the study was a cholesterol level *lower* than 5.2 mmol/L (200 mg/dL). Although published in 2003, this study was completely ignored as a major adverse side effect of cholesterol-lowering drugs, which aim to get everyone's cholesterol down much lower than 5.2 (200).

Deep vein thrombosis (DVT)

DVT is a condition where clots (thromboses) form in the deep veins of the legs, which may then travel to other parts of the body. If the clot goes to and blocks a major blood vessel – in the lungs or heart, for example – it can have fatal consequences. It is euphemistically called 'economy class syndrome' because it was first reported in people who sat for long periods in the economy section of aircraft on long-haul flights. More recently it has also been reported in people who sit for long periods at their office desks.

When my wife and I flew out to Singapore in 1962, we had never heard of DVT. There we were, sat on an aircraft for 24 hours with not the slightest knowledge of such things. But, in those days, neither had anyone else. Planes were slower; they were also smaller, with less room to move around; and we sat for much longer. So why didn't we get DVT in those days? Why is it that DVT only reared its ugly head in the last decade or so?

The reason was probably because of what we ate in those days. The answer to DVT is not necessarily to move about more, do special exercises and wear anti-DVT stockings. These all may reduce the risk, but they don't address the cause: a carb-based 'healthy' diet. All one needs to do to prevent DVT is eat less carbohydrate-rich foods.

Peripheral artery disease and intermittent claudication

Peripheral arterial disease (PAD), whether symptomatic or not, is a condition where the arteries of the legs and feet are wholly or partially blocked. It affects between 10% and 25% of people over the age of 50. PAD is most commonly caused by blood clots and clogged arteries but may reflect the existence of another condition such as arteritis, aneurysm or embolism. In recent years, it has become evident that PAD is an important predictor of substantial coronary and stroke risk. A 10-year study conducted at the University of Minnesota found factors which increased the risk of PAD. No, not raised blood cholesterol, but raised levels of glucose and insulin in the blood.[39]

Intermittent claudication is a cramping pain most often felt in calf and leg muscles which is induced by exercise and relieved by rest. It is the result of partial or complete blockages of the leg arteries. Leg pulses are often absent and feet are often cold. A complication of diabetes, claudication leading to gangrene is the most common reason for leg amputation. Reducing blood glucose levels has been found to be very effective in alleviating this condition.[40] And the best way to do that is with a low-carb diet.

Strokes

The risk of recurrent stroke is increased in people with impaired glucose tolerance according to Dr Sarah Vermeer and co-workers at Erasmus Medical Center, Rotterdam.[41] Compared with patients who had normal glucose levels (5.8-7.7 mmol/l), stroke risk was nearly doubled in those with impaired glucose tolerance (7.8-11.0 mmol/l) and nearly tripled in patients with diabetes (greater than 11.0 mmol/l).

A high glucose load after a carbohydrate-rich meal also has adverse effects in healthy people according to a study conducted at the University of Gothenburg, Sweden. Here, scientists found that a high-carbohydrate meal had significant effects in humans: after such a meal, there was a marked alteration in the pattern of the circulatory responses to psychosocial stress, characterized by a much reduced increase in the diameter of blood vessels and a rise in systemic vascular resistance and systolic blood pressure.[42]

High blood glucose levels and consequent high blood insulin levels produce two effects that are responsible for inducing strokes.[43-45] They are: increased thickening and stickiness of the blood, which tends to clot and block the blood vessels, and the increased permeability of the capillary walls leading to the smaller blood vessels and capillaries leaking and rupturing.

Many studies have demonstrated that a breakdown of the *endothelium*, the inner lining of arteries and veins, occurs early in the insulin-resistant state and can predict future cardiovascular events. Similarly, insulin resistance also increases the risk of adverse cardiovascular outcomes. In July 2004, Dr Willa A. Hsueh and colleagues at the Division of Endocrinology, Diabetes and Hypertension, University of California at Los Angeles, reviewed evidence that improving the function of the endothelium with a variety of drugs could prevent both cardiovascular disease and diabetes.[46] However, as raised glucose levels are an independent risk factor for stroke in people both with and without diabetes,[47] by reducing the levels of insulin in the blood, a low-carb, high-fat/protein diet does the same job naturally, making unnatural drugs redundant.

Considering the strong link between obesity and hypertension, it's easy to understand why there has been such a steep rise in hypertension among Americans in recent years. Obesity has reached epidemic proportions in the US, and the enormously high levels of hypertension among the population appear to follow this trend closely. Some 25% of the adult US population suffers from high blood pressure and the problem is even more widespread among the elderly, of whom 50% are sufferers. Simply put, the heavier we become, the more prone we are to hypertension. This adds to the weight of evidence against our so-called 'healthy' diet.

Aspirin is dangerous

To ward off a heart attack or stroke, middle-aged men are routinely advised by their GPs to take a daily dose of aspirin. Aspirin has been around for a long time and is generally regarded as entirely safe. It isn't. The increased risk of death to a 50-year-old man from taking his small aspirin pill is 10.4 extra deaths per 100,000 men per year.[48] That might not sound a lot, but it is almost identical to the added risk that professional fire fighters face of 10.6 deaths per 100,000 people per year, compared with 0.4 for office workers.[49] The risk is much higher than using a cell phone while driving[50] – and we legislate against that! It's much safer to change your diet.

Conclusion

We have now had over half a century of the cholesterol hypothesis and wasted countless billions of research dollars and pounds, yet we have still to achieve what cattle-herders in Kenya can do merely by possessing a cow for food – achieve freedom from heart disease.

There is widespread dissatisfaction with the cholesterol idea, with more and more doctors seeing it for the fiasco it really is. However, many members of the medical profession and academicians have such a lot invested in the 'fat-causes-heart-disease' paradigm that it would now be professional and academic suicide for them to admit the truth.

But you don't have to put up with it; you can do something about this mess, yourself. The evidence has demonstrated that it is not animal fats and cholesterol which increase the risk of a heart attack, but glucose and insulin in the blood. And glucose and insulin are raised only when we eat a so-called 'healthy' carbohydrate-based diet. So, to protect against cardiovascular diseases, merely reduce your intake of fruits, bread, pasta, and cereals and replace them with foods such as fatty meat, eggs, fish, butter and cream.

Chapter Twenty-Two

The dangers of low blood cholesterol

We are told incessantly that high cholesterol is bad for us. But low cholesterol is far more serious. Cholesterol is an essential compound in our bodies. Low levels of cholesterol are associated with increased total mortality, cancer, Alzheimer's and Parkinson's diseases, antisocial behaviour, depression, suicide, increased susceptibility to infections and other conditions.

> Low concentrations of naturally occurring total serum cholesterol, including those levels in the currently defined 'desirable' range, were associated with poorer cognitive performance.
>
> *Dr Penelope K. Elias*

After all that you have heard about cholesterol, you may be surprised to learn that as you age, your chances of an early death *rise* if your total cholesterol falls. This disturbing finding was discovered more than 20 years ago.[1] It showed clearly that after the age of 50, heart death rates increased by 14% for every 1 mg/dL (0.026 mmol/l) *drop* in total cholesterol levels per year. Individuals whose total cholesterol levels decline by 14 mg/dL (0.364 mmol/l) during 14 years can expect an 11% higher death rate than if the level had remained the same or risen. In a British context, if your cholesterol level drops from 6.0 mmol/l to a 'healthy' 5.0 mmol/l, your relative risk of death increases four-fold. European-wide research on patients with chronic heart failure also found that those who had a higher total cholesterol lived longer. The chance of survival increased by 25% for each increase of 1.0 mmol/l (38.5mg/dL) in total cholesterol.[2]

The Japanese confirmed these results with a study conducted at

Kyushu University. This concluded that '[Total cholesterol] level reduction from 240-259 mg/dl [6.2-6.7 mmol/l] to 160-199 mg/dl [4.2-5.2 mmol/l] leads to an increase in total mortality rate in the Japanese population.'[3] The figures from this study of 55,000 men and women aged between 35 and 70 shown in Figures 22.1 and 22.2, should provide a reason for those who are trying to get their cholesterol down to reconsider that decision. You can clearly see that CHD was not affected greatly by changing blood cholesterol levels in either men or women. But low cholesterol levels were quite obviously undesirable as far as all other causes of death were concerned, death rates amongst those with *low* cholesterol levels being much higher across the board.

Recovery from existing heart failure also takes longer if you have low cholesterol. In an analysis of 1,134 patients with heart disease, low cholesterol was associated with worse outcomes and lower survival rates, while high cholesterol improved survival rates.[4] This study also showed that high cholesterol among patients was not associated with high blood pressure, diabetes, or coronary heart disease.

So if your doctor tells you that your cholesterol is high and he wants to put you on cholesterol-lowering drugs, you might like to reflect on the fact that taking them may well shorten your life – particularly if you are approaching or above the age of 50.[5] Which all rather makes a nonsense of the cholesterol hypothesis. But then, cholesterol is only a 'risk factor' for CHD; it doesn't cause CHD; it merely shows some statistical association with various coronary events. In this respect it is similar to several hundred other 'risk factors.' A diagonal earlobe crease and premature

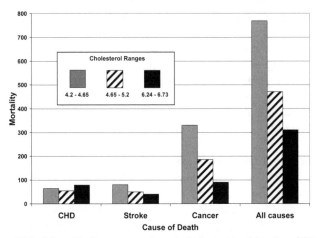

Figure 22.1: Mortality by cause and total cholesterol – Men (aged 35-70)

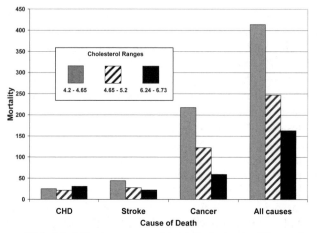

Figure 22.2: Mortality by cause and total cholesterol – Women (aged 35-70)
(Graphs compiled from data in Reference 3)

baldness are also 'risk factors' for heart disease but plastic surgery or a hair transplant won't extend your life – and neither will lowering cholesterol.

High cholesterol protects against heart disease risk

Strengthening the evidence against the 'cholesterol myth' are other findings which suggest that high cholesterol levels also protect against atherosclerosis. There is a growing amount of evidence for a hypothesis that the first step in the formation of atherosclerosis is an inflammatory response to some injury of the arterial wall caused by damage to that wall, perhaps by an infectious bacterium or virus. As we will see later in the chapter, low levels of cholesterol harm the body's immune system. Putting these two factors together shows how a high cholesterol level could actually protect against atherosclerosis. This would also explain why, although most cardiovascular diseases are seen after the age of 60, the elderly with high cholesterol have *fewer* heart attacks than those with low cholesterol.

Low cholesterol increases stroke risk

Stroke is defined as the sudden rupture or blockage by clotting of a blood vessel to or within the brain. Symptoms can range from minor dizziness or momentary temporary loss of function that is barely perceptible to paralysis or death. Strokes generally used to be confined to the very elderly, but recently have been increasingly seen in younger people.

Asians traditionally eat a diet which is poor in animal products; they have low levels of cholesterol in their blood – and have a very high level of strokes. Japanese scientists believed that their diet could be the cause of their high stroke risk. US scientists, on the other hand, were sceptical of the possibility, believing that there were few if any risks associated with low blood cholesterol. This difference in viewpoint was thought worthy of further investigation to resolve the question.

Because medical trials are expensive, they tend to involve only a relatively small number of people. But there are exceptions. One such arose after the Second World War, when the Japanese diet, influenced by American dietary habits, changed dramatically. From 1958 to 1995 fat consumption increased four-fold and animal protein intake in the form of meat, eggs and dairy products increased by 22%. At the same time, they ate less rice. This was a perfect opportunity for scientists, who noted that this change in diet brought dramatic benefits. During the period, cholesterol levels rose from averages of 3.9 mmol/l (150 mg/dL) to 5.0 mmol/l (192 mg/dL),[6] but the numbers of strokes of both types fell by 85% from 1344 to 205 per 100,000 per year.[7] Deaths from cerebral haemorrhage also declined by 65% in men and 94% in women aged 40-69.[8] Even though blood cholesterol went up, there was no increase in heart disease deaths in either sex. The authors concluded that the benefits to health in Japan were a result of blood pressure fall and a rise in total cholesterol.

A follow-up study by the Institute of Community Medicine, University of Tsukuba, Japan, over a 30-year period, confirmed the earlier findings. By that time, heart disease deaths had also fallen by 20%.[9]

A later study of both men and women aged 35 to 89 years over the period 1984 to 2001 showed clearly that the really beneficial part of the Japanese diet was their increased intake of animal fat and cholesterol.[10] In this study, the risk of a stroke was reduced by almost two-thirds (63%) in those who had the highest intake of animal fat and cholesterol, compared with those with the lowest. Animal protein was not significant – just the fat and cholesterol.

These results were not confined to Japan or even to Asia. In 1997, the results of a follow-up of 350,000 men screened for the Multiple Risk Factor Intervention Trial in the US showed that the excess risk of death from cerebral haemorrhage was six times higher in middle-aged men with low blood cholesterol levels.[11]

Scientists at the Cardiovascular Health Research Unit, Washington University, conducted an analysis of 13 randomized controlled trials to look at the effects of lowering blood cholesterol on diseases other than CHD.[12] They found that while lowering cholesterol resulted in a slight lowering of *non*-fatal strokes, fatal strokes were increased by 32%, and where cholesterol was lowered by a drug, the death rate from stroke rose by a huge 264%.

It is not just numbers of strokes that benefit from higher cholesterol levels; survival rates do as well. A team of doctors at the Acute Stroke Unit, Gardiner Institute, Glasgow, found that: 'After adjustment for known prognostic factors, higher serum cholesterol concentrations were associated with reduced long term mortality after stroke . . . Our data suggest an association between poor stroke outcome and lower serum cholesterol concentration.'[13]

Because strokes and cerebral haemorrhages are rare in younger people, there has been little research done at these lower ages. However, cerebral haemorrhages are now affecting the under-40s. Doctors at the Stroke Clinic, Instituto Nacional de Neurologia y Neurocirugia, Mexico City, looked into this new phenomenon.[14] They found a number of 'risk factors' including smoking, drinking alcohol and raised blood pressure. You might expect that high blood pressure posed the most risk, but that only accounted for 13%. The factor posing the highest risk, at 35%, was a low blood cholesterol level.

Low cholesterol increases ischaemic stroke risk

There is no doubt now that the risk of haemorrhagic stroke is increased by low cholesterol levels, but that still leaves *ischaemic* strokes. Although the effect is similar to a haemorrhagic stroke, the cause is different. For the same reason that heart attacks are blamed on cholesterol blocking coronary arteries, so are ischaemic strokes blamed on a fatty diet. But the theory that eating too much saturated fat increases the risk of a stroke is weak at best.

In 1997, the long-running Framingham study showed that for every 3% more calories from fat, ischaemic stroke risk went *down* by 15%.[11] Confirmation came six years later in yet another study. This time, scientists at the Department of Nutrition, Harvard School of Public Health, studied 43,732 men aged 40-75 years who were free from cardiovascular diseases and diabetes in 1986 and followed them for 14 years.[15] During that period they studied intakes of every conceivable type of fat: animal fat, fish oil, vegetable oil, saturated, mono-unsaturated, polyunsaturated, trans fat, as well as the amounts of each that were consumed. They found that intakes of total fat, cholesterol, or specific types of fat made no difference whatever to the risk of stroke in men.

Low cholesterol increases cancer risk

Countries with diets high in saturated fats tend to have high levels of colon cancer. In 1974 a review of the Framingham data and those from

Ancel Keys' 'Seven Countries Study' was expected to show that the cancer could also be blamed on high blood cholesterol. However, the baffled researchers found the opposite; those with cancer had cholesterol levels which were *lower* than average. In 1989, the Renfrew and Paisley Survey, studying the lowering of cholesterol to prevent heart disease, found that cases of cancer rose as cholesterol levels fell, such that any reduction in the numbers of heart deaths was more than offset by an increase in cancers, mainly lung cancer.[16] This was also the case in the World Health Organization's Cooperative Trial of the cholesterol-lowering drug, clofibrate, which was published in the same year.

We should remember that cholesterol is a vital building block in cell membranes; it is essential for their integrity and stability. It is not an alien substance that must be reduced at all costs. Professor Michael Oliver pointed to the part that cholesterol played in the integrity of body cell membranes, saying:

> 'Normal cell activity depends . . . on membrane function and permeability. This is partly dependent on the balance . . . between cholesterol and saturated and polyunsaturated fatty acids. The possibility that normal membrane function is impaired when there is a disproportionate decrease in cholesterol, with resulting loss of resistance to cancerous change, has to remain on the agenda of the risk/benefits of lowering plasma cholesterol.'[17]

Many epidemiological studies have shown consistently that cancer deaths rise in number as blood cholesterol levels fall. A German study conducted at the Medizinische Universitätsklinik II, Tübingen, investigated blood cholesterol values at the time of diagnosis in patients with Hodgkin's lymphoma and found that they were significantly lower in these patients than in age- and sex-matched people without the disease. They also noted that patients with normal cholesterol values had a five-year survival rate which was two-and-a-half times higher than in patients with low blood cholesterol.[18]

Another study published in 1990 showed that diagnosis of colon cancer was preceded over a 10-year period by a fall in blood cholesterol levels. That doesn't necessarily mean the lower cholesterol caused the cancer. There are three possibilities: that the drop in cholesterol caused the cancers, that the drop in cholesterol was a result of the cancers, or that the fall in cholesterol and the appearance of cancer at that time was merely a coincidence. The scientists looked meticulously at these possibilities and concluded that falling cholesterol was the culprit.[19] The figures are the interesting aspect of this study because the average level at diagnosis of cancer was 5.56 mmol/l (214 mg/dL), yet doctors are trying still to reduce levels of cholesterol in the general population to below 5.0 mmol/l (192 mg/dL). You might like to know that this study also specifically attributed the cancers to low levels of LDL.

Other cancers linked to low cholesterol levels include squamous cell and small cell lung cancers,[20] liver cancer,[21] multiple myeloma,[22] adrenal cancer,[23] lymphoma, acute leukaemia, chronic myeloid leukaemia, chronic myelomonocytic leukaemia, policytemia vera, myeloma, chronic lymphoid leukaemia,[24] hairy cell leukemia,[25] brain cancers[26] and gastro-intestinal cancers.[27]

So what is a dangerously low cholesterol level? Well, it's almost certainly higher than you think. Scientists at the University of Padua, Italy, analyzed cancer deaths in 3,282 men and women aged 65 years or over taking part in the 12-year CASTEL (CArdiovascular STudy in the ELderly).[28] This clearly showed an increase in cancers in people 'with very low cholesterol'. 'Very low' was defined as a level below 4.63 mmol/l (178 mg/dL). This level is close to that found in a study of middle-aged men published four years earlier: 'Serum cholesterol concentrations below 4.8 mmol/l were associated with the highest all cause mortality . . .'[29]

Incidentally, CASTEL showed that men whose body mass index was 22.7 or lower – i.e. the 'healthy' weight range – also had an increased cancer risk.

Not surprisingly, there have been several reviews of the cholesterol-cancer connection. This is of greater concern in cases where cholesterol has been lowered artificially with drug treatment as, in an increasingly litigious society, the person administering the drugs could be blamed and sued for causing the cancer. Drs T. B. Newman and S. B. Hulley of the School of Medicine, University of California, San Francisco, reviewed the findings and implications of studies of cancer and cholesterol-lowering drugs in trials involving both rodents and humans, and listed the drugs and types of tumour found. They noted in their review that: 'all members of the two most popular classes of lipid-lowering drugs (fibrates and statins) cause cancer in rodents, in some cases at levels of animal exposure close to those prescribed for humans.' But they add that: 'Evidence of carcinogenicity [cancer-causing properties] of lipid-lowering drugs from clinical trials in humans is inconclusive because of inconsistent results and insufficient duration of follow-up.'[30] Newman and Hulley concluded that longer-term surveillance needs to be carried out over the next few decades. In the meantime:

> 'the results of experiments in animals and humans suggest that lipid-lowering drug treatment, especially with the fibrates and statins, should be avoided except in patients at high short-term risk of coronary heart disease.'

However, while this surveillance is conducted, anyone taking these drugs is effectively a guinea pig in an uncontrolled trial.

Low cholesterol and other conditions

Low blood cholesterol compromises immune function

Low cholesterol levels are also associated with other, non-heart related deaths and with an increased susceptibility to infectious diseases. A group at the Center for Clinical Pharmacology, University of Pittsburgh, Pennsylvania, found that the immune systems of the men whose cholesterol averaged 3.9 mmol/l (151 mg/dL) were significantly less effective than those of men whose cholesterol was 6.8 mmol/l (261 mg/dL).[31] This finding is not surprising as several studies have shown that cholesterol is necessary for the proper functioning of blood cells – macrophages and lymphocytes – that form part of our immune systems. This could well be another reason why numbers of cases of infectious diseases have recently become more prevalent.

Tuberculosis (TB), a disease thought to have been conquered long ago, is returning. Low levels of cholesterol are common in patients suffering from TB. TB patients with low cholesterol also have higher death rates, particularly those with small (*miliary*) nodules in their lungs. A hospital for respiratory diseases tested whether giving TB patients high-cholesterol meals would be effective in treating their condition.[32] They split patients into two groups. One had meals containing 800 milligrams of cholesterol per day; the other had 250 milligrams of cholesterol per day. By the second week, the number of TB bacteria in sputum was reduced 80% in the high-cholesterol group; it was only reduced by 9% in the low-cholesterol group. High-cholesterol diets now form part of the treatment for TB.

Infections and deaths in surgical patients

Low cholesterol is also linked to increased susceptibility to postoperative infections,[33] and it predicts death and adverse outcomes in hospitalized patients.[34]

A study of patients undergoing surgery for gastrointestinal diseases at the Universita di L'Aquila in Italy, found that: 'Hypocholesterolemia [low blood cholesterol] seems to represent a significant predictive factor of morbidity and mortality in critically ill patients.'[33] Of the patients studied, 35.1% contracted a postoperative infection; three-quarters of these were in patients with cholesterol levels below 2.73 mmol/l (105 mg/dL).

The Department of Surgery, Weill Medical College of Cornell University, New York, found that lower levels of total cholesterol, and of LDL and HDL, occurred early in the course of critical illness and led to the development of a hospital infection. With or without the infection, lower cholesterol was independently associated with a higher death rate.[35]

Many patients in hospitals acquire infections during or after major abdominal surgery. The Department of Surgery at the Catholic University, Rome, Italy, conducted a study to identify factors that influenced mortality in patients who were affected by such infections.[36] The hospital records of patients who had had a variety of abdominal operations and who had acquired an infection such as peritonitis were reviewed. Checking deaths against a battery of blood measurements, the authors of the study found that low cholesterol levels and low protein levels were both 'strongly and independently associated with the outcome.'

Dr Uffe Ravnskov wrote: 'There is much evidence that blood lipids play a key role in the immune defence system. Bacterial endotoxin and *Staphylococcus aureus* α-toxin bind rapidly to and become inactivated by low-density-lipoprotein (LDL).'[37] (*Staphylococcus aureus* is what the 'SA' in MRSA stands for.) Dr Ravnskov also pointed out that: 'Total cholesterol is inversely associated with mortality caused by respiratory and digestive disease, the aetiologies of which are mostly infectious. Total cholesterol is also inversely associated with the risk of being admitted to hospital because of an infectious disease.' So if you have low cholesterol, you are more likely to end up in hospital and you are more likely to contract an infection while there.

Low cholesterol increases depression and suicide risk

Men with low cholesterol have a higher death rate from injury. Although cholesterol-lowering tends to reduce CHD mortality in certain age groups, there is no evidence that it reduces total mortality. In populations with naturally low blood cholesterol there is also a significant death rate from 'non-medical' causes. Why is there this association?

A pilot study into blood cholesterol and depression in schizophrenics found a highly significant interaction between low levels of cholesterol and depression. Extreme lowering of cholesterol with drugs altered the functional state of the 'feel good' hormone, *serotonin*. The authors suggest that: 'the degree of the low cholesterol combined with its duration might be a risk factor for the development of an abnormal mental state.'[38] Dr A. Ryman, writing in the *British Medical Journal*, said: 'Our current understanding of the relation between cholesterol metabolism and psychiatric illness is poor . . . The possibility that a low or falling cholesterol concentration is a marker of risk merits further study.'[39]

A large study at the Cholesterol Center, Jewish Hospital, Cincinnati, Ohio found that cholesterol concentrations below 4.16 mmol/l (160 mg/dL) as well as lower LDL and HDL were much more common in patients with affective disorders such as depression, bipolar disorder and schizophrenia than in healthy people of a similar sex and age.[40]

Dr M. Law added confirmation two years later. 'Treating depression has been shown to increase serum cholesterol concentration . . . Low serotonin concentrations (which accompany and may cause depression) are, not surprisingly, also associated with low cholesterol, people who attempt suicide have low serum cholesterol concentrations, . . . men with declining serum cholesterol concentrations are particularly likely to commit suicide.'[41]

Depression is the main psychiatric illness leading to suicide and there is an observed increase in suicides among those undertaking cholesterol-lowering dietary regimes. A French study concluded: 'Both low serum cholesterol concentration and declining cholesterol concentration were associated with increased risk of death from suicide in men.'[42]

Low cholesterol and antisocial behaviour in adults

Low blood cholesterol is also associated with aggression and antisocial behaviour. In 1992, Dr H. Engleberg proposed a hypothesis to explain this. He suggested that decreases in blood cholesterol affected the balance of the metabolism of fats within the brain and that this could have profound effects on brain function.[43] He showed that low blood cholesterol was found in aggressive people and those with an antisocial personality. These averaged typically 5.04 mmol/l (194 mg/dL). Mental patients with high blood cholesterol of 7.55 mmol/l (290 mg/dL) were less regressed and withdrawn than those with 4.80 mmol/l (185 mg/dL).

There are many clinical studies showing that total cholesterol levels below 4.7 mmol/l (180 mg/dL), which is regarded as 'healthy' goal, are associated with depression, accidents, suicide, homicide and antisocial personality disorder in criminals and Army veterans, cocaine and heroin addicts. It is also associated with high relapse rates after detoxification and rehabilitation.[44]

Low cholesterol and mental illness and crime in children

In the Third National Health and Nutrition Examination Survey (NHANES III) conducted in the US between 1988 and 1994, blood cholesterol levels were measured in 4,852 children aged 6-16 years.[45] Psychosocial development was evaluated by interviewing the mother regarding her child's history of school suspension or expulsion and difficulty in getting along with others. The survey showed that children whose cholesterol was below 3.77 mmol/l (145 mg/dL) were almost three times more likely to have been suspended or expelled from schools than their peers with higher cholesterol levels. The authors concluded that low total cholesterol may be a risk factor for aggression or a risk marker for other biologic variables that predispose to aggression.

Low cholesterol and Alzheimer's disease

Numbers of cases of Alzheimer's disease are currently on the increase. Work in the 1950s found that as we get older, the level of cholesterol in our brains declines.[46] Later studies suggested that this decline may be the cause of brain disorders such as Alzheimer's. In 1991, a paper discussing the relief of Alzheimer's disease, asked that: 'strategies for increasing the delivery of cholesterol to the brain should be identified.' It recommended increasing fat intake.[47]

The Framingham Study added weight to this proposition when it examined the relationship between total cholesterol and cognitive performance.[48] Participants were both men and women who were free of dementia and stroke and who received biennial cholesterol checks over a 16- to 18-year surveillance period. Cognitive tests were administered four to six years after the surveillance period. This showed a significant linear association between the level of blood cholesterol and measures of verbal fluency, attention, concentration, abstract reasoning and a composite score measuring multiple cognitive domains. Participants with 'desirable' cholesterol levels of less than 5.2 mmol/l (200 mg/dL) performed significantly less well than participants with cholesterol levels higher than 6.25 mmol/l (240 mg/dL). Dr Penelope K. Elias from Boston University said that: 'It is not entirely surprising that lower cholesterol levels were associated with moderately lower levels of cognitive function, given [that] cholesterol is important in brain function.'

Low cholesterol and Parkinson's disease

There is much evidence that also suggests a link between low levels of cholesterol and Parkinson's disease. The Rotterdam Study, involving 6,465 people aged over 55 examined over an average follow-up period of 9.4 years, showed that lower levels of total cholesterol in the blood were associated with a significantly increased risk of Parkinson's disease.[49] The highest risk was found with cholesterol levels below 6.1 mmol/l (234 mg/dL). Using that figure as a reference, they found that the risk dropped to 46% between 6.8 (261) and 7.4 (285); and with a cholesterol level above 7.4 (285) the risk was down to only 16%. Strangely, however, this link was only seen in women. No reason for this was given.

Low cholesterol, diabetes and obesity

Because of a heightened interest in people with very low cholesterol levels, several studies have looked at other possible effects. One unexpected finding was that diabetics tended to have lower cholesterol levels than non-diabetics. And those with the lowest cholesterol levels were also more likely to be obese.[50]

Low cholesterol increases kidney disease risk

Low cholesterol and protein levels in the blood also predict a higher death rate in kidney disease patients according to a study conducted at the Department of Medicine, Morehouse School of Medicine, Atlanta, Georgia.[51] While age, gender, and underlying chronic medical conditions did not predict death, both low protein and low cholesterol levels did. This finding was reinforced four years later at the University of California in a study of kidney dialysis patients, which found that patients were more likely to survive if they were overweight and had high blood cholesterol and high blood pressure.[52]

Crohn's disease in children

Low blood cholesterol was also noted in patients with Crohn's disease as a result of lower LDL concentrations than in control subjects at the Gastroenterology-Nutrition Unit, Université de Montreal, Canada.[53]

Low cholesterol and sickle cell anaemia

Sickle cell anaemia is a disease in West Africa in which red blood cells are not the usual round shape but curved like the blade of a sickle. This condition prevents haemoglobin, a protein that carries oxygen around the body, from doing its job. There is some disagreement as to whether sickle cell anaemia also increases the risk of coronary heart disease. Scientists at the Department of Biochemistry and Molecular Biology, School of Medicine, University of New Mexico, in Albuquerque, analyzed the blood serum of children with the disease looking for levels of total cholesterol, HDL, LDL, triglycerides and homocysteine.[54]

They found that both the male and female children with the disease had much lower cholesterol than healthy children of the same ages and sex. Because those with the disease had low levels of cholesterol, the scientists concluded that: 'Collectively, these results indicate that children with SCD [sickle cell disease] in northern Nigeria are not at increased risk of CVD [cardiovascular disease].' But they obviously recognized that this low cholesterol was not as healthy as we think it is, because they continued: 'However, their marked hypocholesterolemia should be a cause of concern about the overall mortality and general well-being.'

Low cholesterol increases death rates in young and old alike

In 1991 the US National Cholesterol Education Programme recommended that children over two years old should adopt a low-fat, low-cholesterol diet to prevent CHD in later life. A table showing a good correlation between fat and cholesterol intakes and blood cholesterol in seven- to nine-year-old boys from six countries was published to support this advice.

What it did not show, however, was the even stronger correlation between blood cholesterol and childhood deaths in those countries. As is clearly demonstrated below, the death rate rises as blood cholesterol levels fall.[55]

Two studies which considered total blood cholesterol levels and mortality in the elderly were published in *The Lancet* almost simultaneously in 1997. In the first, scientists working at Leiden University's Medical Centre found that: 'each 1 mmol/l (38 mg/dL) increase in total cholesterol corresponded to a 15% decrease in mortality . . . In people older than 85 years, high total cholesterol concentrations are associated with longevity owing to lower mortality from cancer and infection.'[56] Similarly, doctors at Reykjavik Hospital and Heart Preventive Clinic in Iceland also studied total mortality and blood cholesterol in men over 80 to show that those with blood cholesterol levels over 6.5 mmol/l (250 mg/dL) had less than half the death rate (48%) of those whose cholesterol level was a 'healthy' 5.2 mmol/l (200 mg/dL).[57]

This relationship between low cholesterol and higher mortality was strengthened by a further study published six years later. The UCLA School of Medicine, Los Angeles, studied the association between blood cholesterol levels and seven-year all-cause mortality.[58] They found that people whose cholesterol levels were below 4.4 mmol/L (169 mg/dL) had nearly double the death rate over the period of those with higher levels. While some of this increase was attributed to inflammation and poor diet, the low cholesterol link was still apparent even after these factors had been allowed for.

Studies in Japan added yet more weight to this argument. Japan is reported to have low levels of death from coronary heart disease but Okinawa has the lowest of all. Yet Okinawa's cholesterol levels are similar to those in Scotland – much higher than the average in Japan. In 1992 a

Table 22.1: Blood cholesterol and mortality in under-5s in six countries. [55]

	Blood cholesterol (mmol/L)	Childhood deaths
Finland	4.9	7
Netherlands	4.5	9
US	4.3	12
Italy	4.1	12
Philippines	3.8	72
Ghana	3.3	145

paper examined the relationship of nutritional status to further life expectancy and health in the Japanese elderly based on three population studies.[59] It found that Japanese who lived to the age of 100 were those who got their protein from meat rather than from rice and pulses. The centenarians also had higher intakes of animal foods such as eggs, milk, meat and fish; significantly, their carbohydrate intake was lower than that of their fellow countrymen who died at a younger age.

These comparisons are important, as Japan might not have the low levels of heart disease deaths that are attributed to it. Although heart disease deaths are reportedly low, deaths from stroke and cerebral haemorrhage are very high. Ancel Keys attributed the lowest levels of heart deaths to Japan in his studies. These findings have been used to support recommendations that we should adopt Japanese eating patterns based on fish and rice. But vital statistics from death certificates are too unreliable for scientific use. One of the recognized facts about Japanese statistics is that the cause of many deaths has not been certified by a qualified doctor. Another is that coronary heart disease was an undesirable cause of death; stroke was a more desirable one as it was thought to be indicative of intelligence in the family. More recent autopsies have revealed that stroke is not as common as once believed and that heart disease is much more common than original figures suggested.[60] This is a good example of why vital statistics used by Keys and others may be unreliable.

However, if we lump deaths from all causes together, we get a figure that cannot be fudged. Comparing average age at death from all causes and food intake, we find that the Japanese who live longest are the ones who eat the most animal products and the least carbs.

The generally held belief that cholesterol concentrations should be kept low to lessen the risk of cardiovascular disease is clearly wrong. In 2001, Dr Schatz, professor of medicine at the University of Hawaii, wrote: 'those with cholesterol levels widely assumed to be healthy had a roughly 35-40% *greater* chance of dying from any cause in the following 25 years.'[61] And in 2004 yet another study suggested that low cholesterol shortened lifespan.[62]

Low cholesterol increases total mortality in the middle-aged

Amongst men in their 40s there does seem to be a correlation between high cholesterol and greater coronary death rates. But here again we find that the *total* death rate is highest in men whose blood cholesterol is lowest – below 4.8 mmol/l (185 mg/dL). These deaths are largely due to cancers and other non-cardiovascular causes.[29] In this age group, while the lowest death rate was seen between 4.8 mmol/l and 5.4 mmol/l (185-208 mg/dL), it rose only slightly as cholesterol concentrations rose above

5.4; it was considerably higher below 4.8.

In 1993 Dr M. G. Dunnigan, writing that both primary and secondary trials had shown a significant number of excess deaths from non-cardiac causes (cancer, violence and suicide). Pointing out that a meta-analysis of 35 randomized controlled trials (RCTs) had little relevance to the non-symptomatic person under 65, he said:

> 'Without definite data on all-cause mortality and with current unresolved concerns about excess deaths from non-cardiac causes in RCTs, decisions to embark on lifelong lipid lowering drug treatment in most patients with primary hypercholesterolaemia depend on the doctor's interpretation of available evidence. . . this varies from evangelical enthusiasm for lowering lipid concentrations to therapeutic nihilism.'[63]

How physicians are fooled

So, with all this information apparently at their fingertips, you might wonder why there is such widespread acceptance of the cholesterol myth in the medical world, and why it is that doctors insist that everyone should have exactly the same cholesterol level. You might also wonder if their oath to 'first do no harm' means anything any more.

The reason is relatively simple to explain. Firstly, there are some 30,000 medical journals published and no doctor can be expected to read all of them. Secondly, wherever heart disease is mentioned in conjunction with cholesterol, out of the many studies that have been published only a mere handful – the supportive studies – are quoted.[64] The vast majority that don't support the myth are rarely mentioned.

This preferential citation has skewed the facts. In addition, pharmaceutical companies who sell cholesterol-lowering drugs produce many publications which broadcast the cholesterol lowering myth to millions. Dr Jerome P. Kassirer, a former editor of the *New England Journal of Medicine*, told readers of *The Washington Post* that major publications such as *Lipid Letter*, *Lipids Online* and *Lipid Management* are all financed by the makers of cholesterol-lowering drugs.[65] These publications which warn relentlessly of the (false) dangers of cholesterol reach millions of medical doctors; they are designed, of course, to persuade doctors to prescribe their cholesterol-lowering drugs. So it isn't really surprising that overworked professionals continue to teach us that cholesterol is dangerous and pharmaceutical companies aggressively push their cholesterol-lowering drugs.

Above are many reasons to reconsider taking cholesterol-lowering drugs. With the latest statins, there are even more. Many compounds that are vital to the body are made via the same pathway as cholesterol, and are also inhibited by statins: Tau proteins, seleno-proteins, co-enzyme Q10 and steroid hormones. Statin therapy affects them all, which is why the drugs are responsible for such a wide range of serious adverse effects.

Conclusion

Dr A. E. Dugdale of the Cherbourg Hospital, St Lucia, Queensland, Australia, looked at the costs and benefits of cholesterol-lowering using 1984 Australian mortality statistics.[66] What he discovered was that the main effect of cholesterol lowering 'is to alter the cause of death'. 'When the lowest quintile of cholesterol levels is compared with the highest, the proportion of deaths from heart disease is almost halved, but the proportion from malignancies [cancers] is almost doubled.' He concluded that:

'A decrease in serum cholesterol of a population by 10%, even if this were possible, would be expensive in money and manpower. The benefits would be small and perhaps not liked by the subjects. We all die . . . heart disease may be preferable to cancer.'

It's a sobering thought. But when we add all the other adverse effects that low blood cholesterol seems to be responsible for and which increase ill health while we are alive, why would anyone want to lower their cholesterol? It is quite obvious that, while there might (or might not) be an increased risk of a heart attack in a man, *if* he is in his 40s and *if* his cholesterol level is very high, for men older than that, and for women of any age, a cholesterol level over 7.0 mmol/l (270 mg/dL) looks healthiest.

In view of this evidence, why on earth are our governments so keen to get everyone on cholesterol-lowering drugs?

Chapter Twenty-Three

Cancer:
disease of civilization

Populations eating traditional diets are remarkably free of cancer, but they soon succumb when they eat our diet. Numbers of cases of cancer have tripled since 'healthy eating' was introduced. This could be because cancers rely on a ready supply of glucose. And that comes from dietary carbohydrates.

Unlike the prevention of many other diseases, the prevention of cancer requires no government help, and no extra money.

Dr Otto Warburg (Nobel Laureat)

Recently, Cancer Research UK placed advertisements on TV in the United Kingdom showing three young girls, one after the other, captioned 'Teacher', 'Lawyer', 'Cancer'. What they were admitting was that, after 50 years and countless billions spent on research, one person in three will get cancer and that: 'Cancer is a major public health problem in the UK with over 250,000 people developing cancer each year and over 150,000 dying of the disease.'[1]

As cancer is so widespread and the subject of so much research effort, it may come as a surprise that, despite the introduction of radiotherapy in the 1920s, chemotherapy drugs after the Second World War and subsequent advances, plus the proliferation of X-ray machines, scanners, computers and other high-tech equipment, not to mention advances in other branches of medicine, the sacrifice of millions of animals (and people) in research, and the billions of dollars, pounds and other currencies spent on studies to broaden our knowledge of how cancers start and how to combat them, we are really no nearer to curing cancer at the beginning of the 21st century than we were at the beginning of the 20th;

and that overall chances of survival haven't really changed all that much in the last 100 years. Indeed, the only significant change is that there are so many *more* cancers now than there were then.

It is one of the great medical myths that, because the medical profession has been so successful in curing other diseases, more people live long enough to get cancer. This is total nonsense. Cancer has little to do with extended longevity – our children get cancer; and other human cultures in which there is no cancer at all live as long as we do.

Cancer is a word we dread. Not so long ago the word was taboo. If you or a member of your family had cancer you kept the fact within the family. It was as if people feared that, if it were known that they had cancer, they would be socially unacceptable. Others seemed to fear that if 'cancer' were mentioned, they might get it too. But then, not so long ago, cancer was a comparatively rare occurrence.

Today all that has changed. We have all become much more aware of cancer recently. For cancer is no longer the rarity it once was; it is a disease that affects us all.

At the beginning of the 19th century about one death in 50 was due to cancer. By the beginning of the 20th that number had almost doubled to one in 27. Thirty years later it had doubled again to one in 12 and by 1960 – another 30 years – it was one in six. Based on statistics in 1992, the American Cancer Society predicted that by the end of the 20th century the number would be one in two. They were not far out: by 2005 more than one person in three got a cancer and that cancer killed one in 3.7.[2]

In 1971, America's President Richard Nixon declared 'War on Cancer' saying: 'The time has come in America when the same kind of concentrated effort that split the atom and took man to the moon should be turned toward conquering this dread disease.' In that year, 635,000 Americans got cancer, 337,000 of them died of it, and about $250 million was spent on cancer research. President Nixon promised a cure by the US's bicentennial in 1976. Since then, trillions of dollars have been invested in cancer research, without success. The war on cancer has been a colossal failure. Chemotherapy, on which most treatment money is spent, is so toxic and ineffective that, according to the late Dr Hardin Jones, Professor of Medical Physics at the University of California at Berkeley, you may live longer by having no conventional treatment at all. After carefully analyzing cancer survival statistics for 25 years, Jones told an American Cancer Society meeting in 1969 that untreated patients do not die sooner than patients receiving orthodox treatment – in many cases they live longer.[3] Although that was 40 years ago, it has never been refuted.

By the year 2000, the numbers of cases of cancer in the US had almost doubled to 1,225,000.[4] We're still assured that a cure may be found any day now – it all depends on how much money is raised for the research. (Scientists have been making those promises, almost word for word, for a century.) And so we keep raising more and more money every year, while the numbers of our friends and family members who fall victim to this hideous disease continue to grow.

In the UK more than 600 cancer charities soak up billions of pounds every year from people who fear cancer and hope that their charity might help them one day. It's a mirage.

The truth is that cancer is a long way from being beaten. The vast amount of time, money and resources spent on drugs, together with innovative advances in highly sophisticated diagnostic machinery, have done practically nothing to alleviate the suffering from cancer. This might be because the cancer industry resists anything that might break their hold on their very lucrative cash cow – particularly anything that might actually work. As Dr Candace Pert wrote in 1997:

> 'I knew even after decades of intense research, there . . . had been no treatment advances beyond the highly toxic drugs developed before 1965. What I didn't know was how fiercely the cancer establishment would resist the efforts of an outsider . . . to come up with new ideas for treatment.'[5]

What is cancer?

My dictionaries all agree on a definition of cancer. It is: 'any malignant tumour arising from the abnormal and uncontrolled division of body cells that then invade and destroy the surrounding tissues.' But that really doesn't tell us a lot.

We know that cancer has no single cause; and we know that it isn't a disease you can 'catch' like flu. It is generally believed that we all have cancer cells within our bodies, probably many thousands of them, but that, in the healthy body, our immune systems deal with them before they develop into tumours. For us to get cancer, then, it seems that some trigger is required which causes a malfunction in one or more cells plus a factor which suppresses our bodies' immune system leaving it too weakened to resist a tumour's growth. That could be a stressful event, an environmental, medical, dietary or emotional crisis, a food or medication – indeed anything which lowers our bodies' defences.

Cancer begins when a cell divides. No matter how many birthdays you have had, very little of your body is more than about eight years old and most is much younger. This is because of a process of programmed cell death (called *apoptosis*) and renewal that goes on throughout our lives. Apart from the obvious signs of parts of the body continually growing –

hair and finger- and toe-nails – most body cells have a programmed life. At the end of that life they die and are replaced. When this happens, a process of cell division called *mitosis* makes new cells. In the process of mitosis, one cell divides to form two cells. First the DNA, the genetic blueprint in the nucleus of the cell which is in the form of a double helix, 'unzips' itself, dividing into two strands, each with half of the original genetic code. Then each of those strands reconstructs the original other half. This 'replication' process produces two identical sets of genetic information and allows the one cell to produce two genetically identical daughter cells. It is in this way that the body is first made, grown during childhood and then, throughout adult life, repaired. If anything disrupts the genetic code when DNA replication takes place, it can lead to mutations and, in some cases, the deregulation we call cancer. The deranged cell may be so genetically damaged that the gene that would normally bring about its death by apoptosis no longer functions. This cell does not die but reproduces itself over and over again to crowd neighbouring cells and form a tumour. As time passes, it may continue to grow out of control and spread (metastasize) throughout the body. It is at this stage that it changes from benign to malignant. This is a dangerous transition for, once a tumour has metastasized, conventional medicine has very little answer for it and the prognosis is bleak.

Causes of cancer

There are as many forms of cancer as there are different types of cell in the body. And it seems there are many agents that can cause a cell to become cancerous. They include viruses, carcinogenic (cancer causing) particles in the air we breathe and the food we eat, ionizing radiation – X-rays from medical machines and gamma radiation from the earth we live on. Even a hard knock, a cut or other source of inflammation can begin a cancer's growth.

Within our bodies we have an extremely competent and effective defence against invasions from outside. Replicated cells are new but they carry on their cell walls the correct code and they are recognized by the immune system as 'Self' – being part of us. Organisms from outside the body carry on their cell walls a foreign code and are recognized by the immune system as 'Non-self' and attacked mercilessly. This attack by the immune system is so powerful that it can completely destroy a transplanted kidney in a very short time. The problem in the case of cancer cells is that they teeter on the brink of Self and Non-self and, as far as the immune system is concerned, it seems that, in many cases, a cancer cell is still regarded as Self, albeit slightly eccentric, and so is allowed to survive and flourish.

This is the problem our immune system faces once a cancer has established itself. It is vital, therefore, to prevent that establishment by avoiding, as much as possible, things that have been shown to start a cancer, promote its growth or compromise our immune systems.

Cancer: a disease of civilization

We have known for a long time that there are enormous differences in incidences of cancer throughout the world. History shows that each type of civilization and each way of life has diseases peculiar to it. While this fact is well recognized by medical historians, its explanation is controversial. Is the reason for the variability of disease to be found in peculiarities of the human constitution, in genetic traits that make some people more susceptible or resistant to the disease, or are environmental factors more important when determining which types of diseases are most common in a given community?

Fortunately, 'the past' still survived until well into the 20th century in the form of many populations that had remained almost completely isolated, and whose mode of life differed profoundly from that of us in the industrialized countries. These primitive peoples could be used as control groups for the study of what modern civilization has done to us.

No cancer – from the Arctic to the Equator

For over a century and a half, medical missionaries, anthropologists and explorers searched in vain for cancer among the primitive peoples they visited. The Inuit have probably been isolated as long as any primitive people. Indeed, many still had a Stone Age culture until just a few decades ago, and they therefore provided excellent material for anthropological studies. Many who studied them remarked that: 'Cancer is not to be found among the Eskimos.' Dr Samuel King Hutton was a board member of the Moravian Mission to Labrador during the first half of the 20th century. Writing of the Labrador Eskimos in 1925, he said:

> 'Some diseases common in Europe have not come under my notice during a prolonged and careful survey of the health of the Eskimos. Of these diseases the most striking is cancer. I have not seen or heard of a case of malignant new growth in an Eskimo. In this connection it may be noted that cookery holds a very secondary place in the preparation of food – most of the food is eaten raw, and the diet is a flesh one; also that the diet is rich in vitamins.'[6]

In his book, *The Northwest Passage*, Roald Amundsen's wrote: 'My sincerest wish for our friends the Nechilli Eskimos is, that civilization may *never* reach them.'[7]

The Inuit were not alone in being free from cancer. Away from western civilization cancer-free societies were ubiquitous. From the tropical frontier Dr Albert Schweitzer wrote in 1957: 'On my arrival in Gabon, in 1913, I was astonished to encounter no cases of cancer . . . This absence of cancer seemed to me due to the difference in nutrition of the natives as compared with the Europeans.'[8]

In 1915, Dr Frederick L. Hoffman wrote an 826-page volume, *The Mortality from Cancer Throughout the World.*[9] Under 'Cancer among Primitive Races' Hoffman reported that:

> 'The rarity of cancer among native races suggests that the disease is primarily induced by the conditions and methods of living which typify our modern civilization . . . cancer is exceptionally rare among the primitive peoples.'

This rarity of cancer in the 19th century was not restricted to primitive populations. In his important book, *Cancer: Civilization and Degeneration*, Dr John Cope discussed the early eating habits of the English and the rarity of cancer at the time. He noted in particular that cancers increased in England as the consumption of meat declined.[10]

Where does the fault lie?

As far as conventional medicine is concerned, the preferred methods for treating cancer are surgery, radiation, or chemotherapy. Cancer cells are removed or their growth slowed. But, significantly, no attempt is made to eliminate the disease by strengthening the body's natural defences. Indeed, chemotherapy and radiation, by severely compromising the immune system, do exactly the opposite. Not surprisingly, many scientists have been profoundly disappointed by the trends in cancer research and their marked lack of success since the end of the 19th century. In the preface to his book, *Cancer: Nature, Cause and Cure*, Dr Alexander Berglas of the Pasteur Institute in Paris, wrote in 1957: 'Over the years, cancer research has become the domain of specialists in various fields. Despite the outstanding contributions of these scientists, we have been getting farther and farther away from our goal, the curing of cancer.'[11]

More than 30 years in the field of cancer research convinced Berglas that the methods of research: 'had the peculiar result of becoming an obstacle to the study of the whole,' and that to continue as they were: 'is not to our advantage.' 'I have come to the conclusion', he wrote, 'that cancer may perhaps be just another intelligible natural process whose cause is to be found in our environment and mode of life.' Berglas was writing particularly of the foods we ate and the way in which they were grown and prepared.

Interestingly, under 'Prediction of Cancer Mortality', Berglas said that the National Cancer Institute of the United States predicted (presumably in 1956) that: '32% of new-born children are expected to contract cancer during their lifetime.' His estimate has turned out to be remarkably accurate. Writing of the contrast between 'civilized' and 'uncivilized' countries since 1900, he said: 'Accounts of regions free from cancer reveal the influence of civilization on the processes of cancer . . . We are faced with the grim prospect that the advance of cancer and of civilization parallel each other.'

Are primitive peoples permanently cancer free?

Primitive peoples have no more immunity to cancers than we have. Once introduced to our 'civilized' foods they succumb to the disease as readily as we do. While there were no known cases of cancer when Dr Albert Schweitzer first went to Gabon, he noted sadly that: 'In the course of the years we have seen cases of cancer in growing numbers in our region. My observations incline me to attribute this to the fact that the natives were living more and more after the manner of the whites.'[8]

But what aspect of our diet causes cancer?

When it comes to possible dietary causes of cancer, frontier doctors wrote apparently contrary views based on their own experiences: when they could find no cancer among vegetarian cultures they were prone to warn against meat; and where no cancers were discovered among meat eaters they tended to caution against mixed or vegetarian diets.

Major General Sir Robert McCarrison, a British army doctor who worked predominantly in the Indian sub-continent, was particularly impressed with the health of the Hunzas, a people who live in a secluded valley in the Karakorum Mountains. He attributed their health to their mainly vegetarian diet. A typical statement appears in McCarrison's *Studies in Deficiency Disease* published in 1921.[12] After quoting the famous Danish nutritionist, Dr Mikkel Hindhede: 'The principal cause of death lies in food and drink,' McCarrison wrote of the Hunza:

> 'My own experience provides an example of a race, unsurpassed in perfection of physique and in freedom from disease in general, whose sole food consists to this day of grains, vegetables, and fruits, with a certain amount of milk and butter, and goat's meat only on feast days . . . Amongst these people the span of life is extraordinarily long; and such service as I was able to render them during seven years spent in their midst was confined chiefly to the treatment of accidental lesions, the removal of senile cataract, plastic operations for granular eyelids, or the treatment of maladies wholly unconnected with food supply.'

But many more have pointed out that, before they started to get cancer in the 20th century, the traditional diet of the Inuit came entirely from animal sources and contained no plant material at all. And, actually, as we will see in Chapter 28 cataract at least *is* connected with a plant-based 'food supply'.

It is suggested that when diseases such as cancer start appearing after people adopt a 'healthy' western diet, it must be because they are living longer. But that excuse is not borne out by evidence. Dr Diamond Jenness, in his book, *The Copper Eskimos*, said: 'Amongst adults, death was nearly always due to natural causes, either old age or the perils that are inseparable from life in the Arctic!'[13] And Dr Henry W. Greist, in his *Seventeen Years with the Eskimos*, speaking of the ancestors of those north Alaskans among whom he was first able to diagnose cancer in 1933, wrote: 'the Eskimo of the far North was healthy . . . He lived to a very great age.'[14]

The answer to the difference in health patterns between primitive and civilized peoples seems to lie in two directions. Firstly, infants are fed in primitive societies as Nature intended them to be fed: at the breast; and secondly, the people live on the unsophisticated – and unprocessed – foods of Nature. McCarrison discussed these at length:

'I don't suppose that one in every thousand of them has ever seen a tinned salmon, a chocolate, or a patent infant food, nor that as much sugar is imported into their country in a year as is used in a moderately sized hotel of this city in a single day . . . enforced restriction to unsophisticated foodstuffs of Nature is compatible with fertility, long life, continued vigour, perfect physique, and a remarkable freedom from digestive and gastrointestinal disorders, and from cancer.'

The food of our developed countries is very different. We are no longer content with such unsophisticated natural foods. McCarrison declared that we 'prefer preserved, purified, polished, pickled and canned' food. He said (about 'civilized' food):

'One way or another, by desiccation, by chemicals, by heating, by freezing and thawing, by oxidation and decomposition, by milling and polishing, he applies the principles of his civilization – the elimination of the natural and substitution of the artificial – to the foods he eats and the fluids he drinks. With such skill does he do so that he often converts his food into a "dead" fuel mass . . . in consequence of food habits they have fostered, normal bodily function cannot be sustained . . .'

That was written over three-quarters of a century ago and, since then the situation has deteriorated even further. Today, relatively few people eat food that hasn't been massively processed and denatured. And, apart from 'five portions of fruit and veg', all the foods regarded as 'healthy' by conventional nutritionists are processed: breakfast cereals, bread, pasta, polyunsaturated vegetable margarines and cooking oils, low-fat dairy products, soy.

Cancer research has hampered progress

Given the fear with which a diagnosis of cancer is viewed, it is not surprising that a great deal of time and resources have been devoted to finding both the cause and a cure. But dogma of one sort or another has hampered progress in both areas.

When Louis Pasteur stated his germ theory of disease in 1862, it was greeted with derision. In 1874, when Joseph Lister acknowledged that his success with aseptic surgery was due to Pasteur's theory, all that changed. From that moment all diseases, including cancer, were thought to be caused by micro-organisms. That belief was strengthened when three scientists, Moreau, Loeb and Jensen, showed that cancer cells could be successfully grafted from one species to another. In *Cancer: Civilization and Degeneration*,[10] John Cope talks of the way in which these two discoveries derailed the research on cancer.

Until the beginning of the 20th century the search for the causes of human cancer was wide. It was studied as it existed in the consulting room, at the bedside, in the operating theatre and in the post-mortem room. And 'not only pathology, but physiology, anthropology, zoology, botany were made to contribute material, and so also were history, chemistry and statistics.' After the two discoveries, Cope told how he believed it all went wrong:

> 'It would be difficult to exaggerate the expectations which were aroused by the progress in scientific method implied by these two events. Towards the end of the century the opposition with which Pasteur's work had at first been received gave place to a tendency to look for micro-organisms as the cause of every disease; and so it naturally came to pass that the methods of experimental laboratory research, which had proved so successful with cholera and tuberculosis, were made use of to throw light on the nature and origin of cancer.'

The discovery around the turn of the 20th century that cancers could be grown artificially in laboratory animals seemed to make the investigation of cancer easier. Laboratory mice grow cancers much more quickly than do humans and they were expendable in a way that a doctor's patients were not. The researcher could use the mouse as he would a test-tube or flask, and throw it away when done with it. It looked like the solution to the cancer problem. And so laboratories were built all over the civilized world; huge sums of money were spent; the lives of many scientists were devoted to the quest; and whole libraries of magazine articles and books testified to the scientists' patience, industry and ability. 'And now,' wrote Cope in 1932, 'after all these years of noble toil, not even the most sanguine research worker can point to anything that can by any stretch of the imagination be termed a solution of the problem which the researchers set out so confidently to answer.'

In 1931, Dr William Henry Woglom, a great American laboratory cancer researcher, put the results more decisively than most when he summed up the achievements of cancer research, saying that so far as human beings were concerned he was unable to point to any sign of progress whatever.

The May 1955 edition of the *Danish Medical Bulletin* carried a paper on the Danish Cancer Registry by the registry's director, Dr Johannes Clemmesen, who evidently felt, as Cope did, that cancer research had swung too far towards animal experimentation.[15] This artificial production of cancers in multitudes of small animals was directed toward discovering, if possible, either before or after they die, how to slow down or stop the deadly cancers inflicted upon the creatures with the laudable purpose of finding out how to alleviate or cure malignant disease in humans. Its deplorable actual result, said Clemmesen, was that: 'in fifty years and after hundreds of millions spent', their skills had not improved even sufficiently to prevent the ever-increasing numbers of cancers. Like Cope, Clemmesen felt that this swing away from human research was a retrograde step. He urged scientists to make active use of: 'the collection of information on the distribution of malignant disease, among various ethnological groups in different regions, in relation to any relevant local factors' – which was exactly what the medical missionaries had been urging for decades.

Now, over 50 years on, it still hasn't happened and we suffer even more cancers.

Cope didn't question the quality or quantity of effort put into laboratory cancer research. What surprised him, I think, was that those engaged in cancer research seemed not in the least discouraged by their total lack of success. 'On the contrary,' he said, 'they seem full of conviction of the imminence of some discovery which will reward them for their industry and patience' while out of a veritable mountain of more than a third of a century's labour, nothing had emerged other than 'a cancer-bearing mouse.'

Cope believed that experimental cancer research had become so isolated and so entrenched that, without being aware of it, researchers almost instinctively regarded those who criticized them or questioned their authority, or adopted other methods of working, as being positive enemies. This attitude, of course, stifles innovation and lateral thinking. Cope said that: 'It must ever be held as one of the worst evils of laboratory cancer research that . . . it is responsible for holding up for a generation one of the greatest and most promising advances of the nineteenth century.'

It has now held research up for another century as well, as all of the above is as true today as it was when Cope wrote it. If Cope was right, and I see no reason to doubt it, we are still approaching the problem of cancer in entirely the wrong way. But there is hope; there is something we can all do to reduce to a minimum our chances of suffering from cancer. It lies in the way cancers use energy.

Cancers are sugar junkies

It's now more than 70 years since Otto Warburg, PhD, won the 1931 Nobel Prize in medicine for discovering that cancer cells have an energy metabolism that is fundamentally different from healthy cells. The crux of his Nobel thesis was that malignant tumours frequently exhibit an increase in *anaerobic* metabolism compared with normal tissues. In other words, they don't like oxygen.[16] The significance of this is that fat and ketone bodies as a source of energy require oxygen while glucose doesn't. And that in turn means that cancer cells are dependent on glucose for growth. All cells can use glucose, but cancer cells consume as much as four or five times more than normal, healthy cells. In fact, cancer cells seem to have great difficulty surviving without glucose.

A study carried out by Johns Hopkins researchers found evidence that some cancer cells are such incredible sugar junkies that they will self-destruct when deprived of glucose.[17] 'The change when we took away glucose was dramatic,' said Dr Chi Van Dang, director of haematology. 'We knew very quickly that the cells we had altered to resemble cancers were dying off in large numbers . . . Scientists have long suspected that the cancer cells' heavy reliance on glucose – its main source of strength and vitality – could also be one of its great weaknesses.'

Normal body cells can use fat and ketone bodies derived from fats metabolized aerobically for energy. The waste products of the process are carbon dioxide and water. The process by which cancer cells derive their energy is one of anaerobic fermentation of glucose, with lactic acid as a waste product. The lactic acid produced is then transported to the liver where it is processed into glucose, ensuring the cancer cells have a constant supply of energy.

This pathway for energy metabolism is very inefficient in that it extracts only about 5% of the available energy in the food supply and the body's calorie stores. The cancer is wasting energy, and the patient becomes tired and undernourished. This cycle increases body wasting,[18] which is one reason why as many as 67% of cancer patients die from malnutrition (*cachexia*).[19]

In addition to being dependent on glucose, most tumours also have abnormalities in the number and function of their mitochondria.[20] These abnormalities prevent the tumour cells from using ketone bodies, which require functional mitochondria for their oxidation.

The famous 19th-century cancer specialist, Dr Stanislaw Tanchou, presented the first formula for predicting cancer risk in a paper delivered to the Paris Medical Society in 1843.[21] It was based on grain consumption and was found to calculate cancer rates in major European cities very accurately. The more grain consumed, the greater the rate of cancer.

Can low-carb diets prevent cancer?

If cancers cannot survive without glucose, surely it follows that a low-carb, high-fat diet is likely to prevent a cancer starting. Just that piece of knowledge might stop all the heartbreak, pain and misery that cancer causes.

Two of the most common cancers are breast cancer – which, incidentally, is not confined to women – and lung cancer. In the context of blood sugar and cancer risk, it may be significant that UK research suggests that people with coeliac disease – and who do not eat wheat and other cereals – have only about one-third the risk of either of these cancers.[22] This adds more weight to the evidence that carbs increase cancer risk.

Furthermore, an epidemiological study in 21 industrialized countries in Europe, North America and Asia, revealed that sugar intake is a strong risk factor that contributes to higher breast cancer rates, particularly in older women.[23] Another four-year study at the National Institute of Public Health and Environmental Protection in the Netherlands found that cancer risk associated with the intake of sugars, independent of other energy sources, more than doubled for cancer patients.[24]

As cancers need glucose so much, cutting off the source of that energy is similar to cutting off the cancer's blood supply.

Insulin and cancer

Blood concentrations of fasting insulin, glucose, cholesterol and triglycerides in non-obese people suffering from colon, stomach and breast cancer were determined and compared with those of healthy non-obese people. Insulin was also measured in tumours and non-cancerous tissues. Insulin and glucose (with the exception of glucose in colon patients) were significantly higher than in healthy people; blood cholesterol and triglycerides levels were lower. Tumours contained 1.9-3.0 times as much insulin, or insulin-like substances.[25] High insulin levels are the result of eating a high intake of 'healthy' carbohydrate-rich foods.

Cancer patients don't need carbs . . .

Cancer therapies should encompass regulating blood-glucose levels. This is best done via diet, supplements, and non-oral solutions for those patients who lose their appetite, with the aim of starving the cancer and simultaneously bolstering immune function. Intravenous feeding, of course, should not use standard glucose-based formulae. One of the biggest obstacles to using this approach in cancer patients in the past was the belief that the brain couldn't function properly without glucose. However, a study published in May 2003 showed that the brain can use ketones made from fats just as other normal cells do.[26] It was also shown nearly 70 years ago that ATP (see Glossary) is delivered from the liver to the brain by red blood cells.[27] So there is absolutely no need to worry about the brain being starved of energy if we cut carbohydrates out of the diet.

A low-carb, high-fat (ketogenic) diet may actually be the best way to attack brain cancers. Just like other body cells, normal brain cells can oxidize ketone bodies as well as glucose for energy; in a similar way to other cancer cells, brain tumours lack that metabolic flexibility and are largely dependent on glucose for energy.[28-34] Although some brain cancers do metabolize ketones, we needn't worry about it as this metabolism is largely for synthesis of fats rather than for energy production.[35 36]

In a recent paper, Drs Thomas Seyfried and Purna Mukherjee of the Biology Department, Boston College, Massachusetts, describe how new therapeutic approaches, which lower circulating glucose and elevate ketone bodies, target brain tumours while enhancing the metabolic efficiency of normal brain cells.[37] Discussing a trial published in 1995 of a low-carb, high-fat diet in patients with brain tumours, the two doctors go on to say that although radiation and chemotherapy had caused severe, life-threatening adverse effects in the patients, they responded remarkably well to the ketogenic diet and experienced long-term tumour management without further chemotherapy or radiation. Then came the bad news which was that, despite the logic of these studies and the dramatic findings, no further human studies or clinical trials had been conducted on the therapeutic effectiveness of the ketogenic diet for brain cancer. Why not? Seyfried and Mukherjee say that:

'The reason . . . may reflect a preference of the major Brain Tumor Consortia for using "hand-me-down" drug therapies from other cancer studies rather than exploring more effective biological or non-chemotherapeutic approaches. This is unfortunate as our recent findings in brain tumor animal models show that the therapeutic potential of the restricted [ketogenic diet] . . . is likely to be greater than that for any current brain tumor chemotherapy.'

In other words, this potentially effective cancer therapy won't be used simply because it doesn't fit with current 'politically correct' medical thinking.

. . . but they can eat some

Cancer patients and those wishing to avoid the disease don't need to cut out all foods that contain carbs. If care is taken the less concentrated carbohydrate foods may still be consumed.

Sugars are considerably worse than starches as far as damage to the immune system is concerned. There is also evidence that the same may apply in the case of cancer. A study of rats fed diets with equal amounts of calories from sugars or starches found the animals on the high-sugar diet developed more cases of breast cancer than those on the high-starch diet.[38] The glycaemic index (GI) can be a useful tool in guiding the cancer patient toward a healthier diet, but it has flaws. It seems advisable based on evidence presented in this book that cancer patients should avoid not only all processed foods whatever their GI, but fresh foods with a GI over 40, and also all fruit. Fresh green leafy vegetables may be eaten freely and some of the starchier root vegetables with a low GI, such as carrot, may be eaten in moderation. Foods from animal sources, with their fat, which have a GI of zero, should, of course, form the basis of all meals.

Meat vitamin is better than plant vitamin

There is a small but ever-growing body of science supporting the potential health benefits of fat-soluble vitamin K in bone, blood and skin health. The European Prospective Investigation into Cancer and Nutrition (EPIC) study added to the list by finding that increased intakes of vitamin K may reduce the risk of prostate cancer by 35%. But there are two forms of vitamin K: vitamin K_1 found in green leafy vegetables and plant oils and vitamin K_2 in cheeses and animal products. The benefits of K_2 were most pronounced for advanced prostate cancer. Vitamin K_1 intake did not offer any prostate benefits.[39]

Conclusion

It seems that the more cancer research has focused on a cure for existing disease, rather than its prevention, the less has been achieved. Despite the countless trillions that have been devoted to alleviating the suffering caused by cancer, we are no closer to a cure now in the first years of this century than we were in the first years of the 20th.

Isn't it about time we concentrated on prevention rather than cure? To this end, the relatively unsophisticated research of the 19th century seems to be far more useful than all the very expensive research of the last 100 years put together.

Unfortunately for anyone who gets cancer, the cancer business is second only to its big brother, petrochemicals, in size. With the obscenely large amounts of money involved it is quite understandable why the cancer cartel have maintained a constant, ruthless campaign to suppress, at birth, any and all attempts to introduce rational therapeutic regimes to deal with this ever-growing disease, as well as any preventative protocol.

It is highly likely that processed foods are a major dietary cause of cancer, particularly as they are inevitably based on cheap concentrated carbohydrates and vegetable oils, and depleted in essential nutrients. Many are those that are promoted today as 'healthy'.

Dr Berglas emphasized that carcinogens in novel foods were not immediately harmful. 'As a rule,' he wrote, 'a relatively long latency period of carcinogenesis, often lasting several years, is observed in man.' Using similar logic, if we revert to healthier practices today, it could still be many years before cancer is eradicated. But we have to start somewhere and the sooner we start, the sooner cancer will no longer blight our lives.

To fight any disease, surely it makes sense to remove anything that might support that disease. So, instead of spending billions developing one form of toxic chemotherapy after another – which by and large don't work – why are we not telling cancer patients: 'Stop eating sugar immediately'? And, as prevention in this case is definitely better than cure, why are we still telling people to eat large quantities of carbohydrate-rich foods?

The refusal of the cancer industry to consider further research into a low-carb, high-fat, ketogenic diet as a treatment for brain cancer, as reported by Drs Seyfried and Mukherjee, is, I believe, utterly reprehensible. It should also be trialled in other cancers, particularly as the standard treatments for cancer have such a dismal record.

There are four aspects of our modern 'lifestyle' that I believe increase the risk of a cancer. The first is a carb-based diet, the second is polyunsaturated vegetable oils and margarines, the third is a low blood cholesterol level, and the last is lack of sunshine. In other words, all the 'healthy' lifestyle changes we are advised to make.

If we really are serious about defeating the scourge of cancer, the only real answer is to prevent it. And as there are (or at least were) many cultures in which cancer is completely absent, we could do a lot worse than to study them and their diets. Books such as Stefansson's *Cancer: Disease Of Civilization*, Price's *Nutrition and Physical Degeneration* and the others mentioned, are invaluable in this respect. They should be required reading for all who profess to practise 'health'. In the meantime, the government and cancer charities should warn about the potential for foods to cause or exacerbate cancers, rather than promote them.

Chapter Twenty-Four

Gut reaction

Being in the front line, the gastrointestinal tract is exposed to the greatest danger if the diet we eat is not suited to us. This chapter looks at how our 'healthy diet' can be harmful and the health problems it can cause.

We got the impression that wholemeal wheat and bran products made people with the condition worse rather than better.

Drs C. Y. Francis and P. J. Whorwell

To anyone holding the view that some foods are unnatural and harmful components of our diet it is quite obvious that the gastrointestinal tract, being in the front line, is exposed to the most danger. The idea of introducing a low-carbohydrate diet as a general mode of therapy for disorders of this system is therefore logical, even if contrary to what is normally advised.

Stomach

Too much acid

Gastric reflux disease or heartburn is caused by a backflow of stomach acid into the oesophagus, a condition that results in inflammation of the oesophagus. Because this acid is produced to break down proteins it is erosive in Nature and can damage the lining of the oesophagus. There are many factors that can lead to the development of acid reflux disease but the most common is incorrect foods.

A clue to culprit foods lies in the fact that gastric reflux is often the first symptom to disappear when carbohydrates are reduced in the diet. However severe, and even if made worse by factors like the backflow of gastric juice into the oesophagus in hiatus hernia, the chances of success are excellent. If patients come back with the complaint that the diet is no longer effective and their heartburn has returned, a closer look usually reveals that carbohydrates have again crept into the diet.

Another clue is that heartburn risk is much higher among people who are overweight.[1] They also suffer more from diarrhoea. Professor Nicholas Talley, from the Mayo Clinic in Rochester, Minnesota, and his team investigated over 700 volunteers from Sydney, Australia. Their data suggested: 'that there is a positive independent relationship between increasing BMI and heartburn . . . that obesity *per se* is a risk factor for gastroesophageal reflux disease.' And obesity, particularly abdominal obesity, is caused by a carbohydrate-rich diet.

Similar results confirming those of Talley's team were found in another study the following year conducted at the Karolinska Institute, in Stockholm, Sweden.[2]

Ulcers

Gastrin, a hormone responsible for gastric secretions, is formed when food enters the stomach. This leads to secretion of hydrochloric acid and the enzymes necessary for digestion in the stomach. When the stomach contents are sufficiently acidified, the pyloric sphincter opens and allows the acid contents to leave the stomach and continue their journey into the small intestine. Here other substances are produced which stimulate activity by the pancreas and also neutralise the acid from the stomach. This also stops production of stomach acid; thus the stomach has a form of self-regulation. Many stomach ulcers are caused by irritation of the stomach lining by high levels of hydrochloric acid, in turn caused by too much gastrin being produced. Carbohydrates especially elicit production of gastrin. Both stomach ulcers caused by high acid levels and duodenal ulcers usually heal if carbohydrates are restricted.[3]

Cirrhosis of the liver

Cirrhosis of the liver is a potentially fatal condition. Many people think of cirrhosis afflicting those who drink prodigious amounts of alcohol. But, in fact, alcohol is only one cause of cirrhosis.

Both experimental and epidemiological studies have shown that alcohol drinkers who eat 'unhealthy' saturated animal fats have no liver injury.[4] It seems it is only when drinkers replace animal fats with 'healthy' polyunsaturated fats containing linoleic acid that problems arise. Linoleic acid, even at levels as low as 0.7 or 2.5% of fat intake, with alcohol, caused fatty liver, necrosis and inflammation.

Omitting cholesterol from the diet has very similar harmful effects.[5]

A major – and increasingly common – form of liver damage is a condition known as *non-alcoholic fatty liver disease* (NAFLD). This can progress to fibrosis and then to cirrhosis. It is estimated that NAFLD affects between 14% and 21% of the populations of Europe and Asia, and 24% of the United States' population. It is more common among adults who are obese or have diabetes.[6] The prevalence of NAFLD with age and with weight in both sexes increases, although NAFLD is more common in males of all ages. Among women, the risk of NAFLD increases after the menopause. Lately, there has emerged a worrying trend as NAFLD is increasingly found in children.[7]

Despite its name, fatty liver is *not* caused by a fatty diet. You may be surprised to learn that 'healthy' starchy foods such as cereals are the prime cause of NAFLD. The French delicacy, pâté de fois gras, is a perfect example of how it develops. The pâté is made from goose livers, but not just any goose livers: they have to be fat ones. To achieve this, the geese are force-fed grain which is high in cereal starch. That is what fattens their livers.

The same thing happens in humans who eat a 'healthy' diet. Dr Jeanne Clark of Johns Hopkins University School of Medicine told delegates at the 54th Annual Meeting of the American Association for the Study of Liver Diseases, of how a study of liver biopsies showed that the high-carbohydrate, low-fat diet often recommended for very obese patients with NAFLD *increased* their risk of liver inflammation as much as seven times compared with patients with the lowest carbohydrate intake.[9] Conversely, she told delegates, high-fat diets appeared to be protective. This confirmed an earlier study in which patients with established alcoholic cirrhosis benefited from a saturated fat diet.[9]

Gallstones . . .

Low-fat diet

Fair, fat and 40. That is the general perception of someone with gallstones. For this reason gallstones, often found in fat people, are usually attributed to a diet high in fats. In fact this is the opposite of the truth: gallstones are caused by eating too little fat rather than too much.

Fats are not soluble in water. Before dietary fat can be digested, it must be emulsified. Bile is used for this purpose. The liver makes bile continuously and stores it in the gall bladder until such time as it is needed. But if a low-fat diet is eaten, that bile remains in the gall bladder.

Gallstones are formed when the gall bladder is not emptied on a regular basis. In people who eat low-fat diets, bile is stored for long periods – and it stagnates. In time – and it is really quite a short time – a 'sludge' begins to form. This then coagulates to form progressively larger stones. The speed with which this happens was dramatically demonstrated in a trial at several American university hospitals.[10] None of the people tested had any sign of gall bladder disease at the start of the study. However, after only eight weeks of low-fat dieting, more than a quarter had developed gallstones. Where they were fed intravenously, half developed gall bladder sludge after just three weeks and *all* had developed it by six weeks. Nearly half of those who developed sludge also formed gallstones.

Missing breakfast also increases the risk of gallstones. In a study of French women with gallstones, it was found that they fasted on average for two hours longer overnight than women without the disease.[11]

Research has also shown that body fat around your middle rather than overall fatness is associated with an increased risk of gallstones.[12] This is no surprise as body fat around the middle is an indicator of the metabolic syndrome, which is caused by eating a carbohydrate-rich, low-fat diet.

The pain of gallstones comes when these are passed through the bile duct with the bile in response to a fatty meal and get stuck.

Wrong-fat diet

A cholesterol-lowering diet in which saturated fats are replaced with unsaturated oils may also increase the risk of gallstones.[13] In a large study looking at changing fats in the diet to control atherosclerosis, the experimental group ate polyunsaturated vegetable oils while the control group ate animal fats. Unexpected by the researchers, they found a positive correlation between the number of high-vegetable-fat meals eaten by the experimental group and the probability that gallstones would be present. There is a high prevalence of gallstones in the US, where the dietary intake of vegetable fat (including plant sterols) has increased during the last half century. It may be important that diets or drugs that lower blood cholesterol may do so by increasing excretion of cholesterol in bile which, in turn, may influence the likelihood of gallstones.

Summary

So, a low-fat or wrong-fat diet appears to cause gallstones. It is eating a high-fat diet, however, that makes them apparent. If you eat a low-fat diet and never eat fat again, then you won't get the pain, even though the stones are there.

If someone suffers from gallstones, a low-fat diet 'prevents' the symptoms, so doctors often suggest such a diet. But it makes the *cause* of the symptoms (gallstones) worse. Doctors are often loath to operate to remove gallstones, so just preventing you knowing about them seems to them to be a good compromise – despite the fact that you will then be miserable and hungry as a result.

. . . and kidney stones

It is a common belief that both uric acid and calcium oxalate stones are more likely to form in the kidneys if you eat a high-protein, low-carb diet than if you eat a higher-carbohydrate diet with more fruit and vegetables. This belief is not borne out by the evidence.

Thirty years ago, kidney stones were shown to be more likely in people who ate refined carbohydrates.[14] I wonder why then the National Institute of Diabetes and Digestive and Kidney Diseases, at the United States National Institutes of Health, was surprised to find that: 'the number of people in the United States with kidney stones has been increasing over the past 20 years.'[15] What is really worrying is that they began that sentence with: 'For unknown reasons.' They also noted that kidney stones strike most typically between the ages of 20 and 40. What change has been made in people's eating habits in the past 20 years? 'Healthy eating' has been introduced.

They continued: 'People who form calcium stones used to be told to avoid dairy products and other foods with high calcium content. But recent studies have shown that foods high in calcium, including dairy foods, help prevent calcium stones. Taking calcium in pill form, however, may increase the risk of developing stones . . . You may be told to avoid food with added vitamin D and certain types of antacids that have a calcium base. If you have very acidic urine, you may need to eat less meat, fish, and poultry. These foods increase the amount of acid in the urine.'

So, *if* you have kidney stones, and *if* you form calcium stones and *if* you have very acidic urine you *may* need to eat less meat. But drinking lots of water will reduce the acidity; this diet is known to reduce the need for antacids; and we don't need calcium supplements as we are eating enough. So where does the problem really lie? You may be interested to know that the National Kidney Foundation, discussing oxalate stones, says: 'The foods with a high content of oxalate are spinach, rhubarb, beets, strawberries, wheat bran, nuts and nut butter.'[16] They don't mention meat at all.

The evidence all suggests that the way to avoid kidney and gall bladder diseases is to eat a diet composed mainly of animal protein and fat.

Kidney failure

Technically termed *renal nephropathy*, kidney disease is an inevitable consequence of the chronically uncontrolled blood glucose and chronically high insulin levels found with type-2 diabetes. Yet one of the most frequently-repeated criticisms of low-carbohydrate, higher-protein diets is that they will allegedly lead to kidney failure. Many studies have shown such a claim to be completely false.[17-20]

The long-running Nurses' Health Study, for example, showed that a high-protein intake was *not* associated with renal function decline in women whose kidneys were healthy at the start of the study. However, high total protein intake, particularly high intake of non-dairy animal protein, did show a borderline significant relationship with declining kidney function in women whose kidneys were *not* healthy at the beginning of the study.[21]

Protein metabolism results in the production of urea, a waste product which must be filtered through the kidneys. While such increases pose no threat to healthy kidneys, damaged kidneys may not be able to process increased amounts of urea safely. Critics of low carbohydrate diets, however, seek to convince those ignorant of the above facts that high protein intakes will damage healthy kidneys.

There is actually no reason for people with impaired kidney function to resign themselves to a life of low-protein, high-carbohydrate fare, with the consequent fatigue, muscle loss and immune impairment. It's no secret that carbohydrates elevate blood sugar levels, which in turn increase glycative activity in the body; and that excess iron has been implicated as a potent free-radical promoter. So Californian researchers placed patients with diabetic kidney damage on a diet in which chicken and fish, which are low in iron, were substituted for red meat, intakes of iron-binding foods, such as dairy and eggs, were increased and total carbohydrate intake was halved. The composition of the trial diet was 25-30% protein, 30% fat, 35% carbohydrate, and 5-10% alcohol. A control group of similarly kidney-impaired diabetics consumed the low-protein diet recommended for kidney patients consisting of 10% protein, 25% fat, and 65% carbohydrate, which is also the ratio recommended for the general population. The results of the trial were impressive: 39% of the low-protein, high-carb control group patients either died or deteriorated to a point necessitating kidney transplant; in the unrestricted protein group, the corresponding figure was 20%.[22]

Evidence suggests that people with signs of kidney dysfunction should opt for iron-poor sources of protein such as poultry, fish, pork, eggs and cultured dairy products together with a low carbohydrate intake, but not so low as to cause ketosis – typically above 30 grams a day.

There is little doubt that a 'healthy' high-carb diet and subsequent high blood insulin can contribute to diabetic patients' deteriorating kidney function; and that insulin treatment in type-2 diabetes patients may cause further injury to the kidney. A low-carb, high-fat diet, with a moderate protein intake, may actually prevent renal failure in type-2 diabetics.[23]

Coeliac disease

Coeliac disease is an auto-immune condition caused by *gliadin*, a fraction of gluten – a natural protein commonly found in many grains, including wheat, barley, rye and oats. In normal, healthy people, gluten is digested like any other protein; in people with coeliac disease, gliadin causes an immune reaction in the body, leading to inflammation and damage to finger-like protrusions called *villi* that hugely increase the surface of the small intestine. This leads to a malabsorption of food with symptoms of diarrhoea and fatty stools. Failure to thrive and grow at normal rates are often the symptoms first noticed in children with coeliac disease.

Coeliac disease is most common among people of northern European descent and it is particularly common in people with blond hair and blue eyes. Although many cases are diagnosed in childhood, coeliac disease can develop at any age.

Recent studies, using specific and sensitive tests, have revealed that coeliac disease is one of the most common lifelong disorders in both Europe[24] and the US.[25] It is thought that most cases go undiagnosed, often because it is assumed that other diseases cause the symptoms or because symptoms are mild. Because so many cases remain undiagnosed the condition carries a risk of complications, including osteoporosis, infertility and cancer.

People with coeliac disease also tend to have an increased risk of developing other auto-immune diseases, such as type-1 diabetes, systemic *lupus erythematosus*, rheumatoid arthritis and thyroid disease. Other conditions that may coexist with coeliac disease include *dermatitis herpetiformis* (an itchy, blistering rash similar to eczema), liver disease and immune system abnormalities.

The medical profession had told coeliac disease sufferers for a long time that they were twice as likely to suffer an early death, and they were in line for lymph cancers, such as Non-Hodgkin's lymphoma. But a study published in 2004 showed this not to be the case.[26] It found that there was a slightly increased risk of cancers compared with people without the condition – but only in the first year after diagnosis. After that first year, people with coeliac disease had a much reduced risk, particularly of the two main cancers: breast cancer was reduced by almost two-thirds, as were lung cancers. Only lymphomas, which are rarer, were increased.

The treatment for coeliac disease is a diet that strictly avoids all foods that contain gluten. This means not only the obvious ones such as bread and pasta, but also packaged foods that contain hidden gluten in unspecific substances such as 'modified starch'.

After diagnosis, therefore, those with celiac disease start cutting down on these foods; consequently, their blood glucose levels would fall. And, as high levels of glucose increase the risk of cancers, merely the change of diet following diagnosis would reduce their cancer risk. This explains why most cancer risks disappear after that first year.

It seems that in the past, most people with coeliac disease were more likely to worry themselves to death with all the bad news doctors were telling them than from the diseases they were supposed to develop. What looked like a major risk has now been reduced to a slight one.

Chronic inflammations of the bowel

There is a spectrum of diseases that affect the small and large intestine which do not appear to have a definite cause. Both Crohn's disease and ulcerative colitis are characterized by chronic inflammation at various places along the gut.

Crohn's disease

Crohn's disease (CD) is a chronic condition that causes inflammation and injury to the small intestine. It typically begins to cause symptoms in young adulthood, usually between the ages of 14 and 24. Why it develops is not clear, although it does seem to run in families. It also seems to follow periods of chronic diarrhoea. CD was first recognized early in the 20th century. Since then the number of cases has increased considerably. Common symptoms of CD are abdominal pain, fever, not wanting to eat, weight loss, and a pain in the lower right quarter of the abdomen.

Once CD begins, it can cause intermittent, lifelong symptoms by inflaming the inside lining and deeper layers of the intestine wall. The irritated intestinal lining may thicken or wear away in spots (creating ulcers) or it may develop cracks (fissures). Inflammation can also allow an abscess to develop. In between attacks, the intestine attempts to heal by recoating itself with a new inside lining. If the inflammation has been severe, the intestine can lose its ability to distinguish the inside of one piece of intestine from the outside of another piece. As a result, it can mistakenly build a lining along the edges of an ulcer that has worn through the wall of the gut, creating a *fistula* – a permanent tunnel between one piece of gut and another. A fistula may even form between the gut and the skin surface, creating drainage of mucus to the skin.

Ulcerative colitis

Ulcerative colitis (UC) is also a lifelong condition. It begins with inflammation of the rectum but can progress to involve much of the large intestine. In a similar way to Crohn's, UC typically begins to cause symptoms in young adulthood, usually between the ages of 15 and 40.

No one knows for sure what triggers the inflammation in ulcerative colitis. It is thought that it may begin with a virus or a bacterial infection, and that the body's immune system malfunctions and stays active after the infection has cleared. In this kind of auto-immune problem, the bowel is injured by the body's own immune system. UC is not contagious, even within families, so there is no worry of direct contamination from one person to another.

UC affects the inner lining of the rectum and adjoining colon, causing it to wear away in spots, leaving ulcers to bleed or to ooze cloudy mucus or pus. Other parts of the body seem to be affected by inflammation and can develop symptoms in UC, including the eyes, skin, liver, back and joints.

Treatment

Both Crohn's disease and ulcerative colitis are normally treated with drugs: steroids and antibiotics. Eventually, if the diseases have progressed to a severe stage, surgery is used to remove part of the gut. However, if these diseases are caught before serious damage has been done, both conditions can be treated simply by restricting carbohydrates. An Austrian doctor, Professor Wolfgang Lutz, has treated these conditions successfully for over 40 years. His figures, graphically illustrated below, show clearly that when carbohydrates are limited, both conditions respond very quickly.[3]

I too have found that the benefits of a low-carb diet can be felt very

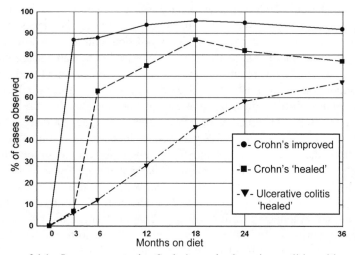

Figure 24.1: Improvements in Crohn's and ulcerative colitis with a low-carbohydrate diet

quickly. Joan, a student in one of my classes, had suffered from UC for 18 years. She told me: 'I am delighted that my daily visits to the toilet have now reduced to once every three or four days! I noticed a difference very soon after changing my diet and it has continued.'

A thought: dietary fibre is a primary cause of ulcerative colitis. Ulcerative colitis increases the chances of getting colon cancer many times over. Yet, to prevent colon cancer, we are told to consume more fibre.

Irritable bowel syndrome (IBS)

IBS is a common but poorly understood disorder that causes a variety of bowel symptoms including abdominal pain, diarrhoea and/or constipation, bloating, gassiness and cramping.

While these symptoms may be caused by a number of different bowel diseases, IBS is usually diagnosed only after your doctor has ruled out the possibility of a more serious problem. Its severity varies from person to person. Some patients experience intermittent symptoms that are just mildly annoying, while others may have such severe daily bowel problems that IBS affects their ability to work, sleep and enjoy life. In addition, symptoms may change over time, such that an individual may have severe symptoms for several weeks and then feel well for months, or even years. Under normal circumstances, most people are never cured of IBS but all that may be needed is a reduction in carbohydrate intake. It is amazing how quickly this can work.

The role of fibre

Prior to the mid-20th century, dietary fibre, which was then called 'roughage', was regarded as harmful. In people with gut disorders such as diverticular disease, the advice was to avoid bran and adopt a low-fibre diet. Later, the notion that constipation was central to human disease gave rise to some quaint practices and a huge breakfast-cereal industry. Population studies in East Africa seemed to show a protective effect of fibre[27] and high-fibre diets became the fashion. Dr Dennis Burkitt and colleagues were concerned with colon cancer, diverticular disease and constipation. By implication IBS was also included in this group. And so high-fibre diets became the standard treatment for the condition, even though the effectiveness of this treatment had never been tested.

So by the 1980s, fibre had been a popular way to treat IBS for about 10 years, despite there being several studies between 1976 and 1985 which showed no convincing effect of any benefit from bran on overall symptom patterns. In 1987, doctors at St Bartholomew's Hospital, London, set out to test its efficacy by conducting a trial of bran in IBS.[28] Two groups of patients were fed either high-bran biscuits or low-bran biscuits as a placebo for three-month periods, and then the two groups were swapped for a second three months. Naturally the patients weren't told which biscuits they were getting, although some may have guessed. The overall responses indicated that bran was not helpful. While IBS in both groups improved, there was no significant difference in IBS symptoms between the two groups. In 1994, doctors at the University Hospital of South Manchester, UK, looking at the weight of evidence so far, said: 'we got the impression that wholemeal wheat and bran products made people with the condition worse rather than better.' So they, too, did a trial – and found that their impressions were correct. They concluded that their evidence suggests: 'that the use of bran in irritable bowel syndrome should be reconsidered' as there is a: 'possibility that excessive consumption of bran in the community may actually be creating patients with irritable bowel syndrome by exacerbating mild, non-complaining cases.'[29]

The weight of all the evidence suggests that bran, wholemeal bread and wholemeal cereals are more likely to cause IBS than they are to cure it. Also, because it is indigestible, bran ferments in the gut and can induce or exacerbate flatulence, distension and abdominal pain.[30] And it is the same story with diverticular disease.

Fruit may also cause IBS

A study, presented by Young Choi and colleagues from the University of Iowa to the American College of Gastroenterology, built on previous research showing that between one third and one half of patients suffering from IBS symptoms, were actually fructose intolerant.[31]

The team initially tested 80 patients suspected of having IBS for fructose intolerance, and confirmed the condition in 30 (37.5%). Those 30 were then instructed on how to eliminate fructose from their diet and, after a year, 26 were interviewed to assess their symptoms. The team reported that in patients who complied with the fructose-restricted diet, symptoms such as abdominal pain, bloating and diarrhoea were significantly reduced, as was the prevalence of IBS itself. Symptoms remained unchanged in patients who did not comply with the diet.

Diverticular disease

Diverticulosis and diverticulitis are conditions very common among older adults in developed countries. Since 'healthy eating' was introduced, the number of cases in developed countries has increased by over 50%. Diverticular disease is one of the five most costly gastrointestinal disorders in the US. Thirty years ago, the proportion of people who died from diverticular disease was decreasing; during the past 20 years annual rates of admission and surgical intervention have increased by 16%.[32]

Diverticulosis develops in weak spots along the walls of the colon, typically in the part on the left side of the abdomen. In response to pressure, small, balloon-like pouches called *diverticula* may poke outward through the weak spots. At this stage, most people have no symptoms. The trouble starts when a *diverticulum* is filled with faeces which ferment. This causes the more serious *diverticulitis* (inflammation of the diverticula) which can infect the colon wall and cause bleeding. At this stage hospital care generally is required and surgery may be recommended in specific circumstances.

Normally, a high-fibre diet is recommended as part of the treatment for this and all conditions affecting the gut. And therein lies the problem. In an article on the subject in *The Lancet*,[30] the editor wrote: 'Bran is on the defensive. There is little direct evidence that increasing the intake of fibre by itself has any beneficial effect on health. The notion that people should tolerate the unpalatability of bran and its unpleasant side-effects because it will prevent diseases . . . is founded on shaky evidence.'

There is one other consideration. Bran and other cereal fibres make faeces loose and soft – and this has been shown to *increase* the risk of colon cancer.[33]

The answer is to avoid cereal bran.

Constipation

Constipation is another condition for which fibre, and bran in particular, is recommended. In my experience, although it can be helpful occasionally, there are better solutions. I, as well as some studies, have found that fibre, particularly cereal fibre, may actually increase the risk of constipation. For example, although it is supposed to travel through the gut at a faster rate, it does not always do so and it has been shown to cause blockages.[34] Good remedies are coconut oil, higher fat intake or green leafy vegetables. Another way to prevent constipation is to have the right breakfast. As Dr K. W. Heaton wrote in 1989: 'For many people the next port of call after breakfast is the lavatory, thanks to the "gastrocolic reflex" being especially active at this time of day. For anyone with a tendency to constipation this is an extra inducement to cultivate the breakfast habit . . . The strongest stimulus is fat so, perhaps, bacon and eggs have something to be said for them after all!'[11] Yet another good way is to ensure that you drink sufficient water – a minimum of 2 litres (3½ pints) a day.

Constipation after change of diet
Constipation is a frequent complaint when people who have eaten a high-

fibre diet adopt the low-carb diet recommended here. But that does not mean that the new diet is at fault. Constipation is really caused by their previous diet. What happens is this. You eat food and the waste is moved along the bowel by circular muscles in rather the same way as a worm moves (it's called *peristalsis*). However, if you eat a high-fibre diet, the fibre itself forces waste through and peristaltic action is made redundant. After a while it stops working. Now you change to a low-fibre, more natural diet, and your bowel muscles have forgotten how to work as they should, so you get constipated.

But the muscles will recover if you keep eating properly (low-carb, high-fat). While they catch up and get working again, increasing salads or raw vegetables might help them; drinking more water will also help. What you should *not* do is go back to the high-fibre regime that caused the problem in the first place.

Detox your gut

The digestive systems of carnivorous and herbivorous animals operate in quite different ways: the former is specifically adapted to digest animal proteins and fats, while the latter has developed to process plant materials.

Whereas the bacterial fermentation of plant starches and fibre, with the production and absorption of short-chain fatty acids, contributes between 60% and 90% of all the energy requirements in plant-eating animals, the colonic fermentation in humans is of minor importance. If the intestine has a normal length and function for nutrition, the human colon has little function other than conservation and the absorption of water.

Plant cell walls are composed of cellulose. This indigestible fibre constitutes a large proportion of the plant. When we eat plant materials, the cellulose passes through the stomach and small intestine to end up in the colon (large intestine) in an undigested state. Other carbohydrates, even though they have been processed to some extent, also end up in the colon. What happens to them is of considerable importance.

The bacterial flora living in the intestines of herbivores are quite different from those in carnivores.[35] Digestion in a herbivore is continued in the colon by a process of bacterial fermentation. It is a vital part of a herbivore's digestive system, designed to get the most out of what is a pretty poor source of nutrition. But no useful digestion takes place in our colons. All our digestion takes place in our stomach and small intestine, and our digestion is close to 100% efficient when we eat foods of animal origin. So what is left is only a small amount of pure (if that is the right word) waste. Within our colon are – or should be – proteolytic (meaning they break down protein) bacteria that live on proteins and fatty acids, breaking them down in a similar way to the proteolytic enzymes that digest proteins in the small intestine. In the colon, these bacteria attack any protein and fat that has escaped digestion and convert these substances into amino acids, glycerine and conglomerates of amino acids called proteoses and peptides – exactly the same process as happens further up the gut. But these bacteria are also capable of operating on carbohydrates. And when this happens, acid and gas are produced.

A pure carnivore should eat no plant material, so there should not be any carbohydrate in its colon to support fermentative bacteria. With no fermentative bacteria to produce acids, the proteolytic bacteria thrive in a healthy alkaline environment.

Civilized man, however, does not restrict his diet to just meat and fat. He also eats carbohydrates which ensures that a lot of indigestible carbohydrate, in the form of vegetable, fruit and cereal fibres, as well as a proportion of other carbohydrates, reaches his colon. This changes the gut flora considerably.

Unfortunately, medical science is still not very knowledgeable about such details in human beings, although it is certain that changes are produced when sugar replaces starch; much greater changes occur when carbohydrates replace proteins and fats in the diet.

Even a small amount of carbohydrate in the colon will support a colony of fermentative bacteria; if there is a large amount of the more indigestible carbohydrates such as bran and raw vegetation from salads, the fermentative bacteria will thrive until they can be overwhelming. As the production of acid in the colon soars, the resultant environment becomes hospitable to yeasts, moulds and other fungi. These too are avid fermenters and, as their numbers also increase, the colonic environment becomes more and more acid. But this environment does not suit the beneficial proteolytic bacteria which should be there, so they die off leaving the harmful fermenting bacteria unopposed. This leaves the colon both irritated and irritable. We start to see diarrhoea and other signs of digestive distress.

The individual knows nothing of the bacterial change that has taken place. All he is concerned with is that his stools are getting smellier, sloppier and more acid, and his rectum is itching and burning.

At the same time, the irritable colon disturbs the rest of the digestive tract. The stomach becomes gassy and the small intestine speeds up the transport of the food within it. The various vegetable fibres, which are difficult to digest at best, are speeded through to the colon with even less digestion than before. And as absorption of nutrients into the body takes time – and that time is now reduced – even more reach the colon. This provides an even better environment for the fermenting bacteria; they proliferate, and things go from bad to worse.

Prehistoric man undoubtedly consumed some plant foods. But it was only in neolithic times, after they had been made edible by boiling or other forms of cooking with fire, that they were used in any real quantity.[36] Right up to Roman times, vegetables, even salad vegetables, were invariably served cooked. While poorer plebeians were described as eating raw plant foods such as chicory, lettuce, endive and garlic, aristocratic Romans certainly didn't – unless they needed a laxative.

The eating of raw vegetables died out throughout the Middle Ages, being used only as a purgative. Renaissance Italy seems to have reintroduced the salad trend, but even then salads consisted of cooked, then cooled, vegetables and fish.

The use of raw plant foods other than as a laxative or purgative, is a very modern fad. And it may not be a very healthy one.

What really is a 'detox' diet?

One of the concepts that alternative health professionals believe in is 'cleansing' or 'detoxifying'. It can happen when you add a super-supplement to your diet, or when you eliminate bad stuff you used to eat or drink. We are familiar with the concept for drugs and alcohol, but not so much for foods and other lifestyle habits.

It is dietary carbohydrates alone that cause intestinal distress of varying degrees in carnivores and humans. What we should eat is a non-irritant type of diet: one in which carbohydrates can be eaten, but in such a way that they don't play havoc with the intestinal flora. We need some form of diet that detoxifies the gut.

Because of incorrect or insufficient knowledge, 'detox' diets all seem to be based on raw vegetation or juicing of vegetables and fruit. Quite what the rationale for this is I have no idea because, as I have shown, such a diet is actually quite toxic to the large intestine. And science has shown that a drink of ordinary tap water is far more effective than the various expensive products sold for detoxing.

As far as the intestine is concerned, our diet should be one that does not irritate it. This means, first of all, excluding laxatives such as prunes, figs and rhubarb; it means avoiding sharp, scratchy wastes such as bran; and it also means not juicing raw plant material and fruit, as this, perversely, is one of the best ways to cause all this agony.

To absorb the most carbohydrate in the small intestine and, thus, prevent it from getting to the colon in large quantities, it is necessary to break down the cell walls so that the digestive enzymes can get at and digest the nutrients inside. Juicing does not do this. Looked at through a microscope, even after juicing, plant cells are seen quite plainly to be intact, merely floating about in the fluid portion of the plant. In this form they are just as indigestible as they were in their original whole raw form.

By drinking a glass of orange juice or carrot juice, it is easy to imbibe five or six fruits and, in this way, to greatly increase the amount of carbohydrate in the diet – which is the very last thing one should do.

Tinned fruit juices are in a different category, as the heat used during the canning process does tend to break down the plant cell walls. But as these juices are generally drunk first thing in the morning, they enter the digestive system quickly, pass through it just as quickly and end up in the colon virtually unchanged – a perfect medium for the fermentative bacteria and their friends. Canned juices are also frequently sweetened, which is not healthy.

There is only one way to set the balance right again and that is to eat little that will allow undigested carbohydrate material to reach the colon. And this is possible. Synthetic diets composed of pure amino acids, fatty acids and glucose, which need no digestion and leave no residue, will halt the production of acid in the colon and restore the correct balance.[37] But trials on volunteers showed that could take up to three months of very strict dieting to achieve this result, and it had to be conducted in a hospital background.

A more realistic way is to reduce the amount of carbohydrate in your diet to a minimum. And avoid at all costs such material as bran or other vegetable and fruit fibre which cannot be digested, as this will certainly end up feeding the very bacteria you are trying to get rid of.

Too much insulin causes colon cancer

So fibre isn't particularly helpful with most diseases of the gut. As I explained in Chapter Seven, there is little to support the contention that lack of fibre causes cancer. However, a similarity in risk factors for insulin resistance and colorectal cancer (CRC) led to the hypothesis that markers of insulin resistance, such as high levels of insulin, glucose, fatty acids and triglycerides in the blood were energy sources and growth factors in the development of CRC. Scientists at the University of Toronto, Canada, set out to examine the individual and combined effects of these circulating factors on cells of the colorectal lining.[38] Their study showed that high levels of blood glucose did not increase cancer risk, but the high levels of insulin as a result of high blood glucose levels did. They concluded: 'These results provide evidence for an acute role of insulin, at levels observed in insulin resistance, in the proliferation of colorectal epithelial cells in vivo.'

High-fat dairy reduces colon cancer

High-fat dairy products do not raise insulin levels; and they have other anti-colon cancer attributes according to a study conducted at the prestigious Karolinska Institute in Stockholm. The Swedish Mammography Cohort study looked at long-term, high-fat dairy food consumption and colorectal cancer in 60,708 women aged 40-76 for nearly 15 years. They found that colorectal cancer was reduced by over 40% in women who ate four or more servings a day of high-fat dairy foods such as whole milk, full-fat cultured milk, cheese, cream, sour cream, and butter, compared with women who consumed less than one serving per day.[39]

To phew or not to phew

Most of us don't go around smelling the droppings of animals or even our own. But those who live in the country and walk the fields will probably have noticed that where cows are kept out to grass, their droppings either don't smell or have a not-unpleasant smell. The same is true of all other animals that eat their natural diet – including carnivorous animals. Compare this with the noisome smell you are likely to carry into the house if you walk in some dog dirt in a city street. This is because domestic pet dogs don't eat a natural diet.

The same is true of humans. Do you pass wind? When you do, does it tend to clear the room? When you go to the lavatory, do you have to open the window and suggest that the next person might be wise to wait a few minutes before 'going'?

My family and I don't. When we go to the lavatory, we use one piece of toilet paper to discover that we didn't need it – our stools leave us cleanly. There is little or no smell other than a faint, vinegary aroma.

Polycystic ovary syndrome (PCOS)

Polycystic ovary syndrome is one of the most common endocrine disorders, affecting approximately 10% of women of reproductive age. Originally considered a gynaecological disorder, PCOS is associated with a wide range of endocrine and metabolic abnormalities, including insulin resistance.[40]

Affected women are at an increased risk of developing gestational diabetes and type-2 diabetes, and there is an association with cardiovascular risk factors including obesity, high blood pressure, and thickening of the artery walls.

What causes PCOS is unclear. However, there are strong indications that dietary sugars play a major part. In view of the proven links with diabetes and cardiovascular disease, a causal link with the carbohydrate-based 'healthy' diet is very persuasive.

PCOS is a disease that is better prevented than cured. Correct diet (low in sugars – and that includes fruit) is probably the healthiest way to prevent it.

Chapter Twenty-Five

Deficiency diseases

I have suggested that reducing our intake of carbs is advantageous. But might cutting out carbohydrate-rich foods like bread, pasta, breakfast cereals and rice and reducing our intake of other plant foods put you at risk of deficiency diseases? The evidence suggests that the opposite could be true.

> Perhaps one reason for the wide acceptance of the suggestion that fibre is an important, if not essential, dietary component is that it had the enthusiastic support of commercial interests.
>
> *Professor John Yudkin*

So far I have suggested that reducing our intake of carbs is advantageous, but you will be told by nutritionists that 'cutting out a whole food group' will put you at risk of deficiency diseases. Current recommendations suggest that we should increase our intake of 'whole grains' and soy is promoted as a useful source of protein, a healthy replacement for the meat we are told to eat less of. As usual, they have it the wrong way around.

While foods from animal sources contain all the nutrients our bodies need, soy, cereals and, to a lesser extent, other foods of vegetable origin all contain anti-nutrients, built into them by Nature to protect them from predators. As a consequence, many contain toxins that, if not adequately fermented or cooked, have adverse effects on us, not only as poisons but also by inhibiting the absorption of many minerals and other nutrients.

Osteoporosis

By the end of the 1980s, post-menopausal women in Britain stood a one in two chance of suffering from osteoporosis (brittle bone disease) and one in five of them died as a direct result.[1] That was twice as many fractures as there were in the 1950s,[2] and numbers are still increasing.

Yet there are many cultures in the world where postmenopausal women are fit, active and healthy right up the end of their lives. Central American Indian women, for example, live for an average of 30 years after the menopause but they don't get osteoporosis, they don't lose height, they don't develop a dowager's hump and they don't suffer fractures. A research team analyzed their hormone levels and bone density. The team found that their oestrogen levels were no higher than those of white American women – in some cases they were even lower. Bone density tests showed that bone loss occurred in these women at the same rate as their US counterparts.[3] So why didn't they suffer fractures?

To understand this, it is important to understand the nature of bones. Bone might appear to be static, but it is a living tissue which undergoes constant renewal and replacement. At any given time, in every one of us, there are up to 10 million sites where small segments of old bone are being dissolved and new bone is being laid down to replace it.[4]

Bone-forming cells are of two different kinds: *osteoclasts* and *osteoblasts*. The job of osteoclasts is to find old bone that is in need of renewal. They dissolve bone and leave behind tiny unfilled spaces. Osteoblast cells then move into these spaces in order to build new bone. In this way, bone heals and renews itself in a process called *remodelling*. It is imbalances in this remodelling process that contribute to osteoporosis: when more old bone is eaten up than new bone is laid down, bone loss occurs.

The process of remodelling continues throughout our lives. But after the age of about 50, although the rate increases, the bone-building osteoblasts become less and less capable of completely refilling the spaces made by the osteoclasts.[3]

The correct term for low bone density is *osteopenia*, literally 'bone poverty'. Density is only one factor in osteoporosis and the fractures that result from it. Another, which tends to be forgotten, is the micro-architecture of the bone. As osteoclasts absorb more bone than is rebuilt, the micro-architecture becomes fragile, making the wrist and hip more vulnerable to fracture. Vertebrae don't really fracture or crack, they collapse, causing loss of height, and if enough vertebrae collapse, a 'dowager's hump' is created.

The medical definition of osteoporosis used to be 'fractures caused by thin bones'. In 1991, it was redefined as 'a disease characterized by low bone mass and micro-architectural deterioration of bone tissue which lead to increased bone fragility and a consequent increase in fracture risk.'[5] However, there is a problem with defining osteoporosis as a disease rather than a fracture because low bone mass is only a 'risk-factor' for osteoporosis, not osteoporosis itself. It's like defining heart disease as having high cholesterol rather than having a heart attack. Needless to say, this new definition has increased the number of women and men who 'have osteoporosis'.

Just measuring bone density can be misleading, for not everyone with low bone density will get fractures. Asian women, for example, tend to have low bone density yet very few bone fractures; and if you ingest fluoride, your bone density will be higher – but so will your fracture risk because the incorporation of fluoride makes the bones more brittle.

The general assumption has been that once bone reaches a certain level of thinness, it becomes subject to fractures more easily. Now that more is known about bone physiology, it is clear that this is not the full story. Bone does not fracture due to thinness alone. Leading bone expert, Dr Susan E. Brown, states: 'Osteoporosis by itself does not cause bone fractures. This is documented simply by the fact that half of the population with thin osteoporotic bones in fact never fracture.'[6]

Lawrence Melton of the Mayo Clinic noted as early as 1988: 'Osteoporosis alone may not be sufficient to produce such osteoporotic fracture, since many individuals remain fracture-free even within the sub-groups of lowest bone density. Most women aged 65 and over and men 75 and over have lost enough bone to place them at significant risk of osteoporosis, yet many never fracture any bones at all. By age 80, virtually all women in the United States are osteoporotic with regard to their hip bone density, yet only a small percentage of them suffer hip fractures each year.'[6]

So why are there many more women now with broken bones than in the past? It is suggested that it may be nothing more than the change in definition. However, that doesn't alter the fact that the numbers of bone fractures in both women and men have increased since 'healthy eating' was introduced. And that may provide a clue. Parkinson's disease is also associated with an increased risk of falls. Several studies found decreased bone mineral density values at the femoral neck and lumbar spine in patients with Parkinson's disease. Limited exposure to sunlight and consequent inadequate vitamin D is a factor in both Parkinson's and bone conditions, as other aspects of our 'healthy diet' may be.

How can one avoid osteoporosis?

The recommended way to prevent osteoporosis is to increase your intake of calcium, usually by drinking low-fat, calcium-fortified milk. But a lack of calcium causes *osteomalacia* (see below), *not* osteoporosis. This is a common misconception which may be counterproductive. Many studies have shown that calcium supplementation could actually make the condition worse. As osteoporosis is caused by a weakening of the protein matrix of the bones, the best preventative measure is not calcium supplementation but a high-protein diet.

So it should not be a surprise that the overwhelming majority of epidemiological studies show low bone density to be more closely associated with low *protein* intakes, and high bone density with high protein intakes.[7]

Bone density varies widely in different individuals. It is determined by the peak amount of bone you started with and the rate of its loss. That is why it is important to eat plenty of bone-forming foods and do weight-bearing exercise to build up bone density when young. It is too late to do either of those things when symptoms appear in your 70s.

In England alone, nearly two decades ago, a fifth of all orthopaedic beds were already occupied by patients with broken hips. The direct hospital costs alone amounted to more than £160 million a year.[8] And that figure did not include other breakages, personal costs and, of course, the pain and hardship brought on by the disease. Is it coincidence that the incidence of osteoporosis has increased by about 10% a year for the past two decades as we have been told to reduce our consumption of meat, and to replace this with fibre-rich cereals?

Protein and bone health

In certain sections of the nutritional world, there seems to be a belief that if we eat animal protein this will cause our bones to lose calcium. This question is of particular interest in the light of palaeolithic diet research for two reasons. The first is because estimates of the levels of animal protein in the hominid diet during at least the last 1.7 million years of human evolution (from the time of *Homo erectus*) are much higher than considered prudent in some sectors of the nutritional research community today; the second is because the fossil evidence shows that palaeolithic humans had a higher bone mass that would have been more robust and fracture-resistant than modern western humans' bones.

Studies published in the 1980s of people eating a high-protein diet also detected no calcium loss even over a long period of time, provided that meat was eaten with its fat.[9] And subsequent studies confirmed that:

- meat eating does not adversely affect calcium balance;[10,11]
- protein actually promotes stronger bones;[12]
- men and women who eat the most animal protein have better bone mass than those who avoid it.[13,14]

Increasing protein intake also helped elderly patients who were taking vitamin D and calcium supplements. Drs B. Dawson-Hughes and S. S. Harris of the Calcium and Bone Metabolism Laboratory, Tufts University, Boston, Massachusetts, tested associations between protein intake and change in bone mass density in 342 healthy men and women aged 65 or over who had completed a three-year, randomized, placebo-controlled trial of calcium and vitamin D supplementation.[15] They found that higher protein intake was significantly associated with a favourable three-year change in total-body bone mass density in the supplemented group but not in the placebo group.

My wife, Monica, is the only woman I know who has lived on a meat-, eggs- and cheese-based, protein-rich diet for most of her life. In 2004, she had a bone scan as part of a national survey. At the age of 66 she had the bone density of a woman half her age.

Are protein powders the culprits?

What is significant in the various studies of protein intake and bone density is that the studies which purported to show protein intake caused calcium loss were *not* conducted with real food but with isolated amino acids and fractionated protein powders of the sort used by low-carb dieters and athletes.

The reason why these amino acids and fat-free protein powders caused calcium loss while the fat meat diet did not is because protein, calcium, and minerals require the fat-soluble vitamins A and D for their assimilation and utilization by the body. When protein is consumed without these factors it upsets the normal biochemistry of the body and mineral loss results.[16]

True vitamin A and full-complex vitamin D are found only in animal fats. Furthermore, saturated fats that are present with meat are essential for proper calcium deposition in the bones.[17,18]

Another nutrient that helps promote good bone health is vitamin B_{12}, found only in foods from animal sources. In a three-year study from Wageningen University in the Netherlands, researchers monitored B_{12} levels and bone mineral density in 615 men and 652 women with a mean age of 76. Results showed that men with low levels of B_{12} had almost four times the numbers of fractures compared with those having normal levels, and women with the lowest levels of B_{12} had almost three times the bone loss and fractures compared with women with the highest levels.[19]

It should be no surprise, therefore, that vegan diets have been shown to place women at the greatest risk for osteoporosis.[20,21]

Lastly, insufficient sunlight and consequent lack of vitamin D is another risk factor for osteopenia and osteoporosis.[22] These days, with the strictures against sunbathing, vitamin D deficiency affects all age groups, not merely the elderly. While hip fractures are commonly attributed to osteoporosis, it may not be the cause. As I explained on page 183, only a quarter of women with broken hips had osteoporosis. What the others had was very low levels of vitamin D. Women over the age of 35 should consider taking as much as 4,000 International Units (IU) daily to help prevent osteopenia, the bone weakening that leads to breakages.

Drug treatments for osteoporosis

However, rather than use diet and sunlight, osteoporosis is routinely treated with the drug, *Fosamax* (alendronate). While this does increase bone density, it doesn't prevent fractures.[23]

Arthritis

There can be few if any who have not suffered from pain in their lower backs at some time in their lives. Back troubles are some of the most common complaints seen in a doctor's office. In each year, about 2% of any general practitioner's patients consult him with backache.

Beverly had suffered intermittent mild to severe lower back pain for over 10 years. She told me that within a week of starting eating the way I recommend, she found that her pain cleared up completely. She said: 'It only comes back when I have slipped off the wagon. I put it down to wheat, as my odd foray into chocolate land doesn't seem to bring it on.'

This case illustrates a simple case of cause and effect as, apart from studies of ancient peoples, clinical trials have also shown that carbohydrates, particularly cereals, in the diet may cause arthritis.[24] They may also be responsible for other conditions.

Arthritis, a common plague of modern society, exists in two major forms:

- *osteoarthritis*, which is caused by wear and tear and, consequently, is generally present only in the middle-aged or elderly; and
- *rheumatoid arthritis*, which may be present at all ages.

Osteoarthritis has been found in the most ancient skeletal remains of humans and animals. But evidence of rheumatoid arthritis has not been identified earlier than about 2750 BC, a time when consumption of cereal grains had become widespread.

Osteoarthritis

Osteoarthritis tends to accompany osteoporosis. Researchers at Wayne State University School of Medicine in Detroit tested the hypothesis that women with arthritis had a lower bone density.[25] They found a significant decrease in bone density in the legs of female patients with relatively mild osteoarthritis of the knee whether or not they had osteoporosis based on a spine bone density measurement. Osteoarthritis is known to be more prevalent in those who are obese.[26] It's not surprising that joints protest at having to support a heavier body.

Rheumatoid arthritis

Rheumatoid arthritis is never found in animal remains. Neither has it ever been found in skeletal remains of corn-eating peoples, such as Central American Indians. But it has been found to be present equally in all races and cultures eating wheat, rye and oats. This finding suggests that rheumatoid arthritis is a gluten-induced condition similar to coeliac disease.[27]

Today, arthritis and other rheumatic conditions are among the most prevalent diseases and the most frequent cause of disability.[28] An American mortality and morbidity report published in 2001 estimated that some 43 million Americans had rheumatoid arthritis in 1997. This was up from 35 million in 1985 – an increase of nearly a quarter. All age groups were affected, including the working-age population, and prevalence increased with age. Prevalence was higher in females overall and for each age group. There is no reason to suppose that the situation is any different in Britain and other industrialized countries.

But in a survey of North American Indians in 1932, Dr Weston Price looked specifically for the presence of arthritis in the more isolated groups. He found not one case, neither did he hear of a case. However, he said: 'at the point of contact with the foods of modern civilization many cases were found including ten bed-ridden cripples in a series of about twenty Indian homes.'[29] One five-year-old boy had been in bed in hospitals with rheumatic fever, arthritis and an acute heart involvement for two and a half years. His mother had been told that her boy would not recover, so severe were the complications. She asked for Dr Price's assistance in planning a nutritional program for her boy. He tells us:

> 'The important change that I made in this boy's dietary program was the removal of the white flour products and in their stead the use of freshly cracked or ground wheat and oats used with whole milk to which was added a small amount of specially high vitamin butter produced by cows pasturing on green wheat. Small doses of a high-vitamin, natural cod liver oil were also added. At this time the boy was so badly crippled with arthritis, in his swollen knees, wrists, and rigid spine, that he was bedfast and cried by the hour. With the improvement in his nutrition which was the only change made in his care, his acute pain rapidly subsided, his appetite greatly improved, he slept soundly and gained rapidly in weight.'[30]

Rheumatoid arthritis is a complex auto-immune disease involving numerous environmental and genetic components, and similar to a number of other auto-immune diseases is found more often in coeliac patients.[31]

Many studies of arthritic patients have demonstrated elevated antibody levels for gliadin (a protein found in gluten).[32,33] While no large clinical trials have been undertaken specifically to examine the effectiveness of gluten-free diets in the treatment of arthritis, there are numerous case studies reporting alleviation of arthritis symptoms with grain-free diets.[34-37]

The other half of Dr Price's protocol – adding fat – is also supported by a recent study which showed that improving the ratio between omega-3 and omega-6 fatty acids by eating fish oils and other omega-3 rich oils is of benefit.[38] It was not necessary to eat a lot, however. The reported total intake of omega-3 fatty acids in the intervention group was 3.1 grams per day, and of this, 1.2 grams were of EPA and DHA. That is just over half a teaspoonful in total. It is important not to overdo this.

It is also worth noting that cardiovascular disease morbidity and mortality are increased in patients with rheumatoid arthritis and much of the excess cardiovascular disease morbidity appears to be due to atherosclerosis.[39] This could be a pointer to a common causative factor between the two diseases, although it could also be that conventional arthritis treatment increases cardiovascular risk.

Vilhjalmur Stefansson's experience

The anthropologist, Dr Vilhjalmur Stefansson, didn't always take his own advice. As an explorer, he had lived on a no-carb diet for many years and believed in it. However, from about 1927 to 1955 he ate a conventional western diet. Over time he put on weight – to a maximum of 184 lbs (83.6 kg). To manage his weight, Stefansson tried cutting down on calorie intake for some years but only lost 5 lbs. He also had noticed that he was developing a stiffness in one knee. This gradually worsened and, by the time he was 75, Stefansson also had increasing soreness in both his hip and shoulder joints. Eventually, in 1955, he decided to revert to the 'Stone Age' all-fat-meat diet he had used on his Arctic explorations. It worked. Not only did he lose his excess weight, the diet cured his arthritis. Stefansson's wife, Evelyn, remarked:[40]

> 'As his knee stiffened, he began to go up and down stairs one step at a time. One day, some months after the start of our meat diet, he found to his surprise that he could use both legs with equal facility in climbing the stairs. Astonished, he proceeded down. When he had reached the foot of the stairs, without pain or stiffness, he shouted for me to come and see.'

Stefansson added:

> 'I did indeed shout for Evelyn, because I had just discovered something that I had not forecast to her because I had not foreseen it. The recovery of not only my stiff right knee but of all my joints, blessedly including my typing fingers, had been "magical." '

Stefansson lived on his 'Stone Age diet' until his death in 1962 at the age of 83, with no further problems with his joints.

Other conditions

Taking starch, and the bran and phytic acid which often accompany it, out of the diet has been shown to improve or prevent the following conditions: ankylosing spondylitis,[41] rickets[42] and osteomalacia, colon cancer,[43] Alzheimer's disease,[44] iron deficiency anaemia,[45] depression, anorexia,[46] low birth weight,[47] slow growth,[48] mental retardation,[49] amenorrhoea, the late onset of menstruation, retarded uterine growth[50,51] and menstrual dysfunction.[52]

Conclusion

One truly healthy aspect of a low-carb way of eating is that it generally means cutting down on cereals such as bread and pasta. This has the advantage that reduction of cereals also reduces the amount of phytic acid consumed, without you having to do anything else. Many people give up bread altogether. This isn't necessary but, if you do eat bread, make it white bread. Although white bread will have lost some of its nutritional value, on balance it may be healthier than wholemeal bread because of the lack of phytates – and it does have that added calcium.

There may be a limit under which bran is not harmful – but we have no ready way to know what that limit is. Therefore, it is much safer for you to avoid bran than to try to gauge what your safe limit might be. If you feel the need for fibre, there is an easier way: get your fibre from green leafy vegetables and don't eat bran, wholemeal bread and unfermented soy.

Chapter Twenty-Six

Diet and the brain

The food we eat has a wide range of effects on our body systems. As the brain uses one fifth of all the energy used by the body, it seems logical to suppose that it could be affected by incorrect diet. This chapter looks at the deleterious effects of 'healthy eating' on many brain functions and at the mental health problems that can result.

Low concentrations of naturally occurring total serum cholesterol, including those levels in the currently defined 'desirable' range, were associated with poorer cognitive performance.

Dr Penelope K. Elias

The food we eat has a wide range of effects on our body systems. So it seems logical to suppose that the brain could also be affected by incorrect diet.

Apart from water, our brains are about three-quarters fat. We need a steady intake of fats for our brains to function properly – and that intake must be of the right fats. Also, while our brains account for only about 2.5% of our body weight, they use about 20% of our bodies' total energy. For these reasons, food intakes and fluctuations in energy levels can have a profound effect on how our brains are formed as infants and how well they perform later in life, as well as affecting our behaviour and emotions.

The food we eat can have many effects on the brain. Carbohydrates engender a feeling of well-being and induce sleepiness; but they also have a wide range of other effects. For example, sugar can:

- cause hyperactivity, anxiety, concentration difficulties, and crankiness in children;[1]
- also cause drowsiness and decreased activity in children;[2]
- adversely affect children's school grades;[3]
- cause an increase in delta, alpha and theta brain waves, which can

alter the mind's ability to think clearly;[4]
* and, in addition, cause depression.[4]
* many neurological illnesses are also associated with cereal grain consumption as well as sugar;[5]
* nearly one out of every five paediatric patients with type-2 diabetes also has a brain-development disorder, psychiatric illness or behavioural disorder.[6]

This last factor tends to support a link between diet and these diseases. The sad thing is that instead of correcting these children's diets, psychotropic medications are often prescribed. Dr Lorraine E. Levitt Katz, paediatric endocrinologist with Children's Hospital of Philadelphia, noted that: 'We started seeing pediatric patients who had gained a tremendous amount of weight while they were on some of the newer atypical antipsychotic agents.'[6] This drug treatment seems only to make the situation worse by increasing weight gain and insulin resistance.

Changing eating habits away from carbohydrates and damaged fats and towards healthy fats and protein may prevent many increasingly common conditions from hyperactivity in children to Alzheimer's disease in adults.

Memory and cognitive ability

Under normal circumstances, the brain uses glucose as its main metabolic energy source. You might expect, therefore, that higher levels of glucose in your blood would mean that your brain would operate more efficiently. This is not the case. Scientists at the University of Wales found that a rapid rise in blood glucose from eating a 'healthy' carbohydrate-rich breakfast had a damaging effect on cognitive performances such as verbal memory in young adults during the four hours following it.[7] On the other hand, people performed much better after a meal that caused glucose levels to rise more slowly. This has implications for other conditions, particularly where the brain and memory are concerned.

A Boston University research team concluded that not having enough cholesterol could also cause a measurable deficit in mental functioning. Their findings showed that when the lowest-cholesterol group was compared with the highest-cholesterol group, who had blood levels of 6.25-9.9 mmols/L (240-381 mg/dL), the lowest-cholesterol group were as much as 80% more likely to perform poorly on tests of similarities, fluency, attention, and concentration.

Autism and ADHD

Autism

Over 500,000 children in the UK are autistic with four times as many boys as girls affected. Autism in children is characterized by few or no language and imaginative skills, repetitive and self-injurious behaviour and abnormal responses to human and environmental stimuli. The cause is not known, and some attribute this condition to a genetic trait. However, Professor Jean Golding of Bristol University points out that there has been a huge increase in numbers of cases of autism in the last 20 to 30 years. So it is likely that the recent large increase is due to environmental factors. Some autistic patients have been shown to have increased antibodies to gluten and casein;[8] however, the amelioration of symptoms in response to gluten-free diets has been equivocal.[9]

ADHD: A Demand for a Healthy Diet?

Attention-Deficit Hyperactivity Disorder (ADHD) is diagnosed from a collection of symptoms and signs that seems to get in the way of a child being educated, as well as such things as excessive risk-taking and an inability to filter the relevant from the irrelevant. These behaviour patterns can be very trying for both parents and teachers. The usual first noticed sign is a child who is inattentive or uncontrollable in class. ADHD is a new 'disease', and the question is: where did it come from? Neurologist, Dr Fred Baughman, gives us an answer: 'They made a list of the most common symptoms of emotional discomfiture of children; those which bother teachers and parents most, and in a stroke that could not be more devoid of science or Hippocratic motive – termed them a "disease." Twenty-five years of research, not deserving of the term "research", has failed to validate ADD/ADHD as a disease. Tragically – the "epidemic" having grown from 500,000 in 1985 to between five and seven million today – this remains the state of the "science" of ADHD.'[10]

There are no objective diagnostic criteria to determine if a child has ADHD. Criteria were decided by majority vote in a committee of the American Psychiatric Association. This is not science. Nevertheless, a huge and entrenched psychiatric treatment and research empire has mushroomed around ADHD and medical care for ADHD has grown into a huge industry. Today, American schools spend $1 billion a year on psychologists working full-time to diagnose students; $15 billion has been spent on the diagnosis, treatment and study of ADHD. There is no pretence to cure the problem.

Typical diagnostic 'symptoms' are:

- **Inattention** – easily distracted and unable to concentrate for long;

failing to pay attention to details; making careless mistakes; rarely following instructions carefully; losing or forgetting things such as toys, or pencils, books and tools needed for a task.

- **Impulsiveness** – blurting out answers before hearing the whole question and having difficulty waiting for their turn.
- **Hyperactivity** – restlessness, fidgeting with hands or feet, or squirming; running, climbing or leaving a seat in situations where sitting or quiet behaviour is expected.
- **Low boredom threshold.**

A teacher or school administrator is usually the one who suggests that a child see a doctor (psychiatrist or paediatrician) whom they know will put the child on the 'chemical cosh', Ritalin, or a similar drug. According to statistics supporting the Americans with Disabilities Act, as many as 10% of the US population have symptoms of ADHD and, even with drug treatment, it frequently persists into adulthood. These drugs are indiscriminate; they alter brain chemistry in ways other than just quieting children. And the side effects can be serious and very long lasting.

The most common finding in children with ADHD is hypoglycaemia (low blood sugar), and that, as I explained on page 276 is caused by a 'healthy' carbohydrate-based diet. When individuals have a low blood sugar response, the body releases adrenaline (epinephrine) to raise blood sugar levels. In children, this may cause them to act aggressively.

Dr Benjamin Feingold, a paediatrician in California, noticed that many hyperactive children become excited after eating foods containing high concentrations of salicylates. These occur naturally in many fruits and vegetables and are especially concentrated in grapes, raisins, nuts, apples, and oranges. A study performed at the Hospital for Sick Children in London, published in the British journal, *The Lancet*, demonstrated that most children with severe ADHD are salicylate sensitive. [11] This study also noted that 90% of these children have additional food allergies. These included allergies to, cow's milk products, corn (an additive in many foods), eggs, wheat and soy.

Other lines of research point to high levels of seed-sourced omega-6 fatty acids such as are found in polyunsaturated margarines and cooking oils, which unbalance omega-6 to omega-3 ratios;[12] and a number of chemical food additives.

The weight of evidence suggests that cutting out processed 'convenience' foods which contain these elements will avoid almost all the probable causes of ADHD. ADHD could really be 'A Demand for a Healthy Diet'. A change of diet is much better than a course of drugs.

However, if you want to make your child shorter than his peers, give him three years of medication for ADHD. The growth rate of children who are medicated for ADHD tends to decrease, and they never catch up after such treatment, according to the results of a National Institutes of Mental Health study.[13]

Depression

According to the World Health Organization, depression is one of the most important diseases in the world. There are now three times as many prescriptions for anti-depressive drugs in the UK as there were just 12 years ago. Research conducted by the WHO highlighted the prevalence of depression in modern society.[14] Assessing the 10 most important disorders in developed countries, WHO found that, in terms of years lived with disability, major depression, termed 'unipolar major depression', was the most important disorder. In addition, 'bipolar disorder', a condition in which periods of depression alternate with periods of mania, ranked sixth on the list. To put that in context, diabetes was 10th. In respect of lost years due to premature death, 'unipolar major depression' ranked second only to cardiovascular diseases. And the situation is getting worse.

The number of young people diagnosed each year with bipolar disorder, also known as manic depression, has increased significantly over the past decade: annual visits to doctors by young people with bipolar disorder increased from 25 in every 100,000 youth visits in 1994 to 1,003 in every 100,000 youth visits in 2003.[15] The number of visits by adults with bipolar disorder also increased significantly over the same period.

Are you feeling tired or depressed? You've all seen the adverts on TV for pick-me-ups, perhaps in the late afternoon: eat a biscuit, chocolate bar or other source of sugar. These advertisements rely on people's belief that a resulting rush of sugar into the bloodstream will give them a mental boost, that it will make them feel good and more alert. There have been many studies of the effects of these different meal patterns and different foods. Some tested and measured subjective things such as fatigue, vigour, anger, hostility, confusion, anxiety and depression. In all of these tests, those who ate carbohydrate-based meals reported worse scores in all classes except anxiety, where there was no difference. In other, objective tests of alertness, auditory and visual reaction times, and vigilance, carbohydrate eaters again came off worse.

There is certainly evidence that eating sugar or other carbohydrate foods has the ability to improve your mood. The role that glucose is known to play in supplying the cells of the body with energy has led to the assumption that an enhanced source of metabolic energy is associated with feeling subjectively more alert and energetic. But in fact, much of the evidence is that consuming carbohydrate has a hypnotic effect. In other words, it makes you feel good by making you more relaxed and sleepy, rather than more alert. This is the reason why many dieticians recommend a carbohydrate meal in the evening – it helps you sleep.

But with depression, if you are tired, you really don't feel like doing anything: it's an effort to get up, work, play, interact with people, get meals, and so on. And under these conditions, carbohydrate meals have exactly the opposite effect from what you might expect. They make you relaxed and slow your reaction times; protein/fat meals make you feel awake, bright, alert and quick-thinking and, crucially, lift depression.

Suicide and violence

Depression is the main psychiatric illness that predisposes to suicide. The anti-cholesterol lobby would have us believe that the lower your cholesterol, the healthier you are. But a French study concluded that: 'Both low serum cholesterol concentration and declining cholesterol concentration were associated with increased risk of death from suicide in men.'[16] This confirmed many previous epidemiological and clinical studies which had described an association between lower blood cholesterol and increased suicide risk.[17]

If your cholesterol is too low, your risk of mood disorders, depression and violence is increased. During trials to lower levels of cholesterol in the blood, a tendency towards more suicides and violent deaths became obvious. In 1991 Canadian investigators examined this trend.[18] Adjusting for age and sex, they found that those whose cholesterol was below 4.27 mmol/l (164 mg/dL) were six times more likely to attempt suicide than those with cholesterol above 5.77 mmol/l (222 mg/dL).

This was confirmed by a study conducted at the Psychiatric Clinic, Charles University of Prague.[19] Patients in this study who had attempted a violent suicide had significantly lower cholesterol levels than patients with non-violent attempts and the control subjects. The authors said: 'Our findings . . . are consistent with the theory that low levels of cholesterol are associated with increased tendency for impulsive behaviour and aggression and contribute to a more violent pattern of suicidal behaviour.' They concluded: 'These data indicate that low serum total cholesterol level is associated with an increased risk of suicide.'

Lower cholesterol also means more violent suicides. A recent study measured the cholesterol content of cortical and subcortical tissue of brains from 41 male suicide completers and 21 male controls. It showed that violent suicides had lower grey matter cholesterol content overall compared with non-violent suicides and controls.[20]

Polyunsaturated fats are recommended to lower cholesterol levels. Yet a 2006 study found that people with a high intake of polyunsaturated vegetable margarines and cooking oils, which were unbalanced with respect to omega-3 fatty acids, were *more* likely to commit suicide.[21] Another of the many studies examining the effects of omega-3 and omega-6 fatty acid levels on suicide and violence reported finding 'a striking correlation' between the greater consumption of omega-6 linoleic acid from seed oils over the period 1961 to 2000 and the growing number of homicides in the US, UK, Australia, Canada and Argentina.[22]

And there may be yet another dietary aspect. A team from the Medical Research Council, led by Professor David Barker, traced suicide rates in 15,500 Hertfordshire men and women whose birth records were available since 1911.[23] They found that men and women who committed suicide tended to have low rates of weight gain in infancy, which may also be caused by a carbohydrate-rich, nutrient-poor diet.

Others have found less anxiety, less aggression and less stress after switching to a low-carbohydrate, high-fat dietary regime.[24]

Depressing drugs

The pharmaceutical industry has a huge vested interest in people with psychiatric conditions as a market for their drugs. According to the *New York Times*: 'Vermont officials disclosed Tuesday that drug company payments to psychiatrists in the state more than doubled last year, to an average of $45,692 each from $20,835 in 2005 . . . Overall last year, drug makers spent $2.25 million on marketing payments, fees and travel expenses to Vermont doctors, hospitals and universities, a 2.3 percent increase over the prior year.'[25] The *Times* found that psychiatrists who took the most money from makers of antipsychotic drugs tended to prescribe the drugs to children the most often.

Dr Andrew Mosholder, an expert with America's Food and Drug Administration, reviewed 24 studies involving 4,582 patients taking one of nine different antidepressants. They showed that the drugs nearly doubled the risk of suicide among children and young adults. The FDA barred him from publishing his findings, but they were leaked to the press in 2004. In 2006, Mosholder's study was published.[26] It makes for extremely worrying reading. More worrying, perhaps, is that the FDA's principal role is guardian of public safety, yet it suppressed this evidence for two years. How many children during that time took their own lives?

Epilepsy

Epilepsy today is generally controlled with anti-epileptic medications. Occasionally surgery and nutritional strategies are also used. Despite these, up to 30% of epileptic attacks are not adequately controlled. Yet since 1920 a carefully calculated diet, very high in fat, low in protein, and almost carbohydrate free, has proven to be very effective in the treatment of difficult-to-control seizures in children. Although Johns Hopkins Medical Center in the US has continued to use it with great success,[27] this diet was generally discontinued for the control of seizures as new drugs were developed.

It is not clear what mechanism of action accounts for reports of decreased seizure activity while using a ketogenic diet in which about 90% of the calories in the diet came from fats. But it works. Drs Lefevre and Aronson of Northwestern University Medical School, Chicago, analyzed 11 published studies and one unpublished study.[28] The results of their review are shown below:

The range of patients who:

Became completely seizure free	7–33%
Had more than 90% reduction	22–56%
Had more than 50% reduction	29–100%

Although there were some adverse effects, such as gastrointestinal symptoms, in up to half of the children, these only lasted for a short time and were probably the result of the diet being so different from what the children were used to.

In 2008, the *Guardian* reported that 'Giving drugs to children with epilepsy is often ineffective and can have terrible side-effects. But there is an alternative – a high-fat food plan that dramatically reduces seizures.'[29] It's good to know that the medical profession is catching up with what is going on!

It's not just for children

A small study of 11 adults – nine women and two men – conducted at Jefferson Medical College, Philadelphia, and published the previous year, had shown that this diet works for adults as well.[30] After eight months of follow-up, three patients had a 90% seizure decrease, three patients had between 50% and 89% decrease in seizure frequency, and one patient had less than 50% seizure decrease. The other four patients discontinued the diet. The authors said: 'The ketogenic diet shows promise in both adult generalized and partial epilepsy' and recommended further study.

But what will further study achieve? This regime has been used successfully for over 80 years and it conforms almost exactly to the diet advocated here for the prevention and alleviation of many other conditions. With millennia of epidemiological evidence and a wealth of clinical study to back it, there is no reason to suppose it has any inherent dangers.

Unlike drug treatment.

Research presented at the American Academy of Neurology's 59th Annual Meeting in Boston on 28 April to 5 May 2007 found that children of women who took the epilepsy drug, *Valproate*, during pregnancy were at a greater risk for lower IQ.[31] According to the study, 24% of the children of mothers who took Valproate had an IQ in the mental retardation range. The study also found that children with higher levels of Valproate in their blood had lower IQ scores.

Epilepsy and schizophrenia

Several studies, have found that patients with epilepsy tend to have a higher prevalence of schizophrenia-like psychosis compared with the general population. The authors of a population-based Danish study of 2.27 million people which reported 'a strong association between epilepsy and schizophrenia or schizophrenia-like psychosis' said that the 'two conditions may share common genetic or environmental causes.'[32] It may be significant that this study showed that the type of epilepsy didn't affect the likelihood of schizophrenia. The risk increased with increasing admissions to hospital for epilepsy treatment, and particularly with increasing age at the first admission for epilepsy. Is it a coincidence that most hospitals treat epilepsy with drugs and a 'healthy' diet?

Schizophrenia

In the 1960s, Dr F. Curtis Dohan noticed that in regions where gluten consumption was common, the rate of schizophrenia was substantially higher than in places where gluten consumption was absent: places where people relied on sweet potato, rice or millet rather than wheat, rye, barley or oats, for example. Subsequent research, involving biopsies and including experiments by others, led Dohan to conclude that diagnosed schizophrenics did not typically have the same type of damage to the villi of the small intestine as people with coeliac disease, but a gluten-sensitive subset of schizophrenics processed gluten and the casein in dairy foods in a way that exposed their brains to certain very potent psychoactive substances that are now known to exist in those foods.

In his first published clinical trial, at a Veterans' Administration hospital, Dohan tried removing gluten-containing cereals and dairy from the diets of people diagnosed as schizophrenic while they were on a locked admitting ward; they went back on a regular gluten-containing diet once they moved to the open wards.

The patients at the hospital who were on the gluten-free diet while on the locked ward were discharged almost twice as quickly as those who were on a high-gluten diet. Dohan writes: 'The average time until discharge for the discharged CFMF [cereal-free, milk-free] patients (77 days) was 55 percent of that of the discharged HC [high cereal] patients (139 days).'[33]

Between 1966 and 1990 more than 50 articles regarding the role of cereal grains as a cause of schizophrenia were published. Dr Karl Lorenz conducted a meta-analysis of them and concluded that: 'In populations eating little or no wheat, rye and barley, the prevalence of schizophrenia is quite low and about the same regardless of type of acculturating influence.'[34]

This supported earlier clinical studies which had shown that schizophrenic symptoms improved on cereal-free diets and worsened upon their reintroduction. [33,35,36]

Schizophrenia and low fat intake

This evidence also ties in well with other dietary research along parallel lines. If people eat more of one thing, they necessarily eat less of another. For this reason, a high-carb diet is likely also to be a low-fat diet, and there is a growing body of research data which suggests that schizophrenia may be the result of an abnormal fatty acid composition of the brain. In a controlled study of fatty acids in patients with schizophrenia, doctors at the University Department of Psychiatry, Northern General Hospital, Sheffield, noticed that arachidonic acid and docosahexaenoic acid (DHA), were particularly low. These fatty acids are plentiful in meat and fish fats respectively, but not found in vegetable oils. Finding that: 'A strong correlation exists between schizophrenia and deficiencies in fats,' they said: 'that diets generally low in fat might worsen schizophrenia or even bring on the condition among those already predisposed to it is hard to ignore,' and suggested this: 'opens up novel and exciting therapeutic possibilities' for dietary treatment of schizophrenia – with a low-carb, high-fat diet.[37]

Antisocial behaviour and crime

Many have observed the links between civilization, including diet, and the increase in antisocial behaviour.[38] As long ago as 1937, Edward Lee Thorndike of Columbia University wrote that: 'Thinking is as biological as digestion,'[39] implying that a defect-free brain is required if we are to think coherently.

Meanwhile, as we saw in Chapter Twenty-Two, low blood cholesterol is also associated with aggression and antisocial behaviour.

Several other recent scientific investigations have also linked criminality to diets high in sugar and carbohydrates in adults. Jails are notorious for their problems with defiance of authority and bad behaviour. It's not surprising, I suppose: jails are full of criminals. Nevertheless, trials have been conducted into the effects of changing diets on inmates. And the results? 'Antisocial behaviour in prisons, including violence, are reduced by vitamins, minerals and essential fatty acids with similar implications for those eating poor diets in the community.'[40] The importance of a complete diet is difficult to overstate.

Sugar and antisocial behaviour

In the Third National Health and Nutrition Examination Survey (NHANES III) conducted in the US between 1988 and 1994, blood cholesterol levels were measured in 4,852 children aged six to 16.[41] Psychosocial development was evaluated by interviewing mothers about their children's history of school suspension or expulsion and difficulty in getting along with peers.

The survey showed that children whose cholesterol concentration was below 3.77 mmol/L (145 mg/dL) were almost three times more likely to have been suspended or expelled from schools than their peers with higher cholesterol levels.

Perhaps again we can learn from history. In the 1940s a New York doctor named Joseph Wilder found that low blood-sugar levels in adults produced mental symptoms such as depression, anxiety, irritability, slow mental processes, dullness and difficulty in making decisions. The effects of low blood-sugar in children were considerably more serious.[42]

Children with this condition would be neurotic, psychopathic and have criminal tendencies, suffer anxiety, run away, be aggressive and destructive. Dr Wilder wrote: 'In its simplest form, it is the tendency to deny everything, contradict everything, refuse everything at any price . . . It is no wonder that a considerable number of criminal and semi-criminal acts have been observed in children in hypoglycaemic (low blood-sugar) states, ranging from destructiveness or violation of traffic regulations all the way to bestiality, arson and homicide.' The low blood-sugar/criminality link has since been confirmed many times.

Despite this, speculation still persists about whether sugar consumption affects behaviour in children. In 1986 a study investigated the effect of sugar on the behaviour of preschool children.[43] On separate mornings each child received six ounces of fruit juice, sweetened on one morning with sugar and on the other with an artificial sweetener. The children were observed for an hour and a half following the drinks, during which time they were given alternating 15-minute sessions of work on structured tasks and 15-minutes of free play.

Following the sugar drink the children's performance in the structured testing sessions went down, and they demonstrated more 'inappropriate behaviour' during free play, mostly 45 to 60 minutes after the drinks.

This study provided strong objective evidence in young children of a rather subtle, yet significant, time-dependent behaviour effect of dietary sugar. The actual cause was a state of hypoglycaemia in the children caused by an overproduction of insulin as a response to the sugar load. But *all* dietary carbohydrates can cause hypoglycaemia if they form the major part of a meal.

Today, children are eating more sugar and high-carbohydrate foods than ever before in history – and, judging from reports in the press, committing more crimes at ever younger ages. Dr Wilder realized that low blood-sugar was not caused by low intake of sugar, but by the reverse. He said: 'Apparently, too copious feeding of sugar may, in the long run, cause an over-function of the islet cells of the pancreas and increase the tendency to hypoglycaemia; on the other hand, there are cases in which a diet extremely poor in carbohydrates and sugars may improve or even cure the condition.'

The 'healthy' dietary guidelines developed for adults are being extended to children, and 'healthy' meals are promoted in schools to curb obesity. But with the roles of carbs in hypoglycaemia and of serum cholesterol in the neurodevelopment of children so poorly recognized, the result could well be the reverse of that intended.

The point is that criminality increases because, despite the rhetoric, we are *not* tough on crime and its causes at all. If we were serious about wanting to reduce crime, one of the first things we would do is consider seriously revising 'healthy eating' advice.

Alzheimer's and Parkinson's diseases

The decline in mental functioning as we get older, which is becoming increasingly common, is accepted as sad and heartrending, but 'normal': an inevitable consequence of old age. But this decline need never happen and should never happen. Senility and its associated conditions are yet more examples of modern diseases which are very rare in primitive society and which are probably largely preventable in ours.

Alzheimer's disease (senile dementia) and Parkinson's disease, which only really appeared in the last century, are the two most prevalent age-related degenerative brain disorders in western societies. The degeneration of synapses and death of nerve cells are defining features of both. In Alzheimer's disease, neurons in the brain regions that control learning and memory functions are selectively vulnerable. In Parkinson's disease it is the dopamine-producing neurons in the brain regions that control body movements that selectively degenerate.

Studies of post-mortem brain tissue from Alzheimer's and Parkinson's patients have provided evidence that the conditions have similar causes to other diseases discussed in this book. Recent data suggest that both diseases can manifest systemic alterations in energy metabolism (increased insulin resistance and deregulation of glucose metabolism, for example). Importantly, evidence is emerging that dietary change can prevent these devastating brain disorders of ageing.

Alzheimer's disease

Alzheimer's disease makes up 55% of dementia cases in the UK, according to the Alzheimer's Society, and over 800,000 people in the UK currently suffer the affliction. Although normally a disease of the elderly Alzheimer's is increasingly seen in younger people. It is also seen in people with other 'healthy' diet related conditions. Not surprisingly, the number of people with Alzheimer's has more than doubled since 1980.

For example, there is a disproportionate number of cases of deteriorations of memory, cognition, speech memory, working memory and visual-spatial skills among diabetics compared with non-diabetics; diabetics also have a two- to three-times increased risk of Alzheimer's compared with the general population.[44,45] Population studies indicate that Alzheimer's disease is much more prevalent in diabetics across the world. Stolk and colleagues at Erasmus University Medical School, Rotterdam, say that: 'These findings are more compatible with a direct effect of insulin on the brain than with an effect through an increase in cardiovascular risk factors.' High-carbohydrate diets could lead to Alzheimer's disease through chronic over-exposure of cells to insulin signalling, which accelerates cellular damage in cerebral neurons,[46] and can cause insulin resistance.[47]

For nine years a research team followed 824 Catholic priests and nuns, 127 of whom had diabetes.[48] One hundred and fifty-one of them went on to develop Alzheimer's. Two thirds of them were diagnosed diabetics. Researcher Zoë Arvanitakis found that insulin in the blood stimulates a protein called 'tau' which tangles brain cells into Alzheimer knots.

In a commentary in the medical journal, *The Lancet*, Dr Mark Strachan reviewed research showing that, while normal levels of insulin have a significant effect on improving memory, high levels are associated with a significant *decline* in memory function. This suggests that the malfunction associated with insulin resistance leads to cognitive dysfunction because of insulin's inability to carry out its proper function.[49]

Adding weight to a diabetes link, recent studies have indicated an association between Alzheimer's disease and central nervous system insulin resistance. Northwestern University researchers suggested that Alzheimer's disease may actually be a third form of diabetes.[50] This was confirmed in 2008. In a longitudinal study, impaired acute insulin response at midlife was associated with an increased risk of Alzheimer's disease (AD) up to 35 years later suggesting a causal link between insulin metabolism and the pathogenesis of Alzheimer's disease.[51]

Insulin and insulin receptors in the brain are crucial for learning and memory, and it's known that these components are lower in people with Alzheimer's disease. In the brain, insulin binds to an insulin receptor at a synapse, which triggers a mechanism that allows nerve cells to survive and memories to form. The research has shown that a toxic protein called *amyloid beta-derived diffusible ligand* (ADDL), found in the brain of Alzheimer's patients, removes insulin receptors from nerve cells, and renders those neurons insulin resistant. It is this substance that causes the plaques found in Alzheimer's disease.

The brain also produces an enzyme called *insulysin* which protects the brain by degrading ADDL. But insulysin is active on two competitors, ADDL and insulin, with a much greater affinity to insulin than ADDL. The more insulin circulating in the blood the less insulysin is available to clean up the ADDL, which is then left to aggregate and produce the Alzheimer's plaques in the brain. If we eat so much carbohydrate that insulin levels sky-rocket, we get no degradation of ADDL due to the high insulin levels.

Evolutionary pressures

Alzheimer's could also be related to evolutionary factors. A gene, the *apoE4 allele*, for example, is nearly three times more frequent among Alzheimer's populations than the general population.[52] Table 26.1 illustrates that populations with a long history of agriculture have much lower frequencies of the apoE4 allele than are found in long-time, hunter-gatherer populations.[53] In consequence, populations with a long history of agriculture have more successfully weeded out the gene than northern Eurasian populations. This may be the reason why we with our inappropriate diet are now succumbing to these diseases.

Healthy diet and Alzheimer's

Starchy foods may be as much the cause of Alzheimer's disease as they are of diabetes. A report showed that a diet rich in saturated fats and low in carbohydrates can actually reduce levels of a brain protein, *amyloid-beta*, which is an indicator of Alzheimer's disease in mice with the mouse model of Alzheimer's disease.[54] The authors believed that insulin and a related hormone, *insulin-related growth factor-1* (IGF-1), are the key players. They said: 'Insulin is often considered a storage hormone, since it promotes deposition of fat but insulin may also work to encourage amyloid-beta production.'

Table 26.1: ApoE4 allele in selected populations

Agriculturalists		Hunter-gatherers	
Greek	6.8%	African Pygmies	40.7%
Turks	7.9%	Papuans	36.8%
Mayans	8.9%	Inuit	21.4%
Arabs in N. Israel	4.0%		

This study runs counter to others which purported to show that high-fat diets had a negative effect on Alzheimer's. However, in an accompanying editorial, Dr Richard Feinman, editor of the journal *Nutrition and Metabolism*, explained that: 'Most studies of the deleterious effects of fat have been done in the presence of high carbohydrate.' In which case, isn't it conceivable that it is dietary carbs and not fats that are the causal factor?

Parkinson's disease

Parkinson's disease seems to have similar causes to Alzheimer's disease, although it affects only about one-tenth as many people as does Alzheimer's. Its symptoms include muscle rigidity and tremor of the hands, which can become increasingly difficult to control as the disease advances, particularly with the development of motor complications, such as end-of-dose wearing off and uncontrollable movement following long-term therapy.

Lack of sunlight also seems to be a major cause. In an excellent paper, a father and son team presented considerable evidence that vitamin D deficiency is a cause, and possibly the major cause, of Parkinson's disease.[55] The researchers reviewed a 1997 case report in which a patient with Parkinson's disease steadily improved when treated daily with 4,000 IU of vitamin D. There are several lines of evidence which note that chronically inadequate vitamin D intake in the United States, particularly in the northern states and particularly in the elderly, is a significant factor in the development of Parkinson's disease.

Low cholesterol is also implicated in Parkinson's disease.

Treatment

The brain uses a disproportionately large amount of energy for its weight. It is usually thought that it needs to get this directly from glucose. However, strictly chemically-speaking, neurons appear to source their energy not from glucose but from carboxylic acids, which are mostly derived from fatty acids, converted to ketones. While there appears to be an obligatory reliance on glucose to sustain normal function of the brain as a whole, this may be because neurons cannot normally survive without the support of glial cells, which may only run on glucose.[56,57] Thus, the brain survives during periods of prolonged fasting by using energy derived ultimately from stored triglycerides (body fats), the glucose being derived from the glycerol the triglycerides are bound to.

During the 1990s, diet-induced high blood levels of ketones were found to be effective for treatment of several rare genetic disorders involving impaired use of glucose or its metabolic products by brain cells.[58] Other work also found that ketones protect neurons from a heroin analogue which induces Parkinson's disease, and a protein fragment which accumulates in the brain of Alzheimer's patients.[59] More than that, addition of ketones alone increased the number of surviving neurons, which suggests that ketones may even help neurons grow.

We know that ketogenic diets are very effective treatments for many other chronic degenerative medical conditions. The evidence is that the Alzheimer's and Parkinson's diseases may also be successfully treated and, more importantly, prevented, with a low-carbohydrate, high-fat, ketogenic diet.

Amyotrophic lateral sclerosis

Amyotrophic lateral sclerosis (ALS) is a rapidly progressive, invariably fatal neurological disease that attacks the nerve cells (*neurons*) responsible for controlling voluntary muscles. The disease belongs to a group of disorders known as *motor neuron diseases,* which are characterized by the gradual degeneration and death of motor neurons. ALS is one of the most common neuromuscular diseases worldwide, and people of all races and ethnic backgrounds are affected. ALS most commonly strikes people between 40 and 60 years of age, but younger and older people also can develop the disease. Men are affected more often than women.

Several lines of research have shown that high levels of blood cholesterol – particularly LDL – protect against ALS, and increase survival.[60] Researchers warn against lowering LDL with statins as these are able to decrease nutrient availability to muscle which might contribute to neuromuscular junction damage and motor neuron death.[61,62]

On the other hand, another 'heart disease risk factor', 'homocysteine levels were significantly increased in patients with amyotrophic lateral sclerosis (ALS) compared with healthy controls.'[63] High levels of homocysteine are found in people whose vitamin B intakes are insufficient.

Conclusion

The mental conditions outlined were rare in our society before the start of the last century, and still are completely absent in traditional cultures.

Although there may be many contributory factors, particularly with a condition such as depression, the fact that there was such an alarming rise during the last century points to a change during that century being responsible for their increases. Much of the research points to diet as the cause and the aspects of diet most implicated, yet again, are too much carbohydrate, too little fat and not enough sunshine.

Possibly the most worrying aspect of the findings is that our leaders are likely to be more influenced by the establishment into reinforcing 'healthy' lifestyle practices. Government ministers and those who advise us on nutrition are likely to be eating the diet that they promote. Given the profound effect upon brain function that such a diet can have, particularly on cognitive function, I am concerned that those who advise and rule us may not be totally competent – and neither may many of those who vote for them!

Chapter Twenty-Seven

Multiple sclerosis

This chapter looks exclusively at one of the most distressing conditions to afflict us. Although the causes of MS are unknown, we discuss compelling evidence that our 'healthy' lifestyle may be a major contributory factor.

> I never again saw any increase of spasticity in patients with multiple sclerosis that I put on the diet.
>
> *Professor Wolfgang Lutz*

Soon after my book, *Eat Fat, Get Thin!*, was published in 2000, I received a letter from K. E., a woman in her early 30s with multiple sclerosis (MS). In the letter she thanked me for the book because she felt so much better and her symptoms had regressed since adopting the low-carb, high-fat diet I recommended.

Until then, I had given little thought to MS in the context of nutrition. Now I started to consider it more. I soon learned that MS first appeared about 175 years ago, and its prevalence had steadily increased from that time. In other words, MS is another modern disease. So could it, too, be caused as a result of incorrect diet? As K. E.'s symptoms were apparently helped by her change of diet, it seemed possible that this was so.

What is MS?

Multiple sclerosis is a chronic, usually progressive disease of the central nervous system in which the immune system attacks and destroys the structure of nerve cells degrading their function. Normally affecting young and middle-aged adults, MS is one of the most common neurologic diseases with two million people affected worldwide.

Think of the body's nerves as electrical cables carrying signals around the body. Just as the electrical wiring in your house has to be insulated to stop the wires shorting across, nerves are insulated with a fatty wrap called the *myelin sheath* in a similar way. In MS gradual destruction of this myelin occurs in patches throughout the brain or spinal cord (or both), interfering with the nerve pathways.

There is compelling evidence that MS is an auto-immune disease. It is characterized by chronic inflammation and damage to myelin sheath tissues in the central nervous system (CNS).[1] This means it is the result of the immune system attacking specific tissues in the body. In this respect it is similar to many other diseases such as coeliac disease and rheumatoid arthritis. Damage to the myelin sheath allows improper interaction between the nerves in the brain and spinal cord which, in turn, affects the functions of these nerves. As the condition can affect any nerves, all of which perform different functions, the disease has a wide and scattered range of symptoms. Typical of these are:

- Unsteady gait and shaky movements of the limbs;
- Rapid involuntary movement of the eyes;
- Defects in speech pronunciation;
- Spastic weakness.

The patient is also beset by recurrent relapses and remissions so that any treatment which seems to be of benefit in the short-term could be merely the result of an unrelated remission. For this reason the testing of potentially successful treatments can be a long drawn-out process.

Causes of MS

There have been suggestions that MS is caused by all manner of things from a genetic defect to allergic reaction to something in our environment. None has proved particularly satisfactory – but they do provide clues.

Is MS a genetic disorder?

To answer this question, pairs of identical twins were studied in high risk areas: Europe and North America. This research indicated that in only 20% to 30% of such twins did both have MS.[2,3] But this is still higher than the 2% of affected twins among non-identical twins. The twin data also convincingly show that, in high prevalence areas, only just over half of individuals who are genetically capable of getting MS actually contract the disease. This means, in turn, that almost half the people in high prevalence areas who have the genes for MS don't get it. As women are 50% more likely to get MS than men, this might also reflect a genetic dimension. These facts suggest that rather than there being one dominant gene which determines susceptibility, many genes may be involved, each having a small influence.[4]

Environmental cause for MS?

The geographic distribution of MS suggests that it is a disease of civilization. It occurs mainly in the US, Canada, western Europe, New Zealand and Australia. In these areas the prevalence is between 50 and 100 cases per 100,000 of the population. In low-risk areas, such as the West Indies, the prevalence is only five to 10.[5] It has been suggested that this distribution is in part due to a genetic factor because all the high-risk areas are dominantly populated by individuals of European origin.[6] But this seems unlikely as, within Europeans, there is a noticeable north/south gradient with MS being more prevalent in higher latitudes; and there are also significant differences in the numbers of cases of MS within individual countries which are not related to differences in ethnic origin.

That the primary cause of MS is something in the environment rather than just a genetic trait has been suggested by several observations:

- There was a sudden increase in prevalence of MS in the Faroe Islands following World War II occupation by British troops.[7]
- Residency in Hawaii increases the risk of MS for those of Japanese descent while simultaneously decreasing the risk for Caucasians.[8]
- Immigrants to London from areas of low risk such as south-east Asia, Africa and the West Indies, have a low prevalence of MS but their British-born children have the same high prevalence as the indigenous British.[9]

Summary of evidence

Taking all that evidence together, it appears that certain people have a genetic make-up that makes them *more susceptible* to succumbing to MS but, for them to get the disease, they have to be subjected to at least one dominant environmental factor. As MS is found all over the world, this factor must be common to most of the world, but it must also be much more prevalent in 'western' industrialized areas of the world. Thus there are a number of potential causes to consider – industrial pollutants, pesticides, chemical food additives, individual foods, and more. These can be divided into two main areas:

- **Indigenous factors such as climate, sunlight, altitude.** I think that all of these can be ruled out simply by the Faroe Islands' experience. Nothing changed there other than other people coming to the islands. It has been suggested that the dramatic increase following the Second World War could have been caused by a virus brought in by the troops. But there is no evidence that MS is transmitted by any infectious agent: despite a very concerted effort to find a specific MS virus or bacterium in the central nervous system of people with MS, none such has ever been found.[10] A recent study did show that higher levels of vitamin D have a protective effect;[11] however, another found that the protection applied only to non-whites.[12]

- **Transportable factors: heavy metals, pollution, sanitation, diet.** The first three of these can, I think, also be rejected. The most convincing reason for this conclusion is the greatly increased prevalence of MS in Japanese people living in Hawaii versus in Japan whereas these factors are much more common in Japan than in Hawaii. The Faroe Islands data, as well as the much higher prevalence of MS on the Canadian Prairies than in the highly industrialized area of southern Ontario, also are not compatible with these factors.

Foods and MS

So what does that leave? The one obvious potential factor is diet. And, as MS follows a similar trend to many other diseases which have a similar cause, this is not an unreasonable assumption. There is also strong evidence which, although not perfect, is hard to ignore:

1. Diets vary throughout the world. Such variations could account for the differences in prevalence between cultures and also account for the differences between areas with different climatic conditions and growing conditions – the north/south divide.
2. Adults who emigrate are more likely to maintain their customary diet whereas their children are more likely to consume more of the food of the new country. Thus diet could explain the differences in MS prevalence between immigrant parents and their offspring.
3. Diet could also explain the differences between identical twins. Twins will almost certainly have similar dietary habits while young, but their diets could change significantly when they leave home, marry and have their diet influenced by someone else.
4. And areas with high rates of MS do tend to have similarities in terms of diet. They are all western 'civilized' countries which eat dairy products, cereal grains, processed vegetable fats and other highly processed foods.

The idea that diet could be the cause of MS is strengthened if we look at specific populations where there are marked differences.

1. Diet explains the apparent paradox whereby MS in Hawaiians of Japanese ancestry differs so much from that of Caucasian Hawaiians. Japanese who immigrate to Hawaii eat more of the sorts of foods eaten in the US, and fewer of their traditional foods. This could account for their increased burden of MS. On the other hand, the diet of

American Caucasians in Hawaii will change in the opposite direction with fewer of the mainland's fast foods, thus lowering their risk. In this way, diet provides a good answer to the Hawaii paradox.

2. Diet can also explain the differences in the prevalence of MS in the Faroe Islands during the last half of the 20th century. The occupying forces brought their own rations and dietary customs with them. Food was imported for the troops and this would inevitably have found its way into – and changed – the local diet, particularly that of the youth.

3. Newfoundlanders eat much more fish and less dairy and cereal grains than do prairie Canadians. The island people have much less MS than their plains-dwelling compatriots.

4. Lastly, the diet of the high-risk areas – Britain, North America, western Europe, Australia and New Zealand – has changed significantly over the last century or so. This trend gathered momentum during the latter half of the 20th century, as did trends in the prevalence of MS. The two trends seem inextricably linked.

Thus diet does, indeed, provide a solid and reasonable explanation for MS and its environmental roots. It also explains, and is entirely compatible with, the non-transmissible characteristic of MS. Dr G. C. Ebers of the Department of Clinical Neurological Sciences, University of Western Ontario, noted: 'In sum these data strongly indicate that the environmental factor is affecting the population risk. Accordingly, factors which influence large populations such as diet . . . deserve careful reconsideration.'

So what in our diet could be the cause?

The question now is: what element or elements in our diet could be responsible for MS? For the answer, it seems reasonable to look for what has changed over the last century or so.

The major changes during the period have been:

- an increase in some forms of dairy products;
- a substantial decrease in animal fat intake;
- a huge increase in processed polyunsaturated vegetable oils and margarines; and
- an increase in cereal grains.

In other words, a change towards what is now euphemistically called 'healthy' eating.

Several statistical studies have found clear relationships between wheat and dairy products and the prevalence of MS.[13-17] These are both likely candidates as they are 'new foods' as far as human evolution is concerned, and both are known to cause allergic reactions. But there are other foods mentioned in these references as being possible contenders which do not fit into these categories. Dr Malosse and colleagues,[17] and Drs Agranoff and Goldberg also indict animal fats.[14] I think we can safely rule these out as we have been eating such fats since the dawn of our species and there has been a decrease in their intake as MS rates have increased.

Is it milk?

The dairy connection, however, is not so clear-cut: Malosse and colleagues found a highly significant correlation between liquid cow's milk and MS prevalence, and a low, but still significant, correlation with cream or butter consumption. However, they found no correlation for cheese. They say: 'These results suggest that liquid cow milk could contain factor(s) – no longer present in the processed milk – influencing the clinical appearance of MS.'

Although allergic reactions are triggered by proteins, from the Malosse group's data it's likely that the milk sugar, lactose, could be a culprit: lactose is at its highest level in liquid milk; there is a much smaller amount in cream; and there is none in cheese as it has been converted to lactic acid by the fermentation process. Thus lactose fits the findings perfectly – except for one small anomaly: there is practically no lactose in butter.

Many peoples with low levels of MS in their native lands are peoples without an evolutionary history of dairy use; such as the populations of south-east Asia and Africa. These people do experience an increase in the disease when they migrate to western countries where milk is drunk. But milk cannot be the only causal factor, as the prevalence of MS has increased in populations who *do* have an evolutionary history of milk drinking – unless, that is, the problem lies in the way that milk is treated today: pasteurization or homogenization perhaps? Milk has been one of Man's foods since pre-history, particularly in more northern regions. Since refrigeration and preservation by pasteurization of sweet milk is a product of 19th- and 20th-century technologies, its consumption until then was limited to sour milk, yoghurt, cottage cheese, or aged cheeses. The infant at its mother's breast was probably the only human to receive sweet milk in significant quantities prior to Graeco-Roman times. So it is certainly possible that changes wrought by heat treatment could be a contributory factor.

Or wheat?

Wheat, however, is in a different class altogether. In the higher latitudes, the first cereal to be cultivated was oats. Wheat is a relative newcomer which was grown mainly in warmer regions of northern Africa and south-east Asia until imported to England by the Romans. But, again, wheat has been eaten for a very long time. If something in wheat is the cause, then it must be something introduced more recently. And there is such a thing: not the nutrients in the natural wheat itself necessarily, but changes in the way wheat is processed.

Amy McGrath's findings

Dr Amy McGrath, an Australian historian, had no end of trouble with her daughters.[18] To say they were hyperactive would be an understatement, and they had all sorts of physical illnesses. When they married and had daughters of their own, these children had similar symptoms. Dr McGrath determined to find the cause. She experimented, wrote to experts, and travelled the world for more than 30 years in her quest. What she found was that bread is no longer manufactured today in the way it used to be, and that this could have had hidden consequences due to its allergic potential.

Apparently the change in conditions of work, specifically the hours of shift-working introduced after the Second World War, meant that bread was no longer fermented overnight. Instead it was rushed through the raising process using 'improvers' to fluff up the loaf. The result was a very different bread, chemically, from the pre-war traditional loaf.

Dr McGrath hypothesized that the reason her family couldn't tolerate modern bread was the large quantities of unchanged maltose it contains. She found that when she had bread made using the old-fashioned *long dough* which removed the maltose, her children's symptoms disappeared as if by a miracle, even though the same ingredients were used.

Dr McGrath discovered that 'primitive' peoples don't eat raw plants:

- Australian aborigines, Melanesians and Polynesians cook vegetables at high temperatures, steaming them or baking them in earth ovens.
- South-east Asians seldom eat raw vegetables or brown rice. Vegetables are usually well cooked. Rice is soaked for hours, then drained, the water being thrown away. The rice is then boiled in fresh water, baked or fried. The husks or bran are fed to the pigs. Brown rice, they say, is indigestible.
- Indians often cook foods for a lengthy time.
- Greeks soak and boil beans for several hours.
- West Africans process corn for days.
- Taiwanese farmers boil sweet potatoes before feeding them to pigs.
- The Native American Hopi pick corn green and dry it to make bound niacin available.

We don't do any of these things. In our 'fast-food' culture, bread goes from raw materials to finished product in about one-and-a-half hours. And that doesn't allow time for its toxic properties to be neutralized by the fermentation process.

As Dr McGrath puts it, it seems that there is a lot of traditional wisdom that has been passed on from generation to generation simply by trial and error: people have found that certain procedures render food less toxic and harmful and therefore more nutritious. But in our haste for 'fast' convenience foods, we have thrown centuries of hard-earned wisdom out of the window.

I suspect strongly that Dr McGrath is correct. I, too, have had trouble with bread in my home country, England, for many years. However, when I holiday in Portugal, I have found that I can eat the locally made *pão caseiro* with no problems whatsoever. This solid, spongy bread with an off-white colour is still made in the centuries-old traditional way: proved and allowed to ferment for several hours overnight, before being baked.

Low cholesterol and MS

Back in the 1950s it was noticed that people with MS tended to have lower levels of cholesterol than healthy people.[19] Over the last couple of decades the focus of dietary advice has been aimed at lowering people's cholesterol levels across the board. As cholesterol plays such an important part in the brain and nervous system, a possible relationship between low blood cholesterol and MS is another avenue worth exploring.

Diet for MS

The veteran Austrian doctor, Wolfgang Lutz, started to work with low-carb diets for his patients in 1957. After seeing the remarkable benefits in other conditions but unable to convince his colleagues of the correctness of his ideas, it seemed to him that the only way he could convince them would be to prove its success in a so-far 'incurable' disease. In collaboration with neurologist, Professor Dr Kurt Eckel, Lutz conducted a systematic investigation of the effects of carbohydrate restriction on MS.[20] The two doctors' patients on the trial were put straight onto a diet very low in carbohydrates: 20-30 grams per day at most. The menu they suggested to these patients was approximately as follows:

- For breakfast, two eggs with bacon, a cup of cream and a cup of black coffee;
- For mid-morning snack, cheese with butter;
- For lunch, meat or fish (cooked with butter or lard), vegetables, and sometimes for dessert, a small helping of stewed fruit, low in sugar, or a sweet omelette with a small quantity of jam;
- In the evening, cold cuts of meat, cheese, butter, and mayonnaise.
- Patients were not allowed to eat bread or anything that contained cereal flour.

- For drinks, patients were permitted unsweetened grapefruit and tomato juice, tea and coffee without sugar, soda water and a moderate amount of alcohol.

Dr Lutz told me: 'Apart from a transient constipation that we put down to the comparative lack of roughage in the new diet, these patients generally managed the actual dietary changeover without difficulty and soon gained an appetite for more fat. However, response to the diet was not beneficial to all participants in terms of the course of the disease itself, for whilst there were some very encouraging results, sadly the condition of a few of the participants worsened.'

The experience taught Lutz three very important lessons. The first of these was that it could take time for the body to accomplish what is really a major change in energy supply. When someone switches from a very high to an extremely low carbohydrate diet, the body's metabolism, which has been used to obtaining a great deal of its energy from glucose, now has to get used to burning fat as its main fuel. It seems, said Lutz: 'that, even in our innards, habits linger! I think that, initially, I underestimated the nervous system's need for the carbohydrate to which it was habituated and that I overestimated its ability to switch quickly to the burning of fat.'

The second lesson he learnt was that, because it can take time for the body to switch fuel supplies, it is important not to reduce carbohydrates too fast. Some people manage the transition in a few days, for others it may take several weeks or even several months. In the trial, it was those patients who were the most ill to start with who had most difficulty adapting to the new diet and who were most likely to worsen with the changeover.

The third lesson was that, for certain people and for certain diseases in addition to MS, it was important not to reduce carbohydrates below a specific amount, as this could cause unnecessary complications. In the trial, some patients with MS thrived on a very low amount of carbohydrate but it troubled others.

Lutz, therefore, abandoned the radical approach he had started out with, and adopted a more moderate procedure. From that point on, he said: 'I never again saw any increase of spasticity in patients with multiple sclerosis that I put on the diet. Thereafter, results were consistent and, time after time, confirmed the real value of treating multiple sclerosis by carbohydrate restriction.'

In that early trial of 36 patients, no success was achieved with patients who'd had the disease longer than five years, or who were already experiencing progressive and continual decline. But the results were very positive with people who had had the disease for a shorter period. Patients who had been diagnosed within the previous six months were consistently helped by the diet, as were those who had had the condition less than five years and whose illness came in stages: these people either gained full or almost full remission or, at the very least, they improved to how they had been before the last step down. So, amongst the 36 people on the diet at that time, there were a few 'miracle cures' – patients who 'took up their beds and walked'. Lutz and Eckel knew of several patients who had kept to the diet and were still free of relapse, many years later.

Lutz was not an MS specialist. However, he had a total of 53 patients, all of whom he treated with a very low-carb diet. He says:

'The amount of improvement one can hope for does depend on the situation at the beginning of treatment. Obviously, whatever the illness, certain things are no longer changeable. With multiple sclerosis, once the brain and bone marrow are so infiltrated with scary foci that a nerve of any length has no chance of reaching its destination without losing its isolation (and therefore its conductivity), one can only hope for limited improvement. If, before starting the diet, patients can no longer walk, if there is already paralysis of the bladder or bowels, then the hope of a return of lost functions is only slight and often the most one can hope for is to arrest decline. But this arrest in further decline, in my experience, one may indeed hope for.

'In all the time since I adopted a gradual approach to carbohydrate reduction with multiple sclerosis patients, I have not witnessed deterioration in the condition of a single person that kept to the diet, only improvement in so far as this was still possible. How I wish that I could convince neurologists of the value of carbohydrate restriction in the treatment of multiple sclerosis. All too often there is a general defeatism that surrounds this condition, and especially as regards diet, as the following case history illustrates.

'At a clinic in Vienna, a young girl was told that no special diet was necessary. She received all the usual therapeutic measures, but in spite of this, her condition continued to deteriorate. She came to me and I put her on my low carbohydrate diet. Almost immediately she started to show signs of considerable improvement; after six months, the patient was practically free of symptoms and all her paralysis and sensory disturbances had disappeared. Two years later she telephoned me to ask if she could go to Morocco with her boyfriend. A year later still, her mother rang to ask whether I thought pregnancy would be harmful to her daughter. I heard that after 3 years on the diet she had stayed well and was still doing fine.'

Dr Lutz's protocol was to reduce the amount of carbohydrate in the patient's diet gradually from their accustomed amount to a certain level, usually not less than 110 grams. Then, step by step, each month he would reduce the amount by about 12 grams, until reaching the level of carbohydrate that was required for long-term daily use: about 70 grams a day.

Dr Jan Kwaśnieski's experiences

Lutz is not alone in pioneering low-carb diets in MS or having success with it. In Poland, Dr Jan Kwaśnieski had similar success over some 30 years with a total of 212 patients: 131 women and 81 men. He told me that someone with MS can expect the following benefits:

1. A full cure from the disease, which often happens provided the disease has not been of long duration. On occasion, a cure has been possible in individuals suffering for as long as five years.
2. A halt in the progression of the disease – always.
3. An improvement in the physical condition and a reduction of disease symptoms, to a varied extent.
4. An elimination (practically total) of new attacks of the disease provided the diet is continued indefinitely.
5. Achievement of the highest degree of resistance to all sorts of infection.

For this disease, however, Dr Kwaśnieski recommends not just a very low-carb, high-fat diet with proportions similar to those on page 240, but also one that includes animal brains. He points out that good results in the US have been achieved with sausages which incorporated brains. Unfortunately, since the BSE scares of the 1980s, brains are no longer available in Britain. A shame really, not just for the treatment of MS, but because, as a client of mine said after sampling them on holiday in France: 'They're yummy!'

Conclusion

MS is considered by conventional physicians to be incurable. It is treated with drugs that are mostly palliative. However, the evidence from both population and clinical observations strongly suggests that, whatever stage the disease has reached, it may be halted with diet alone. The evidence also strongly suggests that, if it is less than five years from first diagnosis, there is a possibility that the condition can be reversed and the patient can lead a normal, symptom-free life.

The treatment is the diet recommended in Chapter Sixteen as far as proportions of carbohydrates to protein to fat are concerned, together with the removal of all products made with cereals (wheat, oats, rye, barley, rice) and processed liquid milk. Regular sunbathing may also help, particularly for Caucasians.

Chapter Twenty-Eight

The signs of 'healthy eating'

There are many other signs of 'healthy eating', including acne, bad teeth and short sight. This chapter looks at this wide range of conditions, many of which are clearly visible as they affect the face, and gives evidence for 'healthy eating' being the culprit.

> I think we could halve the number of people going blind with macular degeneration if we could change their diet, cut out the vegetable oil.
>
> *Dr Paul Beaumont*

Lastly, I want to look at some conditions, other than being overweight, that mark you out (to anyone who knows the signs) as a 'healthy eater'.

Acne

There is no classic acne case. Those who suffer from acne are of different ages, different backgrounds and different lifestyles. What they share is their frustration with the condition of their skin. They all want to know why this is happening to them.

In westernized societies, acne is a universal skin disease. It afflicts 79% to 95% of the adolescent population. Indeed, acne during teenage years is now so widespread it is considered 'normal' in developed nations. But it also continues into adulthood: 45% to 54% of adults older than 25 years still have acne and in up to 12% of men and 3% of women it persists until well into middle age. In adolescence it may be considered a nuisance; it is considerably less well tolerated in adulthood.

However, it is noticeable that nations who do not consume a 'western diet' do not suffer the problem. A study by Dr Loren Cordain and his team looked at the prevalence of acne in two non-westernized populations: the Kitavan Islanders of Papua New Guinea and the Aché hunter-gatherers of Paraguay.[1]

Of 1200 Kitavan subjects examined, including 300 aged between 15 and 25 years, Cordain and colleagues didn't find one case of acne. It was

---

Case history – E . C.

'I first developed acne aged about 12 – a year or so after the doctors put me on a low-fat diet. It was not unexpected that I would have acne, my father had it badly; my sister, who is 5 years older, also suffered. I was determined not to let it scar me as it had my sister and father, so my doctor was supportive and helpful. Although my GP told me it would probably resolve when I finished puberty, I started with tetracycline and calamine, and went via ultra-violet light treatments, ending up using retin-A lotion, prescribed by the hospital dermatologists. Nothing helped. When I was 19 the university GP refused to prescribe, putting me on the pill instead. No change. I was told that, by the time I was 25 my skin would be clear. It wasn't. I was also "recommended" to have a baby, as this would "most likely" clear my skin. I decided not to try that one! At 30 I was told that, when I went through menopause, my skin would improve wonderfully – what a thing to look forwards to!

'To tell you about the acne itself – I had constant blackheads and disgusting pus-filled angry red spots on my face, back and shoulders. I was impeccably clean – washing my face several times daily and using alcohol impregnated wipes in between and I bathed twice daily as well. I was unable to wear a blouse without a jumper or jacket covering it, as it would be covered in blood and pus if I leaned back against a chair. Bras were always stained. I never wore sleeveless tops, as the spots extended down to a few inches above my elbows. I was a keen swimmer, but the spots made me too self-conscious to swim. Later, when I took up scuba diving, I could wear a t-shirt over the swimming costume in the pool, and a wet suit when in open water. I loathed having my photograph taken.

'When I started a low-carb diet, 4 years (& 10 days!) ago, I had no expectations of any improvement in my skin, but a few months later, a very good friend looked at me and said my skin was looking much better. I hadn't noticed! I tended not to look in a mirror – too many spots again! However, I braced myself, and saw something I had not seen in my adult life. Smooth, unblemished skin! My face was not spotty at all, and there were no blackheads to be seen. My back still had a few bumps, blemishes, and old scars, as did my shoulders, but my face had escaped scarring. My 46-year-old skin is smooth and possibly my best feature!

'I now find that my acne is absent, as long as I stay below around 50 grams carbs daily. I "cheated" for 48 hours at Christmas (about 150 grams total!), and within a week my skin had erupted, and it took until the end of January for it to calm down again. This happens every time I indulge – a visible reminder to stay low carb!'

the same with the Aché subjects they examined for nearly two-and-a-half years: not one case of acne was found.

Cordain and his team attributed the absence of acne in these peoples to their diets. They said: 'The astonishing difference in acne incidence rates between non-westernized and fully modernized societies cannot be solely attributed to genetic differences among populations but likely results from differing environmental factors. Identification of these factors may be useful in the treatment of acne in western populations.'

The significant dietary difference they highlighted was that while western children ate refined sugar- and starch-rich foods, both the study groups ate hardly any cereals or refined sugars. The Kitavans ate primarily fish, fruit, tubers and coconut, and the Aché diet consisted mostly of wild game, the root vegetable sweet manioc, peanuts, maize and rice.

Skin aging

We are told that sunbathing ages the skin; that a fake tan is safer. In a fake tan, chemicals are applied to the skin to produce an effect similar in appearance to a traditional suntan. It does not involve skin pigmentation nor does it need UV exposure to initiate the colour change. The tan is not a dye, stain or paint, but a chemical reaction between the chemicals in the tanning product and the amino acids in the dead layer on the skin surface. This is the same reaction as the browning process during food manufacturing and storage. It is well known to food chemists and is called the Maillard reaction.

As we age, our skin ages with us. The rate at which this happens is governed to a large extent by glycosylation (see page 298), and oxidation. In a similar way to fake tans, the glycosylation and oxidation reactions modify insoluble collagen in both the aging process and if we have diabetes.

To measure the effects of glycosylation, a study, published in the *Journal of Clinical Investigation*, measured Maillard reaction products in skin collagen from both type-1 diabetics and non-diabetic control subjects.[2]

The researchers found that in non-diabetic people, glycosylation of collagen increased by only 33% between 20 and 85 years of age. In diabetic patients, there was a 300% increase. Other measurements for the effects of skin aging were also much higher in diabetics than in non-diabetics. The researchers concluded that: 'These results support the description of diabetes as a disease characterized by accelerated chemical aging of long-lived tissue proteins.' It also means that a high-carb diet will age the skin more quickly. It's not the sun that ages our skin, it's our diet!

Say 'cheese' for healthy teeth

Dr Weston A. Price discovered isolated, non-modernized populations, whom he often went to great lengths to contact, who were immune to tooth decay. He studied what they ate, how they maintained their soil fertility, and related these factors to their tooth decay rates. He found that, despite their having no way of cleaning their teeth, many of the groups had no tooth decay at all. He also identified members of the same cultures who had contact with civilization. They tended to have high levels of dental decay.[3] He noted in particular that in East Africa the mostly-vegetarian Kikuyu had 13 times the rate of cavities of the mostly-carnivorous Maasai, who had probably the best teeth and health of any group. The Maasai ate almost nothing but meat, milk and blood.

Based on his findings, Price devised a dietary regime for his patients which emphasized raw milk, bone broths with meats and vegetables, cod liver oil, butter and ghee, unrefined wheat, and cooked vegetables and fruits. With this he actually *reversed* tooth decay in his patients – and took X-ray pictures to prove it.

Sugars – and starches

It is now no secret that sweets and fizzy soft drinks and fruit drinks increase dental decay rates. But it is less well known to the general public that starches such as bread, pasta and breakfast cereals are worse. Dentists at the University of Gothenburg, Sweden, used a variety of starchy foods: plain potato crisps, sugar-free cheese doodles and sweetened crackers, and measured acidity levels in the mouth together with how long the foods remained in the mouth.[4] They found that, while sugary foods increased mouth acidity more than starches during the first 30 minutes, all three snack foods were worse than sugar after that time. This was because the starchy foods did not cause the eaters to produce so much saliva to clear the starch from the mouth. Cooked starches, particularly potato starch in products such as potato chips, cling longer to the teeth than many sugar foods.

Most research has shown clearly that carbohydrates of all sorts increased decay, but much less work has been done on identifying foods that may have a protective effect. Recent investigations are changing that.

One of the foods that has declined in popularity in recent years is cheese – it isn't perceived as 'healthy' because of the amount of fat and salt it contains. But it looks as if that belief will have to change: evidence suggests that cheese helps to prevent dental decay (caries) if it is the last food eaten in a meal. A 1991 review of the scientific literature looked at the various theories about why this should be so. Several mechanisms have been proposed:[5] chewing cheese stimulates saliva flow; the alkaline nature of saliva buffers the acids formed in plaque; the increased rate of sugar clearance due to the diluting action of cheese-stimulated saliva. Research has also suggested that chewing cheese might reduce the levels of decay-causing bacteria; the major protein in milk, casein, reduced the amount of calcium leached from teeth by bacteria; and the high calcium and minerals in the casein concentrated calcium and phosphate in plaque.

In 1999, this evidence was confirmed and added to when a team of researchers at the Dental School, Newcastle upon Tyne, gave readers of the *British Dental Journal* a Christmas present. The 25 December edition carried a paper showing that cooked cheese raised the calcium levels in plaque and helped to protect against dental caries.[6]

Lastly, a review by two scientists at the Forsyth Institute, Boston, Massachusetts, showed that milk and cheese could reduce the effects of metabolic acids, and could help restore the enamel that is lost during eating.[7] In one study reviewed by the Forsyth Institute team, cheese eaters experienced 71% less damage to their enamel over time.

The cheese-dental protection picture is a complex molecular ballet, involving the calcium in cheese, an increase in saliva from chewing, and the ability of cheese to restore depleted enamel. Widely vilified like chocolate and wine before it, cheese is now earning a measure of redemption as researchers recognize that even seemingly unhealthy foods often have their good points. A quarter-century's worth of dental studies prove that one of our 'guilty pleasures' actually prevents cavities. Given this information, consumers may be motivated to use cheese to reduce, or reverse the caries-causing effects of 'healthy', starchy foods.

Misaligned teeth and dental arches

As well as dental decay, Dr Price also noticed that the children of people who had been influenced by western dietary ideas had facial and dental arch deformities. These showed up as narrow faces, narrow noses with pinched nostrils, and crooked, misaligned or overlapping teeth. These conditions were all associated with high intakes of concentrated starchy foods, and a greatly reduced use of dairy products.

Look around you today, and see how many children and even young adults wear ugly braces on their teeth in an effort to correct the problem. But these do not solve other problems such as restricted breathing through narrow nasal passages.

'Healthy diet' and the eyes

Our eyes were developed for an environment very different from that of today. In prehistoric times we needed to be able to perceive a predator or other danger throughout our lives. With no doctors or opticians, our eyes had to last. And, judging from studies of peoples who still eat a 'stone-age diet' today, their eyes did a very good job for a whole lifetime. But many of us are plagued from birth to old age with a variety of sight defects. This is because the type of food we eat now has a profound effect on our eyes.

Myopia (short-sightedness)

Have you noticed how many children wear glasses these days? Myopia, or short-sightedness, is very common. There has been a dramatic increase in myopia in developed countries over the past 200 years. In the US and Britain myopia affects around 25% to 35% of people of European descent and up to half or more of Asian descent.

For many years myopia in children was thought to be caused by excessive reading. This was because rates were typically less than 2% among populations with no formal education and who didn't read books. Other research found that myopia afflicted as many as one in three children brought up in towns and cities and where they went through a course of formal education. These observations combined were used to justify the conclusion that myopia must be caused by reading. Wearing glasses became synonymous with intelligence. In mid-20th century films, brainy children were always portrayed wearing glasses.

But then anomalies were noticed. There were places in the world where myopia was rare despite there being compulsory education programmes (for example, incidences of myopia are 10% in Germany and 95% in Japan[8]); children who skipped school or who had no formal education in civilized societies also had high rates of myopia. And focusing on reading did not explain why the levels of short-sightedness were low in societies that adopted western lifestyles but not western diets.

Except for the past few thousand years, since the advent of agriculture, all our ancestors were hunter-gatherers. It was a lifestyle in which accurate distance vision was essential for survival.[9] In Nature, all mammalian and bird species tend to be long-sighted or *emmetropic*, which means that they can see any object further than six metres clearly without any effort needed to focus. They rarely develop myopia. This makes evolutionary sense. If we did not have compensatory mechanisms for myopia and were left to mere palaeolithic resources, it is likely that short-sighted individuals would not survive for long. Clear distance vision is required for escape from predators, location of food, recognition of other species members and awareness of environmental dangers and benefits. Consequently, any gene or genes that favoured myopia would be lethal and rapidly eliminated by natural selection. That rules out a genetic defect as a cause of short-sightedness.

It was just possible that the discrepancies in susceptibility to myopia might have been due to genetic differences, but studies showed that when groups migrated from primal living to a more urbanized existence, rates of myopia shot up within a single generation. That was too quick to be a genetic mutation and so completely ruled out a genetic susceptibility. It seemed that myopia occurred only when new environmental conditions associated with modern civilization were introduced into the hunter-gatherer lifestyle.

This is confirmed if we look at hunter-gatherer populations today. Again we find little evidence of myopia where these peoples eat their traditional diet. Of some 3,624 eyes examined in a 1936 study of 20- to 65-year-old hunter-gatherer tribes-people in Gabon (then French Equatorial Africa), only 14 (0.4%) were classified as myopic.[10]

Similarly low rates for myopia were reported amongst Angmagssalik Inuit in 1954:[11] an examination of 1,123 eyes, found only 13 (1.2%) to be myopic. But things were to change. In 1969 scientists compared the eyes of older and younger Inuit and found an astonishing difference between the two groups.[12] Testing the right eyes of 131 adults over 41 years of age, the scientists led by Dr F. A. Young discovered only two myopic eyes amongst them. But over half – 149 out of 284 – of the right eyes of 11- to 40-year olds were myopic. Most of the older Inuit had grown up and lived most of their early lives in isolated communities with a traditional Inuit lifestyle and little or no schooling, whereas their children and grandchildren had grown up in Barrow, Alaska, and had had compulsory American style schooling. This was the reason, the scientists thought, for the huge difference in incidence of myopia between younger and older Inuit. It was simply that the younger ones had had to learn to read.

But they were wrong. The Inuit have been studied in great depth. Vilhjalmur Stefansson wrote in 1919 that both women and men engaged in work which could strain the eyes in a similar way to reading with such occupations as sewing and tool making for hours on end in dimly lit snow houses during the long arctic winter yet did not develop myopia.[13]

In 1966, Dr E. Cass suggested the reason for myopia in younger Inuit was that they had been born and brought up in an increasingly western dietary environment; they ate imported cereals, bread, potatoes and sugar rather than the fish and seal meat that their elders had eaten as youngsters.[14] It was this, he suggested, that might have caused the rapid increase of myopia noted in these aboriginal people.

In 2002 a group of scientists led by Professor Loren Cordain, an evolutionary biologist at Colorado State University, published a review of the scientific literature.[15] They looked at 229 hunter-gatherer tribes and confirmed that differences were all down to food. Cordain was clear that cereals were to blame. 'In the islands of Vanuatu,' he said, 'they have eight hours of compulsory schooling a day. Yet the rate of myopia in these children is only two percent.' The difference between them and Europeans was that the Vanuatuans ate fish, yam and coconut rather than white bread and cereals.

Experts interviewed by the BBC had mixed reactions to this review.[16] Dr Nick Astbury, vice-president of the Royal College of Ophthalmologists, told BBC News Online: 'It's an interesting theory, but it needs more evidence to support it,' although he did admit that the reasons for short-sightedness were 'multi-factorial' so diets high in refined starches could play a part. And James Mertz, a biochemist at the New England College of Optometry in Boston, remarked: 'It's a very surprising idea.'

However, Bill Stell of the University of Calgary in Canada said: 'It wouldn't surprise me at all. Those of us who work with local growth factors within the eye would have no problem with that – in fact we would expect it.'

When hunter-gatherer societies changed their primitive existence to a more western lifestyle during the last two centuries, they not only became literate and began reading within one or two generations, they also altered the type of food they had previously eaten. Hunter-gatherer diets typically consist of high levels of protein and fats, and low levels of carbohydrate compared with modern western diets.[17] Even those carbohydrates that are present in hunter-gatherer diets are less concentrated, producing only a minimal rise in blood glucose and insulin levels.

Dr Cordain's team found that although refined cereals and sugars were rarely if ever consumed by groups living in their traditional manner, these foods quickly became dietary staples following contact with western influences. When these societies changed their lifestyles and introduced grains and other carbohydrates, they rapidly developed levels of myopia that equalled or exceeded those in western societies.

How carbs could cause myopia

As well as stimulating the production of insulin, diets high in refined starches such as sugar and cereals also stimulate production of a related compound called *insulin-like growth factor 1* (IGF-1). Too much IGF-1 stimulates excess growth of the eyeball during its development making it abnormally long. And this is the fundamental defect in myopia.

As with so many other conditions, far-sighted scientists suspected diet – and processed carbohydrates in particular. Professor Jennie Brand-Miller of Sydney University linked the dramatic increase in myopia in developed countries to childhood over-consumption of bread.[16] Short-sightedness is extremely rare in societies where the diet does not contain processed carbohydrates. It is also noticeable that short-sighted individuals are more susceptible to other conditions associated with the excessive consumption of sugar or starch: diseases such as diabetes and dental decay.

Confirmation

That diet could be the reason for short-sightedness was confirmed in 1999. It was thought to be uniquely human trait, completely unknown in the animal kingdom – until evidence came to light with a study of domesticated Labrador dogs.[18]

Dogs don't read; that could not be the reason that the Labradors had myopia. But wild dogs do not get myopia; nor are they fed by civilized humans. Domesticated dogs are – and the difference between the wild and domesticated animals is that wild dogs eat meat and Man's best friend is fed on wheat-based dog biscuits. It's exactly the same pattern as was found in the comparisons between the traditional Inuit and their younger offspring.

Myopia is a modern trend. Although highly refined sugars and cereals are common elements of our diet today, such foods were eaten rarely or not at all by the average citizen in 17th and 18th century Europe. Their availability to the masses only increased after the industrial revolution, and wheat flour of a low extraction with much of the grain discarded became widely available with the advent of steel roller mills in the late 19th century.

Myopia was not the only condition to increase when this dietary change was made. Studies of hunter-gatherer populations that have recently adopted western dietary patterns frequently show high levels of blood sugar, insulin, insulin resistance, and type-2 diabetes. Conversely, hunter-gatherer populations in their native environments rarely exhibit these symptoms.[19]

Over the last two centuries the carbohydrate content of foods in urban areas of industrialized countries has risen steadily, primarily because of increasing consumption of refined cereals and sugars. The progression of myopia has been shown to be slower in children whose protein consumption is increased.

Taken as a whole, then, the research which suggested that reading was the prime cause of myopia was a bit, well, short-sighted. Conventional dietetic wisdom makes claims for the health-promoting effects of a diet rich in starchy staples such as breakfast cereals. Perhaps they are unable see the effect it is having.

Macular degeneration

It's not just the young whose eyes are helped by eating a low-carb, high-fat diet. There is another condition spreading rapidly throughout western society like a major epidemic – a blindness called macular degeneration. Age-related macular degeneration (AMD) was almost unheard of as late as 1980. Now, affecting millions, it is the second leading cause of blindness in humans.

The *macula* is the area located at the centre of the retina that is responsible for detailed, fine central vision. AMD involves a number of degenerative changes in the macular region, particularly in people with diabetes.[20] And there is no really effective conventional treatment for this condition. It is widely believed that the reason for the continuing rise in the numbers of cases of this disease is because of the increasing size of the elderly population in western countries. But this may not be so.

Polyunsaturated vegetable oils and AMD
It has been suggested that AMD is caused by atherosclerosis in the blood vessels that supply the retina, in a similar way to the mechanism underlying coronary heart disease (CHD).[21] According to this hypothesis, dietary fat components related to CHD may also be related to AMD. As you know, dietary saturated fat, cholesterol, and *trans* unsaturated fats are believed to increase the risk of CHD, and polyunsaturated fats, to reduce that risk. Thus, these specific types of fat were thought to have similar associations with AMD.

Well, it seems to be true that the balance of fats and oils in your diet can affect your vision – but not in the way that was expected. Researchers at the Massachusetts Eye and Ear Infirmary carried out a study of 349 individuals aged 55 to 80 with AMD, and compared their diet with a control group with eye diseases other than AMD.[22] Those who consumed foods high in 'healthy' vegetable oils had more than twice the risk of AMD of those whose intakes were low. People eating the other 'healthy' monounsaturated fats, such as olive oil, also had a 71% higher risk of AMD. But diets rich in omega-3 fatty acids, found in oily fish such as tuna and salmon, were protective against AMD.

This was confirmed in the same year by a much larger study at Harvard Medical School.[23] These researchers also determined that linoleic acid, the principal omega-6 fatty acid in most vegetable oils, as well as oils containing monounsaturated fatty acids, increased the risk of AMD. As antioxidant vitamins have been shown to reduce the risk of AMD,[24] this too adds to the weight of evidence against 'healthy' fats, as these are the only oils to oxidize readily.

The major reason for blindness in Australia 30 years ago was the retinopathy which accompanies diabetes and it was rare to find macular degeneration. Today AMD has overtaken diabetes five-fold and is now the leading cause of blindness in Australia. Is it merely a coincidence that Australians use vegetable oils probably more than any other nation?

Dr Paul Beaumont from the Australian Macular Degeneration Foundation is horrified at the rate macular degeneration has multiplied. 'I've seen an exponential rise from the early 1970s through to the 1990s,' Dr Beaumont said in an interview on Australian Channel Seven, broadcast on 5 July 2004.[25] 'If we look at Japan forty years ago the disease was rare, now it's common.' And he has seen a 10-fold increase in the condition in Australia in the last 30 years. 'I don't think there's any doubt we have an epidemic.'

Dr Beaumont studied particularly the link with polyunsaturated fats. '[The research] showed that people eating vegetable oil got the disease twice as commonly as the people who didn't,' he said.

'Even more convincing was a prospective study where they looked at patients with the disease and those eating too much vegetable oil progressed at 3.8-times the rate of those eating a little vegetable oil.

'You look at bread, they make it on margarine; you look at currants and they've gone and sprayed vegetable oil on them to stop them from sticking; you go and try and get tinned fish and they've put it in vegetable oil.

'So yes, it's become ubiquitous; it's crept right into our food chain and you hardly know you're eating it.'

Dr Beaumont says there should be a consumer health warning on the packages similar to a warning on a cigarette packet: 'VEGETABLE OIL CAN LEAD TO MACULAR DEGENERATION.' 'I think we could halve the number of people going blind with macular degeneration if we could change their diet, cut out the vegetable oil.'

The message is clear that if you want to look after your eyes, cut down on processed foods high in vegetable fats, but eat more fish.

If you don't care much for eating oily fish, there is another answer: eat more eggs. These contain two compounds, lutein and zeaxanthin, which slow the progression of dry macular degeneration and in some patients, improve visual acuity. Over the last couple of decades we have been told to cut down on eggs. That could be a mistake as eggs as well as spinach and broccoli are particularly rich in these two compounds.[26] Studies are showing that restricting eggs from the diet can have harmful effects.[27,28]

But there is one other consideration: 52% of the lutein and 44% of the zeaxanthin is transported by HDL and about 22% of lutein and zeaxanthin is transported by LDL; 20-25% of alpha-carotene, beta-carotene and lycopene is transported by HDL; and 50-57% of these is transported by LDL.[29] So even if you eat a diet high in lutein and zeaxanthin, their uptake and transport into the retina may be adversely affected if you have low cholesterol levels.

Carbohydrates and ARM

Several dietary factors have been linked to age-related *maculopathy* (ARM), the early form of age-related macular degeneration. Because there was reason to think that dietary carbohydrate might play a part in the development of ARM, this was tested as part of the Nurses' Health Study from Harvard University.[30] The researchers found that glycaemic index was related to ARM (specifically to retinal pigmentary abnormalities), whereas total carbohydrate intake was not. But high-GI carbohydrates include 'healthy' carbohydrates such as bread.

Excitotoxins

And there are other factors in modern foods, particularly the pre-prepared foods, which increase the risk of AMD and ARM. Studies in rats have shown that common food additives such as aspartame which many people eat because they've been told to cut down on sugar, and monosodium glutamate, both of which are added to many processed foods, can wreak havoc. Aspartame, for example, breaks down into eye-destroying formaldehyde and methyl alcohol.[31-33] It doesn't help that aspartame is addictive.[34]

Cataracts

Another eye condition that may be caused by the oxidation of polyunsaturated fatty acids is cataract. When damaged proteins gather within one or both of the eye lenses, the resulting area becomes cloudy, or opaque. This is called a cataract. Cataract is the leading cause of blindness worldwide, and about 20 million Americans older than 40 have it.

Cataract is usually attributed to exposure to sunlight while not wearing protective sunglasses.[35] But while it is true that even low exposure to UVB significantly increases risk of cataracts, that happens only if you consume a western-style, junk food diet rich in unsaturated fats and their oxidized products.[36,37] Those who consume a more natural diet do not get cataracts even from lengthy sun exposure.[38]

A community-based ophthalmic survey of Asians and Caucasians aged 40 years and over randomly selected from the patients of four General Practitioners was conducted in Leicester. Age-related cataract was significantly higher in the Asians when compared with the Caucasians and it was found to develop earlier in the Asians. The significant risk factor for age-related cataract in the Asian community in Leicester was found to be their strict vegetarian diet.[39]

Animal studies had suggested a causal role for dietary carbohydrate in the formation of cataracts for many years before. However, few published human studies had evaluated associations with carbohydrate nutrition until recently. A study in 1992 showed that sugars increase cataract risk.[40] Since then several large studies have found that any 'healthy', high-carb diet can increase the risk.[41,42]

Scientists funded by the Agricultural Research Service in Boston, Massachusetts, found that the higher the carbohydrate intake, the higher the odds of developing a certain type of cataract among a group of women aged 53 to 73 years. The women in the study, whose average carbohydrate intake was between 200 and 268 grams per day, were 2.5 times more likely to get cortical cataracts than the women whose intake was between 101 and 185 grams per day. This association was the same whatever the glycaemic index of the carbs eaten. The study concluded that: 'These data suggest that carbohydrate quantity, but not carbohydrate quality, is associated with early cortical opacities, and that neither the quantity nor the quality of dietary carbohydrate affects the risk of nuclear opacities in middle-aged women.'

A Japanese team at Shinshu University Graduate School of Medicine also showed that low levels of cholesterol in the eyes may raise cataract risk.[43] Normally, epithelial cells form a thin, single layer across the eye lens which maintains the lens's transparency. In eyes with cataracts, these cells fail to mature normally. The researchers showed that a defect in cholesterol production alters proliferation of epithelial cells and contributes to the eye lens becoming opaque. These findings may prove important for people taking cholesterol-lowering medications or for those with defective cholesterol production, they said.

One other known cause of cataract is the fluorides used for water fluoridation and toothpastes.[44]

Whichever way you look at it, following current 'healthy' advice is a likely reason for the increase in this condition.

Glaucoma

In 1999 I stayed for three months in New Zealand. While there I met the cousin of a friend in my home village. N. L. was in her late 60s, overweight and diabetic. I suggested that for both conditions she should adopt a low-carb, high-fat diet. And I managed to convince her of its benefits. Several months later, she wrote to tell me of her progress. Not only had she lost weight; she no longer needed her diabetes medication. But more than this, she wrote: 'I had been to my ophthalmologist for a variety of tests . . . First major surprise – the pressure behind my eyes which had for many years been border-line glaucoma, had reduced – excellent result.'

I met N. L. again three years later when she visited England in 2002. Her glaucoma was completely cured without any other intervention.

Affecting around 2% of the population, glaucoma, which involves deterioration of the optic nerve, is the second most common cause of
blindness in the UK and the US.

For years, we were told that glaucoma results from fluid-pressure
build-up in the eye causing the optic nerve to deteriorate. But this theory
turns out to have been based on an incorrect medical model – and found
to be wrong. Now, the experts have given birth to a new theory. According to this, glaucoma is the result of insufficient blood flow due to
agglutination (clumping together) of the red blood cells and waste build-
up in the cells and intercellular fluids. These blood-corpuscle clusters
cannot squeeze through the extremely tiny capillaries in the back of the
eye and so they block them, preventing the eyes from getting the nutrients they need. As glaucoma is more prevalent in diabetics, this makes a
lot more sense and, as it is high levels of glucose in the bloodstream that
cause blood to become 'sticky', it should be no surprise that a low-carb
diet helps both to treat the condition and to prevent it.

Harvard University conducted a study of antioxidant use in glaucoma,
but found no benefit. However, there was a small benefit from lutein and
zeaxanthin found in eggs.

Retinopathy

Retinopathy, which affects the retina of the eye (the layer at the back of
the eye that contains photoreceptors), is a recognized complication of diabetes. It is caused by the small blood vessels that supply blood to the
light-receptor cells becoming damaged or blocked. This in turn is caused
by two aspects of the diabetic condition. One is chronically high levels of
glucose in the bloodstream, which cause single-cell thick capillaries to
begin to leak. This leakage of blood, when near the surface of the retina,
is easily seen by an ophthalmologist when he examines the eye with an
ophthalmoscope. As they accumulate, these small patches of blood may
form small dark spots or 'floaters' in the vision. These may become larger
and block the light from reaching parts of the retina, causing a progressive
form of blindness. In this event, a sudden rupture of the blood vessel may
occur with a consequent reduction in the eye's blood supply.

The other cause is high insulin levels associated with diabetes, again as
a consequence of a 'healthy diet' or orthodox medical treatment, both of
which amount to about the same thing. In this case, the small arteries of
the retina begin to experience a form of atherosclerosis similar to that of
the body's larger arteries. This causes a build-up of plaque on their inner
surfaces and a stiffening of the wall with the consequent reduction of
blood supply to the retina. It also increases the likelihood of a blood clot.
If a blood clot occurs in one of the eyes' larger arteries or at a junction

that supplies a larger part of the retina with oxygen and nutrition, blindness may occur as quickly as in a few hours. Both the venous leakage and the artery blockage are progressive. Although the body tries to repair the damage by growing new arterioles and veins, a process called *neovascular overgrowth*, these new blood vessels tend to be weaker and soon suffer the same fate as the ones they replace. There is also another problem: the new blood vessels tend to form a tangled web that interferes with the light-sensitive photoreceptors. These can also interfere with the optic nerve that transports the visual information to the brain, an activity which can ultimately lead to structural damage in the eyes such as a detached or torn retina. And, of course, loss of sight.

Orthodox treatments include drugs to lower either blood cholesterol or blood pressure and laser treatment may be suggested, but none of these treats the cause. In the case of laser treatment to stop the leakage, as the leakage is progressive and the laser treatment is not, it really isn't a lot of use in the long term.

Dry eye syndrome

Many millions of people in the industrialized countries, predominantly women, suffer from dry eye syndrome, a painful and debilitating eye disease. Dry eye syndrome is characterized by a decline in the quality or quantity of tears that normally bathe the eye to keep it moist and functioning well. The condition causes symptoms such as pain, irritation and a sandy or gritty sensation. If untreated, severe dry eye syndrome can lead to scarring or ulceration of the cornea, and loss of vision. Victims may experience symptoms so severe that reading, driving, working and other vision-related activities of daily life are difficult or impossible.

In the first study of its kind to examine modifiable risk factors, researchers from Brigham and Women's Hospital and Schepens Eye Research Institute, an affiliate of Harvard University Medical School and the largest independent eye research institute in the world, found that the amount, type and ratio of essential fatty acids in the diet may play a key part in dry eye prevention in women.[45]

This study set out to examine how changing dietary habits in America, primarily a shift in the balance of essential fatty acids they are consuming, may be associated with onset of this eye disease. What it found was that a high intake of omega-6 fatty acids, of the type found in margarines, cooking and salad oils, increased the risk of dry eye syndrome. On the other hand, omega-3 fatty acids, found in fish oils and walnuts, reduced the risk, as of course does reducing intakes of vegetable margarines and oils containing excessive amounts of omega-6.

Summary
The evidence speaks for itself. Beginning at birth, and continuing throughout life, a so-called 'healthy' carbohydrate-based diet, and one that also replaces natural fats with processed vegetable oils, poses a significant danger to our eyes.

Incidentally, as I write this, I am 72 years old. Although I do use very low-powered (1.00 dioptre) reading glasses for reading in poor light, I have no need of glasses for anything over about 18 inches (450 millimetres) distant. But, then I have lived on a low-carb, high-animal fat diet for most of my life.

Hearing loss (age related)

Presbycusis, as it is called, is the gradual loss of hearing that occurs as people age. It is the most common hearing problem in older people, occurring in about 25% of people aged 65-75 years and in 50% of those over 75 years. Despite increasing awareness of, and implementation of preventive measures against industrial noise exposure, the condition is increasing in our society.[46] Apart from aging, hearing loss is also associated with other degenerative conditions such as diabetes.[47,48]

Dr Samuel Rosen and colleagues conducted a number of studies in the early and mid 1960s. These led them to the conclusion that: 'diet was an important factor in the prevention of hearing loss.'[49] Since then, a wealth of evidence has been amassed which implicates hydrogenated vegetable oils and trans-fatty acids; the common mechanism of aging, and degenerative disease in general, is now widely believed to be due, in whole or in large part, to free radical damage of such fatty acids.

Other research confirms that diabetes can cause hearing loss – and at a younger age. Dr Hisaki Fukushima of the International Hearing Foundation, Minneapolis, Minnesota and colleagues examined temporal bones obtained at autopsy from patients with type-1 diabetes, average age 37, and compared them with similar bones obtained from healthy people. Diabetics had significant damage to the inner ear. The researchers said: 'The findings in our study suggest that the microangiopathy associated with diabetes affects the inner ear vasculature and causes degeneration of inner ear structures.'[50] Diabetes is a condition where blood sugars are high.

Gout

The prosperous, usually aristocratic, man with the hugely bandaged foot is a caricature beloved of comedy programmes. But gout is a painful and far from a laughable form of arthritis. For decades, gout sufferers have been advised to avoid high purine-containing foods. Purines are the chemicals that form uric acid in the body, which in turn causes painful deposition of urate crystals in the joints. Examples of these are: kidneys, sweetbreads, liver, bacon, beef, pork, duck, shellfish and venison.

However, a study published in 2000 presented a challenge to the 'low-purine, high-carbohydrate' diet usually advised for gout patients. As insulin resistance has been increasingly implicated in the development of gout, and changes in blood cholesterol levels seen in persons with gout are similar to those associated with insulin resistance, an investigation was conducted at the University of Witwatersrand, Johannesburg, South Africa, of non-diabetic men, each of whom had had at least two gout attacks during the four months immediately prior to the study. In the study, each man ate a diet which restricted carb intake and increased fats and protein. They were also encouraged to increase their intakes of fish and poultry, which are relatively high in the purines which are classically avoided in managing gout. After 16 weeks on this diet, not only had the men lost an average 17 lb (7.7 kg) in weight, gout attacks were reduced from an average of 2.1 per month to 0.6 per month. Not surprisingly, the researchers stated that 'current dietary recommendations for gout might need re-evaluation.'[51]

Another cause is the fruit sugar, fructose, both in high-fructose corn syrup and too much fruit.[52,53] So be careful with those 'five portions'.

Conclusion

The signs of 'healthy eating' poisoning are all too obvious. Even if you keep your weight down by low-calorie dieting (going hungry), your face will still bear the marks of bad diet.

The acne may clear up in time, whether you treat it or not. Your teeth, eyes and hearing, however, will not. Spending your childhood eating sweets, fizzy drinks and cheaper margarines will cost you dearly in later life, as dentistry and eye-glasses and hearing aids can be very expensive. Anyone who decides not to change to a low-carb, high-animal fat diet because of possible increased costs would do well to consider this aspect.

Chapter Twenty-Nine

And, finally . . .

Changes have already been made within medical schools to break the shackles of the pharmaceutical industry on health. It is time we took a stand against the misinformation that is making us ill by taking responsibility for our own health.

The superior doctor prevents sickness.
The mediocre doctor attends to impending sickness.
The inferior doctor treats actual sickness.

Huang Dee Nai-Chang (2600 BC)

The 'Big C' – cancer – really frightens us. It's not just that cancer kills us; it's the way it kills us. But there are other, possibly worse, conditions. These are the long drawn-out, often painful or uncomfortable, and unbearable conditions such as multiple sclerosis, Alzheimer's disease and osteoporosis; there are blindness, leg amputations and dialysis for diabetics to look forward to, as well as lesser discomforts experienced by the overweight. As things stand now, practically every one of us living in an industrialized country will suffer not just one, but many of the conditions mentioned in this book. Indeed, one in every three of us will get cancer. Ischaemic heart disease, the disease that current lifestyle advice is primarily aimed at preventing, is positively benign by comparison. We will all die. Given the choice, I would prefer a quick heart attack to years of lingering and painful decay.

These disorders are still absent or rare in populations pursuing a traditional subsistence lifestyle. This should remind us of our original human diet, during millions of years of Ice Ages, with its carnivorous background. This alone should be enough to make any open-minded dietician or clinician stop in his or her tracks and ponder why a food which our species has been eating for millions of years, 'saturated fat', should suddenly become 'bad for us'. Why are we told that new foods such as cereals and bread are preferable? Fat meat has been our main food for most of our existence as a species. Why are we told to avoid it now?

Evolutionary change grinds slowly. Our intestinal organs developed long ago to cope with foods of the time. Practically nothing in our bodies has changed since then – but our foods have. I realize that palaeolithic foods are not easy to obtain now, as food animals and plants have been modified out of all recognition. Cattle, pigs and other food animals are bred to be lean; their feed consists of materials as unnatural to them as ours are to us, in order to make their body fat 'healthier' for us to eat, or to make them grow more quickly. As a consequence, they are getting sicker as well. Plants are selectively bred for calories only – more starches and more sugars; mineral and vitamin contents are a minor concern.

When the natural fresh diet of a primitive lifestyle population is altered by the introduction of processed and refined foods, degenerative diseases appear that have not been seen previously. Some of the most impressive work in this area was done by an epidemiologist, Surgeon General T. L. Cleave, who found that degenerative diseases such as CHD, diabetes and hypertension began to appear only 20 to 30 years after the introduction of processed and refined foods. Fat and cholesterol content of the diet did not play a part.[1] Cleave found no exceptions to this pattern in hundreds of peoples of the world. The only exception I am aware of is in a paper describing changes in an Inuit population where the food supply abruptly changed and 'foreign' food was flown in.[2] The lag time before degenerative diseases showed up shortened to only 10 to 15 years from the usual 20 to 30.

One thing is certain: the lower the Glycaemic Index and Glycaemic Load of any meal, the lower is the risk of a wide variety of conditions.[3] But that means a lower carb content overall; not relying on 'slow-release wholemeal' bread that is certainly little or no better than white bread, and might be worse.

No doubt someone will ask why, in this case, we are living longer than ever before. The answer is that, by and large, we are not. When an improvement in life expectancy is reported in the press, most people really have no way of understanding what is going on. In the past century average life expectancy at birth continued to increase but this was due largely to reductions in *infant* death rates. In 1900 the infant death rate in the US and industrialized countries in Europe was around 100 per 1,000 live births. Today the infant death rate in advanced countries is around five per 1,000 live births. The statistic to look for here is how long people are living after achieving a certain age. For people already aged 40, life expectancy has shown no dramatic improvements as a result of antibiotics and other medical breakthroughs.

If I am right that 'healthy eating' could actually increase the risk of the diseases in this book, then we should be starting to see the numbers of cases of ischaemic heart disease increasing just about now, particularly in younger age groups. And that is exactly what is happening.[4]

Medicine gets far more credit than it deserves. Child deaths from diphtheria, measles, scarlet fever and whooping cough fell dramatically long before the introduction of antibiotics and widespread immunization. The biggest benefits to infant death rates and average life expectancy rates have not come from medicine but from public health measures such as potable water, cleaner food, warmer and drier living conditions and better sanitation.

Food quality, on the other hand, has declined over the last century. The biggest effect of this has to be the development of degenerative diseases as evidenced by increases in childhood obesity and diabetes rates. And most diseases of physical degeneration have little effect on overall life expectancy. They just make people more miserable as they age.

In an attempt to combat the frauds and food adulterations that were common in the 19th century and novel foods and drugs developed in the 20th, various regulatory bodies have been set up to protect the consumer. The US's watchdog is the Food and Drugs Administration (FDA). Despite a budget for 2007 of approximately $1.6 billion, the FDA is failing miserably in its allotted tasks. A confidential report, published in November 2007 for the FDA Science Board, concluded that the FDA's oversight system is dysfunctional and 'in crisis'; that it poses a hazard to public health rather than a safety net.[5] The report gives the FDA failing grades in every aspect of its public mission. The report states that: 'Inadequately trained scientists are generally risk-averse, and tend to give no decision, a slow decision or, even worse, the wrong decision.' The *New York Times* says of the report that it is the latest and perhaps most far-reaching in a string of outside assessments that have concluded that the FDA is poorly equipped to protect public health. The *Times* echoes the words of the report's authors: 'The nation's food supply is at risk, its drugs are potentially dangerous and its citizens' lives are at stake.'

Garret A. FitzGerald, a pharmacologist from the University of Pennsylvania and adviser to the authors of the report, blamed a 'cabal of Congressional majorities and presidential administrations that has serially stripped the agency of assets.' The Alliance for Human Research Protection says that this situation is a deliberate action in order to incapacitate the FDA, accomplished by the unduly pervasive influence of two industries: 'Big Pharma' and 'Big Food'.

Since 1992, user fees – that is money coming from the very food and drug companies the FDA is meant to control – have played a critical part in supporting pre-market review and approval functions of new medical products.

The FDA does not just influence and control food and drugs in the US. Decisions made by the FDA have repercussions around the globe; FDA decisions on the safety and efficacy of drugs and novel foods influence similar decisions made in Britain and other countries.

In Britain we have the National Institute for Health and Clinical Excellence (NICE). This organization, too, is heavily lobbied by drug companies. Although NICE may try to be conscientious, both government and a naïve populace influenced by commercial lobbying put immense pressure on NICE to accede to the drug and food companies' demands.

There have been increases in many diseases in recent years. The British government suggested in December 2007 a range of measures which, it said, would reduce the burden of disease in the UK. But those proposals were an increase in the very things that have been shown to increase the diseases against which they are aimed: the increases in degenerative disease are a consequence of our changing to a 'healthier' lifestyle. Albert Einstein said: 'If you keep doing what you have been doing but keep expecting different results then that is insanity.' Einstein would no doubt judge our government to be insane.

I am convinced that the biggest threat to our health today is the healthcare system itself, aided, abetted and coerced by the pharmaceutical and food industries, and even by our governments. Ever more people are drawn into treatment as a result of unnatural dietary advice. There is an astonishing increase in diagnoses and ever-expanding definitions of what constitutes a disease, with new ones being invented all the time. The British government actually encouraged this with a contract introduced in 2004 which pays doctors to diagnose 'disease'. This resulted in a spectacular 850,000 extra cases of chronic disease being diagnosed in England during 2006, and raised the average doctor's annual earnings by a massive 63%.[6] One can understand doctors making the most of what is, for them, an unprecedented bonanza.

The late Dr Robert Mendelsohn wrote that 'doctors in general should be treated with about the same degree of trust as used car salesmen.' But today that applies more to the nutritionists and dieticians who neglect the evidence and extol the supposed virtues of manufactured, vegetable-based oils which are more akin to the drying oils in old-fashioned paints than to food, while vilifying entirely natural and healthy fats.

A classic example of the stupidity of this obsessive dogma came in June 2007, with the refusal of the Broadcast Advertising Clearance Centre, which approves all UK television advertisements, to allow reruns of one of the most famous TV adverts of all time: 'Go to work on an egg'. This advertisement was blocked on the grounds that eating an egg for breakfast every day is not a 'varied diet'. (I'm sure Lord Strathcona wouldn't agree!) Yet they allow advertisements for sweets, sugar-loaded breakfast cereals, margarines, and similar foods which have absolutely no place whatsoever in a truly healthy diet.

You might think these questions would really give health professionals cause for concern – and for a rethink on their part, before they are called to account for the disaster they have caused. But they don't seem to 'get it'. Not only do they carry on parroting the dogma, they push it even harder. Despite so much clear scientific evidence that 'healthy eating' is neither effective nor healthy, most authorities encourage an even stricter dietary compliance. You might wonder, as I do, how they could have let the present situation degenerate so far without, it seems, questioning the very foundations of their recommendations.

Sadly, the fact that they seem unable to change is not unprecedented. It's a fact that most people when confronted with evidence that they are wrong do not change their point of view or course of action. They justify it even more vehemently. Forget 'five portions of fruit and veg', it's now seven to nine portions. Plus 'three portions of fibre'. Even irrefutable evidence is rarely enough to pierce the mental armour of self-justification. Thomas Kuhn exploring the necessity for scientists to make a paradigm shift,[7] discovered that many found it impossible to make such a change.

Kuhn considered that these observations did not mean that scientists were incapable of admitting their errors even when confronted with the evidence that refuted them; that was not the issue. The source of the resistance by those with long, productive scientific careers was the belief that their current paradigm would eventually prove to be correct, so it was unnecessary to make the switch. In other words, it simply was not possible to force a transfer of allegiance.

Max Planck once remarked: 'A new scientific truth does not triumph by convincing its opponents and making them see the light, but rather because its opponents eventually die, and a new generation grows up that is familiar with it.' Science advances funeral by funeral.

And there is, of course, that other consideration: money. As Upton Sinclair once remarked: 'It is difficult to get a man to understand something when his salary depends on his not understanding it.' It's not that every scientist is greedy, but they do have to make a living. Most scientists today are funded by commercial enterprises: food producers, drug companies, health charities and so on. If the conditions they are (supposed to be) working toward curing actually were cured, their funding would stop and they could be out of a job. The company or charity they work for might also lose its *raison d'être* and all its employees could also be out looking for work. Cynical though I might seem to be by pointing this out, it really is a fact of life. How, for example, would the world's 30,000 medical journals survive if there were nothing new to report every few days?

Teaching also needs to change. Students should be taught to question, investigate and dissect information. The way in which paradigms such as 'healthy eating' are perpetuated appears to lie in the ease with which many students accept what they are taught as fact, rather than researching and questioning for themselves. Isn't learning to think for oneself, rather than just accepting what one is told, a major part of a university education? Although, having said that, you won't be popular these days if do you think for yourself. H. L. Mencken warned: 'The most dangerous man to any government is the man who is able to think things out for himself, without regard to the prevailing superstitions and taboos. Almost inevitably he comes to the conclusion that the government he lives under is dishonest, insane and intolerable.'

People power: we can make a difference

Kuhn concluded that persuasion was more important in changing paradigms than hard evidence. He wrote that if a paradigm is to win over the old dogma, the first thing it must do is gain supporters: people who would carry the word and develop it further. Then, as more and more are converted, the exploration of the new paradigm may continue until, at last, only a few old die-hards remain. I hope that I have persuaded you, dear reader, that 'healthy eating' is a disaster of epic proportions, and that you will spread the word before it is too late.

At this stage I must repeat and emphasize that I do not believe that family doctors are willing accomplices in the current 'wealth-not-health' scams. I believe they are unwitting pawns, unscrupulously manipulated by the drug and food industries, aided by the unthinking, dogmatic reluctance to change on the part of nutritionists and dieticians. As such, doctors are unwitting participants in the fraud.

That, however, doesn't let them off the hook entirely. I gleaned most of the evidence in this book from mainstream medical journals. These are what doctors (should) read. Instead, it seems that both in medical school and after they leave it, the main method by which doctors acquire knowledge is from medical sales reps. The famous British physician, Sir

William Osler, told his peers: 'One of the first duties of the physician is to educate the masses not to take medicine.' That is still a duty that GPs today might consider.

The backlash has started

A move for change has started in the medical world as the pharmaceutical industry's subterfuge is at last being understood. Just after the turn of the 21st century, the American Medical Student Association, which represents 30,000 students, interns, and residents throughout the United States, began a campaign called 'PharmFree' which aims to break the entanglement between the pharmaceutical industry and medical students and the medical profession.[8] The association called for an end to gift giving, free lunches, sponsored education and paid speaking. Medical students were urged to sign a 'PharmFree pledge' to seek out unbiased sources of healthcare information. They even took a recently revised Hippocratic oath, called a 'model oath for the new physician,' which includes the commitments:

> 'I will make medical decisions . . . free from the influence of advertising or promotion. I will not accept money, gifts, or hospitality that will create a conflict of interest in my education, practice, teaching, or research.'

Not that it is all good news. In May 2007, in a 'move to improve global public health', Weill Cornell Medical College students were successful in their efforts to get a generic version of the cholesterol-lowering drug, simvastatin, marketed as Zocor, included on the WHO's list of essential medicines.[9] Students from Weill Cornell's chapter of Universities Allied for Essential Medicines (UAEM) answered the calls of Dr David Skorton, President of Cornell University, and Dr Antonio M. Gotto Jr, Dean of Weill Cornell Medical College, to 'seek new strategies for Cornell to advance public health' across the globe. UAEM comprises a national group of students whose goal is to determine how universities can help ensure that biomedical products, including medicines, are made more accessible in poor countries and further the amount of research conducted on neglected diseases affecting the poor.

'I am extremely proud that the students at Weill Cornell Medical College have had such an admirable influence on global health policy,' said Dr Skorton, who is also a professor of internal medicine and pediatrics. 'Such actions by our students show the promise of their future leadership.'

I, on the other hand, am horrified. How, pray, does drug-pushing 'advance public health'?

But this aberration aside, there are many other small campaigns starting up throughout the health industry to be rid of drug companies' influence. Professional associations, standard-setting bodies, and individual institutions around the world are beginning to disentangle themselves from some of the unhealthy flows of money and influence. These are indications of a desire on the part of concerned doctors to redefine fundamentally the relationships between doctors and drug companies. Aims include: restrictions or prohibitions on drug representatives visiting doctors, on educational events funded by the drug industry and on individuals or organizations with conflicts of interest running accredited continuing medical education. There are also campaigns to end acceptance of all gifts, trips and honoraria for speaking at educational conferences. Professional bodies are trying to reduce reliance on drug company sponsorship and on researchers with conflicts of interest when conducting research. Medical journals are reducing reliance on advertising revenue and sponsored supplements. And there are calls for new national bodies to conduct research driven by public interest and advisory committee members to avoid conflicts of interest. But while most of such organizations now have a code of conduct on relations with industry and conflicts of interest, when the negotiations come down to the wire and money and jobs are at stake, that code of conduct may not be enough to keep a researcher on the straight and narrow.

In December 2006, *The Los Angeles Times* reported the first prosecution of a government employee under federal conflict-of-interest laws in 14 years. Dr Trey Sunderland III, who headed Alzheimer's research at the US National Institute for Mental Health, which is part of the National Institutes of Health, pleaded guilty to criminal conflicts of interest.[10] Dr Sunderland was lucky not to receive a jail sentence; he was ordered to perform 400 hours of community service, submit to two years of probation and to pay the government the $300,000 he took in unauthorized payments from the drug company, Pfizer. You might think this indicates the start of a change in the NIMH – except that Dr Sunderland was allowed to remain a federal employee.

Stop direct drugs advertising

The US and New Zealand are the only industrialized nations to allow direct-to-consumer advertising of pharmaceutical drugs. Far from helping those targeted to become healthier, these advertisements allow pharmaceutical makers to increase sales of often useless, or even dangerous, drugs. It is not surprising that the pharmaceutical industry has boomed while the health of Americans is in a deplorable state. In 2005, more than 200 medical school professors endorsed a statement calling for an end to direct-to-consumer prescription drug advertising. In 2006, following an alert by Dr Leonore Tiefer, Professor of Psychiatry at the

New York University School of Medicine, many US health professionals proposed a Public Health Protection Act, to prohibit direct-to-consumer marketing of prescription drugs. According to the wording of the proposed Act, 'This advertising does not promote public health. It increases the cost of drugs and the number of unnecessary prescriptions, which is expensive to taxpayers, and can be harmful or deadly to patients.' New Zealand is considering similar action.[11]

These are certainly moves in the right direction, but the multinational health industries have many other tricks up their sleeves and will continue to use them. The drug companies are now targeting Britain. Don't forget, this is the world's richest industry; it has no intention of just giving up. There is simply too much money to be made out of illness for them to lie down without a fight.

This was evidenced in late 2007 by an article in the *Journal of the American Medical Association* which showed that drug companies were still investing in their sales-force.[12] Two-thirds of the 125 medical schools and teaching hospitals surveyed were receiving some funding from a drug company, through either research grants, purchase of equipment, or even 'discretionary' funds to buy food and drink for the students. The beneficence continued on an individual level, with 60% of the departmental heads receiving some funding from a drug company.

And there are no moves aimed at banning the advertising of inappropriate and harmful foods.

The problem of monopoly

In 2006 a Swedish doctor was caught teaching her diabetic patients to manage their condition with a low-carb diet. It worked, of course, and her patients felt much better. They were delighted, but her professional governing body wasn't – and her licence to practise medicine was suspended. Why? Because what she was doing didn't accord with what they allowed. The fact that her patients were healthier was totally irrelevant.

Two years later she was acquitted by the official authority (*Socialstyrelsen*). All the major media aired this conflict; there is a rapidly rising understanding that the dietary advice given by the industry-paid professors at the governmental Swedish Food Institute is ill-founded.

When you give one group a monopoly, whether it be the medical profession or a government body, they will always exercise this type of control. The problem is not medicine, *per se*; the problem lies squarely in the fact that we allow one group of people to have complete control over it. It is the way we have allowed the NHS to be governed that lies at the heart of the problem in Britain.

Before the NHS was set up, people were free to choose their own remedies. They could seek out whomsoever they wished to consult – and that would not necessarily be a medical physician. In a free market, people can vote with their feet: a medical professional who pushed useless or harmful drugs would soon be out of business as people would simply stop buying his product; a company that didn't improve its quality would stop trading. Yet the system we have is such that many treatments are banned by law – particularly, it seems, if they really work. The monopoly held by the health industry today ensures not only that useless drugs are all that are allowed to be sold, but also that they command exorbitant prices.

If healthcare were just like any other commodity, obeying the same natural laws of supply and demand, not only would it be much more effective, we wouldn't need so much of it. A free market always strives to give us the highest quality at the cheapest price; a monopoly, which is what we have at the moment, is exactly the other way around.

We hear almost daily about people hurt by medical mistakes. Who carries the can? Nobody. The professionals say they'll learn from their mistakes, that it will never happen again, but it seems it always does. In any other business, the company would be sued out of existence, and its executives possibly charged with corporate manslaughter. The medical profession, however, buries its mistakes – and gets away with it.

So can you go somewhere else? Only with difficulty. There is no free market in health; anyone trying to compete can be in big trouble. For the health professional, the choice is to toe the line or be sued. The consumer has very little choice.

We need a complete change of policy. The only bodies large enough to make that change are governments (and I doubt they will), or us the population. As I mentioned at the beginning of this book, we have it within our own powers *not* to be reliant on the health industry and *not* to become another statistic. Doctors and nutritionists have made theirs the only treatments available, but they can't make us take them or even make us reliant on them.

We are ultimately responsible for our own health

We are being exploited as never before. This has been allowed to happen by those who have a duty to protect us and whom we trust, literally, with our lives. Many over the last century have warned that this was happening. They were ridiculed, dismissed as 'cranks', sacked from their jobs, sidelined, reviled and ostracized as a result. When the situation was less obvious than it is today, the public accepted ill-health as a fact of life. In the last two decades, however, the rapid escalation in the numbers of chronic diseases and the visibility of them means that the evidence can no longer be brushed under the carpet.

Naturally, those responsible blame the individual. It's your own fault, they say. You are eating too much, or eating the wrong things, or not doing this right or that correctly. There may be some truth in this; the food companies also want to make a profit. But you now know, dear reader, that the dietary advice you have been given for over 20 years is the wrong advice. It is encouraged by huge industries that profit from your misfortune.

And it's about time they were brought to account for the harm they have done.

In one respect, however, it *is* our own fault. It is we who blindly accept the propaganda we are fed; it is we who clamour for every new – and ever more expensive – treatment that comes onto the market, without looking at the evidence; it is we who insist on 'the government' putting more and more money into 'health'; it is we who don't realize that we as taxpayers fund such expense. In 2006, the total tax take in the UK reached a landmark figure: £365 billion. That was £1 billion a day; and with a population of about 60 million, that works out at over £6,000 for every man, woman and child in the country. That's £6,000 of your money. The UK is the most highly taxed nation in Europe. While other countries' taxes have fallen over recent years, ours have risen. Today, nearly a quarter of all money earned in this country goes directly to fund profligacy and corruption within the NHS.

We cannot go on like this.

One problem with the NHS is the way it is set up and funded. When large numbers of people pay for and share any common resource, each individual tends to increase his personal use of that resource. But if we all increase our use of it, the resource is overexploited until eventually all the individuals paying for it are ruined. This is a phenomenon termed the 'tragedy of the commons'.[13]

The NHS is such a common resource which is subject to this tragedy. A person with an illness seeking a treatment that produces a benefit, however small, is acting within his rights. If that treatment is expensive, the patient is unaware of it because the cost is spread among all the others. It is this attitude that has allowed the NHS to become a bottomless pit; it is also the attitude which has allowed the NHS to be exploited so callously by the health industry.

There is no question that there is an ever-increasing funding crisis for medical services. This will continue until there is a radical change in the paradigm. As long as the demand for drugs increases and drug prices continue to rise, the pharmaceutical companies' bank balances will get healthier at the expense of your health and bank balance.

The only solution is to change the entire system: to redirect the spending towards care that will build the health of the country and provide people with the energy to be more productive. This was what was expected when the NHS was instituted. By focusing on health and truly preventative strategies, rather than disease treatment after the fact, the total cost of providing medical care could decline dramatically; healthy people require fewer medical resources; they also take less time off work. Theoretically, extra productivity alone should create more than enough additional wealth to pay for all the healthcare that we might need. But cost saving is really a less significant benefit; the major reason to pursue such a goal is that a great deal of pain and misery could be avoided, and people could start to experience what it means to live a life of health and vitality.

Help yourself

We are all victims. It's time that we all helped ourselves by taking a stand against the misinformation pumped out by the health industry, those in power who are too afraid to lose big business, those medical professionals who push drugs they know to be ineffective, and nutritionists who parrot unsupported dogma. It is up to all of us to learn what we need to do to protect ourselves. You won't learn this at school; the propaganda begins with schoolchildren. Today our schools are a major part of the problem; they are little more than government-run indoctrination camps where mis-informed teachers offer nutrition classes to infants. Few if any escape from that indoctrination. No, the key is to educate yourself.

In 1968, a time when medical information was expanding exponen-tially, Dr Lawrence Weed wrote that doctors 'are a guidance system, not a book of knowledge.'[14] Doctors can only do so much. Physicians need reliable and unbiased information sources for an accurate diagnosis of specific diseases, yet they read unreliable or biased medical journals and listen to sales reps. If you have a health problem, try to learn as much about it as you can. In my experience, doctors like their patients to be part of an active partnership. Use your doctor as you would your lawyer – someone from whom to seek advice so that you can make an informed decision. And target the causes; don't let him treat just the symptoms. Ultimately you should make the decisions that affect your life, not your doctor.

Dr Weston Price discovered what health is made of, and proved it. In more than 100,000 miles of travels all over the world, he sought out peo-ple 'who were living in accordance with the tradition of their race and as little affected as might be possible by the influence of the white man.' Regardless of their race, diet or the climate they were a 'picture of su-perb health', with perfect physiques and teeth, no degenerative diseases, and cheerful and happy. That all changed radically in groups of the same peoples who had been introduced to processed 'trade foods' produced in our industrial society.

Price found that it took only one generation of eating such food to destroy these peoples' health and immunity. My hope is that it will take only one generation to restore it.

One last thought: when you are assured by an advertisement for a new, 'better' drug, or a new 'wonder food', that these will save lives, think again. Whatever that product is, I can assure you that it will not. We are not an immortal species; life is a universally fatal, sexually transmitted disease. The best that anything can do is *prolong* our lives. And that might not be worthwhile if our quality of life is ruined. As one woman said to her neighbour over the garden fence: 'The trouble with making all these changes so you live longer is that all the extra years come at the end – when you're old!' She's right: it is during those extra years that we get Alzheimer's disease, cancers and many other distressing and debilitating conditions. My grandmother, who died aged 98, was senile for several of her last years. In one of her lucid moments, she told me that getting old was 'not much fun'. Increasing longevity may make national statistics look good – but many of the effects of a 'healthy' lifestyle can leave you physically and mentally disabled, blind and deaf. It might be nice to live to be 100, but not if you have lost the senses that allow you to appreciate and enjoy it.

There is one other way in which you can make a difference. The next time you are asked to donate to a cancer organization, bear in mind that your money will be used to sustain an industry which has been deemed by many eminent scientists as a qualified failure and by others as a complete fraud. The same goes for most of the other big medical charities. To make a difference in the best possible way, inform these organizations that you won't donate to them until they change their approach to one which is focused on prevention. If we make their present business unprofitable, we really do have the power to change things. These institutions survive only through our charitable donations and our gullibility.

The year, 2008, marks the NHS's 60th birthday. Let us celebrate the occasion by making a concerted effort to turn the present disastrous situation around.

References

Introduction

1. *The Daily Telegraph*, 5 February 2005.
2. Price WA. *Nutrition and Physical Degeneration*. Paul B. Hoeber, Inc. 1939.
3. Hopkins Tanne J. US health spending reaches a sixth of gross domestic product. *BMJ* 2006; 332: 198.
4. Smith C, et al. National health spending in 2004: recent slowdown led by prescription drug spending. *Health Affairs* 2006; 25: 186-196.

Chapter One: Trick to treat

1. Transparency International's *Global Corruption Report 2006*. London: Pluto Press; 2006.
2. Moynihan R. Selling sickness: the pharmaceutical industry and disease mongering. *BMJ* 2002; 324: 886-891.
3. Gillie O, McKee I. Patients put at risk as doctors aid drug firms in sales drive. *Sunday Times*. 29 Jan 1978; 4.
4. http://www.casacolumbia.org/supportcasa/item.asp?cID=12&PID=138
5. Tuffs A. Only 6% of drug advertising material is supported by evidence. *BMJ* 2004; 328: 485.
6. Kauffman JM, McGee CT. Are the biopositive effects of Xrays the only benefits of repetitive mammograms? *Med Hypoth* 2004; 62: 674-678.
7. Moss RW. *Questioning Chemotherapy*, Brooklyn, NY: Equinox Press. 2000.
8. Kauffman JM. Bias in recent papers on diets and drugs in peer-reviewed medical journals. *J Am Phys Surg* 2004; 9: 11-14.
9. Connor S. Glaxo chief: Our drugs do not work on most patients. *The Independent*, 8 Dec 2003.
10. Smith R. Where is the wisdom: the poverty of medical evidence. *BMJ* 1991; 303: 798-799.
11. Armstrong D. Bitter pill: how the New England Journal missed warning signs on vioxx, *The Wall Street Journal*, May 15, 2006; A1.
12. Kleinfield NR. In diabetes, one more burden for the mentally ill. *New York Times* June 12, 2006.
13. Moncrieff J, Cohen D. Do antidepressants cure or create abnormal brain states? *PLoS Med* 2006; 3(7): e240.
14. Healy D, et al. Antidepressants and violence: problems at the interface of medicine and law. *PLoS Med* 2006; 3 (9): e372.
15. Prescription drugs and their potentially adverse effects. http://www.worldhealth.

net/p/4169,4436.html.
16. Wazana A. Physicians and the pharmaceutical industry: is a gift ever just a gift? *JAMA* 2000; 283: 373-380.
17. Chren MM, Landefeld CS. Physicians' behavior and their interactions with drug companies: A controlled study of physicians who requested additions to a hospital drug formulary. *JAMA* 1994; 271: 684-689.
18. Drug firms try to bribe doctors with cars. *The Guardian*, 31 October 2007.
19. Griffith D. Reasons for not seeing drug representatives. *BMJ* 1999; 319: 69-70.
20. Shimm DS, Spece RG Jr. Industry reimbursement for entering patients into clinical trials: legal and ethical issues. *Ann Intern Med* 1991; 115: 148-151.
21. Reed Abelson. Charities tied to doctors get drug industry gifts. *New York Times*, 28 June 2006. (Accessed online 18 May 2008)
22. Fugh-Berman A. Doctors must not be lapdogs to drug firms. *BMJ* 2006; 333: 1027.
23. Ellison S. *Health Myths Exposed: How Western Medicine Undermines Your Health*. 2nd Edition. http://www.health-fx.net.
24. Relaxing the rules. Does the *New England Journal of Medicine*'s decision to relax its conflict of interest policy strengthen or weaken the prestigious publication? *Tufts eNews*. Boston, 19 June 2002.
25. Healy D, Cattell D. The interface between authorship, industry and science in the domain of therapeutics. *Br J Psychiatry* 2003; 182: 22-27.
26. Brownlee S. Doctors without borders. Why you can't trust medical journals anymore. *Washington Monthly*. April 2004. http://www.washingtonmonthly.com/features/2004/0404.brownlee.html.
27. Zuckerman D. Hype in health reporting: "checkbook science" buys distortion of medical news. *Int J Hlth Serv* 2003; 33: 383-389.
28. Collier J, Iheanacho I. The pharmaceutical industry as an informant. *Lancet* 2002; 360: 1405-1409.
29. Bekelman JE, et al. Scope and impact of financial conflicts of interest in biomedical research. *JAMA* 2003; 289: 454-465.
30. Willman D. Stealth merger: drug companies and government medical research. *Los Angeles Times*. 2003 Dec 7: A1, A32-33.
31. Bero L, et al. Factors associated with findings of published trials of drug–drug comparisons: why some statins appear more efficacious than others. *PLoS Med* 2007; 4: e184.
32. Jørgensen AW, et al. Cochrane reviews compared with industry supported meta-analyses and other meta-analyses of the same drugs: systematic review. *BMJ* 2006; 333: 782-785.
33. Anon. Upfront: calling the tune. *New Scientist* 2006; 192: 6.
34. David Rose. Forcing drug companies to publish negative trial results 'is against law'. *The Times*, 27 February 2008.
35. Pitkin RM, et al. Accuracy of data in abstracts of published research articles. *JAMA* 1999; 281: 1110-1111.
36. Dixon B. New opportunity for an old technique. *Lancet Infect Dis* 2003; 3: 454.
37. Figueiras A, et al. An educational intervention to improve physician reporting of adverse drug reactions. *JAMA* 2006; 296: 1086-1093.
38. Healy D. Did regulators fail over selective serotonin reuptake inhibitors? *BMJ*

2006; 333: 92-95.
39. Avorn J. Paying for drug approvals – who's using whom? *NEJM* 2007; 356: 1697-1700.
40. http://www.usatoday.com/money/industries/health/2008-02-20-medical-device-suits_N.htm, accessed 21 February 2008.
41. (No authors listed) Time for a debate on health care in the USA. *Lancet* 2006; 368: 963.
42. Evans R, Boseley S. Drug firms' lobby tactics revealed: documents show how companies try to get new medicines fast-tracked. *The Guardian*, 28 September 2006.
43. Open up NHS to our drug firms, White House demands. *The Guardian*, 14 November 2006.
44. Boseley S. GSK claims victory in battle over drug prices. *The Guardian*, 28 September 2006.
45. BBC News. *Q&A: GPs' pay.* 18 April 2006. http://news.bbc.co.uk/1/hi/health/4918040.stm, accessed 18 April 2006.
46. www.icservices.nhs.uk, accessed 1 September 2006.
47. Siegel-Itzkovich J. Doctors' strike in Israel may be good for health. *BMJ* 2000; 320:1561.
48. Horne, Ross. *Health & Survival In The 21st Century.* HarperCollins Publishers Pty Limited, Australia, 1997. Chapter 11.
49. *Science News,* 28 Oct 1978; 114: 293.
50. Starfield B. Is US health really the best in the world? *JAMA* 2000; 284: 483-485.
51. Wilson RM, et al. The Quality in Australian Health Care Study. *Med J Aust* 1995; 163: 458-471.
52. Motl S, et al. Proposal to improve MedWatch: decentralized, regional surveillance of adverse drug reactions. *Am J Health Syst Pharm* 2004; 61: 1840-1842.
53. Ashcroft DM, et al. Likelihood of reporting adverse events in community pharmacy: an experimental study. *Qual Saf Health Care* 2006; 15: 48-52.
54. Davidoff F. Shame: the elephant in the room. *BMJ* 2002; 324: 623-624.
55. http://www.garynull.com/documents/iatrogenic/deathbymedicine/deathbymedicine1.htm.
56. House of Commons Committee of Public Accounts. *A safer place for patients: learning to improve patient safety; Fifty-first Report of Session 2005-06.* 12 June 2006.
57. Mendelsohn RA. *Confessions of a Medical Heretic.* New York: McGraw-Hill Contemporary; 1979.
58. Mori website, http://www.ipsos-mori.com/polls/1999/bmajan99.shtml
59. (No authors listed) Drug-company influence on medical education in the USA. *Lancet* 2000; 356: 781.
60. Wrench GT. *The Wheel of Health: a study of a very healthy people.* The C. W. Daniel Company Ltd, London, 1938.
61. Boseley S. Concern over cancer group's link to drug firm. *The Guardian*, 18 October 2006.

Chapter Two: What's behind the screens?

1. *A New Contract for General Practitioners.* HMSO, London, 1990.
2. Wilson JMG, Junger G. *Principles and practice of screening for disease.* Public Health Papers No 34. Geneva: WHO, 1968.
3. Rattigan P. *The Cancer Business.* HarmonikIreland, quoting *The Guardian* 29 September 1990. http://www.harmonikireland.com/index.php?topic=cancerbusiness.
4. Registrar General's Mortality (Cause) Statistics, HMSO, London, 2007.
5. State of the Evidence: *What is the connection between the environment and breast cancer?* Breast Cancer Fund and Breast Cancer Action Report, 2004. See http://www.breastcancerfund.org.
6. Skrabanek P, McCormick J. *Follies and Fallacies in Medicine.* Glasgow: The Tarragon Press, 1989.
7. Hibberd AD. Surgery – prolonged survival or cure? In: *Breast Cancer. Treatment and Prognosis.* B. Stoll (Ed), Oxford: Blackwell, 1986.
8. Epstein S, et al. Dangers and unreliability of mammography: breast examination is a safe, effective and practical alternative. *Intl J Hlth Serv* 2001; 31: 605-615.
9. Gøtzsche PC, Olsen O. Is screening for breast cancer with mammography justifiable? *Lancet* 2000; 355: 129-134.
10. Miller AB, et al. Canadian National Breast Screening Study – 2: 13-year results of a randomized trial in women aged 50–59 years. *JNCI* 2000; 92: 1490-1499.
11. Kearney R. Factors affecting tumour growth. *Int Clin Nutr Rev* 1988; 8: 62.
12. Rubin P, ed. *Clinical oncology for Medical Students and Physicians: A Multidisciplinary Approach.* 6th Edition. American Cancer Society and the University of Rochester School of Medicine and Dentistry, 1983.
13. Cronin-Fenton DP, et al. Rising incidence rates of breast carcinoma with micrometastatic lymph node involvement. *JNCI* 2007; 99: 1044-1049.
14. Jørgensen KJ, et al. Are benefits and harms in mammography screening given equal attention in scientific articles? A cross-sectional study. *BMC Med* 2007; 5: 12.
15. Elmore JG, et al. Efficacy of breast cancer screening in the community according to risk level. *J Nat Cancer Inst* 2005; 97: 1035-1043.
16. Baum M. Informed consent may increase non-attendance rate. *BMJ* 1995; 310: 1003.
17. McMenamin M, et al. A survey of breast cancer awareness and knowledge in a Western population: lots of light but little illumination. *Eur J Cancer* 2005; 41: 393-397.
18. Bigenwald RZ, et al. Is mammography adequate for screening women with inherited BRCA mutations and low breast density? *Cancer Epidemiol Biomark Prev* 2008; 17: 706-711.
19. Campion MJ, et al. Psychosexual trauma of an abnormal cervical smear. *Br J Obstet Gynaecol* 1988; 95: 175.
20. Lerman C, et al. Adverse psychologic consequences of positive cytologic cervical screening. *Am J Obstet Gynecol* 1991; 165: 658.
21. Posner T, Vessey M. *Prevention of Cervical Cancer. The Patient's View.* London: King's Fund Publishing Office, 1988.

22. Raffle AE, et al. Detection rates for abnormal cervical smears: what are we screening for? *Lancet* 1995; 345: 1469-1473.
23. Harvey JA. Guidelines, standards, and evidence in cervical screening: a personal view. *Cytopathology* 1998; 9: 2-5.
24. Slater DN. Quality assurance in cervical cytopathology time for a more evidence-based approach. *Cytopathology* 1997; 8: 75-78.
25. Whelan P. Are we promoting stress and anxiety? *BMJ* 1997; 315: 1549-1560.
26. Albertsen PC, et al. 20-year outcomes following conservative management of clinically localized prostate cancer. *JAMA* 2005; 293: 2095-2101.
27. Gavin Phillips. *The Cancer Racket.* Liberty for All Online Magazine. http://www.libertyforall.net/2002/archive/cancer-racket.html.
28. Hopkins PN, Williams RR. A survey of 246 suggested coronary risk factors. *Atherosclerosis* 1981; 40: 1.
29. Bush TL, Riedel D. Screening for total cholesterol. Do the National Cholesterol Education Program's recommendations detect individuals at high risk of coronary heart disease? *Circulation* 1991; 83: 1287.
30. Bachorik PS, et al. Lipoprotein-cholesterol analysis during screening: accuracy and reliability. *Ann Intern Med* 1991; 114: 741.
31. Myers GL, et al. College of American Pathologists – Centres for Disease Control collaborative study for evaluating reference materials for total serum cholesterol measurement. *Arch Pathol Lab Med* 1990; 114: 1199.
32. Moore RA. Variation in serum cholesterol. *Lancet* 1988; ii: 682.
33. Executive Summary of the Third Report of the National Cholesterol Education Program (NCEP) Expert Panel on Detection, Evaluation, and Treatment of High Blood Cholesterol in Adults (Adult Treatment Panel III). *JAMA* 2001; 285: 2486-2497.
34. Majeed A, et al. Prescribing of lipid regulating drugs and admissions for myocardial infarction in England *BMJ* 2004; 329: 645.
35. Ioannidis J, Lau J. Completeness of safety reporting in randomized trials. An evaluation of 7 medical areas. *JAMA* 2001; 285: 437-443.
36. Pedersen TR, et al. High-dose atorvastatin vs usual-dose simvastatin for secondary prevention after myocardial infarction. The IDEAL Study: A randomized controlled trial. *JAMA* 2005; 294: 2437-2445.
37. Golomb BA, et al. Severe irritability associated with statin cholesterol-lowering drugs. *QJM* 2004; 97: 229-235.
38. Silver MA, et al. Statin cardiomyopathy? A potential role for coenzyme Q10 therapy for statin-induced changes in diastolic LV performance: description of a clinical protocol. *Biofactors* 2003; 18: 125-127.
39. Node K, et al. Short-term statin therapy improves cardiac function and symptoms in patients with idiopathic dilated cardiomyopathy. *Circulation* 2003; 108: 839-843.
40. Shepherd J, et al. Pravastatin in elderly individuals at risk of vascular disease (PROSPER): a randomised controlled trial. *Lancet* 2002; 360: 1623-1630.
41. Scandinavian Simvastatin Survival Study Group. Randomised trial of cholesterol lowering in 4444 patients with coronary heart disease: the Scandinavian Simvastatin Survival Study (4S). *Lancet* 1994; 344: 1383-1389.
42. Rosch PJ. Guidelines for diagnosis and treatment of high cholesterol. *JAMA* 2001; 286: 2400-2402.

43. Rosch PJ. Determining optimal statin dosage. *Mayo Clin Proc* 2003; 78: 379, 381.
44. Rosch PJ. Peripheral neuropathy. *Lancet* 2004; 364: 1663.
45. Graveline D. *Statin Drugs – Side Effects and The Misguided War on Cholesterol.* 2006, published by www.spacedoc.net.
46. Davey Smith G, et al. Cholesterol lowering and mortality: the importance of considering initial level of risk. *BMJ* 1993; 306: 1367.
47. Thomas P. The cholesterol controversy. *BMJ* 1992; 302: 912.
48. Most NHS staff say patients are not top priority. *The Guardian,* 9 April 2008.

Chapter Three: How we got to where we are

1. Orr JB. *Food, Health and Income.* London. 1936.
2. McCarrison R. Nutrition in health and disease. *BMJ* 1936; 26 September: 611.
3. Orr JB, Gilks JL. *Studies of Nutrition: The Physique and Health of Two African Tribes.* London: HMSO, 1931.
4. Monckeberg JG. Uber die Atherosklerose der Kombattanten (nach Obdurtionsbefunden). *Zentralbl Herz Gefasskrankheiten* 1915; 7: 7.
5. Monckeberg JG. Anatomische Veranderungen am Kreislaufsystem bei Kreigsteilnehmern. *Zentralbl Herz Gefasskrankheiten* 1915; 7: 336.
6. Enos WF, et al. Coronary disease among United States soldiers killed in action in Korea. Preliminary report. *JAMA* 1953; 152: 1090.
7. Holman RL, et al. The natural history of atherosclerosis: the early aortic lesions as seen in New Orleans in the middle of the 20th century. *Am J Pathol* 1958; 34: 209.
8. McGill HC jr (ed): *The Geographic Pathology of Atherosclerosis.* Baltimore: Williams & Wilkins Co, 1968.
9. Strong JP, McGill HC jr. The natural history of coronary atherosclerosis. *Am J Pathol* 1962; 40: 37.
10. Anitschkow N. On variations in the rabbit aorta in experimental cholesterol feeding. *Beitr Path Anat u allgem Path* 1913; 56: 379.
11. Gofman JW, et al. The role of lipids and lipoproteins in atherosclerosis. *Science* 1950; 111: 166-171, 186.
12. Keys A. Diet and the development of coronary heart disease. *J Chron Dis* 1956; 4: 364-380.
13. Landé KE, Sperry WM. Human atherosclerosis in relation to the cholesterol content of the blood serum. *Arch Path* 1936; 22: 301-312.
14. Mathur KS, et al. Serum cholesterol and atherosclerosis in man. *Circulation* 1961; 23: 847-852.
15. Marek Z, et al. Atherosclerosis and levels of serum cholesterol in postmortem investigations. *Am Heart J* 1962; 63:768-774.
16. Hecht HS, Harmann SM. Relation of aggressiveness of lipid-lowering treatment to changes in calcified plaque burden by electron beam tomography. *Am J Cardiol* 2003; 92: 334-336.
17. Keys A. Atherosclerosis: a problem in newer public health. *J Mt Sinai Hosp* 1953; 20: 118.
18. Cristakis G. Effect of the Anti-Coronary Club Program on coronary heart disease

risk-factor status. *JAMA* 1966; 198: 129-135.
19. Kannel WB, Gordon T. *The Framingham Diet Study: diet and the regulations of serum cholesterol (Sect 24)*. Washington DC, Dept of Health, Education and Welfare, 1970.
20. Ravnskov U. Cholesterol lowering trials in coronary heart disease: frequency of citation and outcome. *BMJ* 1992; 305: 15-19.
21. Miettinen TA, et al. Multifactorial primary prevention of cardiovascular diseases in middle-aged men. *JAMA* 1985; 254: 2097-2102.
22. Strandberg TE, et al. Long-term mortality after 5-year multifactorial primary prevention of cardiovascular diseases in middle-aged men. *JAMA* 1991; 266: 1225-1229.
23. Oliver MF. Doubts about preventing coronary heart disease. *BMJ* 1992; 304: 393-394.
24. Connor W. The acceleration of thrombus formation by certain fatty acids. *J Clin Invest* 1962: 41: 1199-1205.
25. Tholstrup T, et al. Acute effect of high-fat meals rich in either stearic or myristic acid on hemostatic factors in healthy young men. *Am J Clin Nutr* 1996; 64: 168-176.
26. For further details, contact or see: http://www.meatingplace.com.
27. Prior IA, et al. Cholesterol, coconuts, and diet on Polynesian atolls: a natural experiment: the Pukapuka and Tokelau island studies. *Am J Clin Nutr* 1981; 34: 1552-1561.
28. Rose G, et al. UK heart disease prevention project: incidence and mortality results. *Lancet* 1983; 1: 1062-1066.
29. Felton CV, et al. Dietary polyunsaturated fatty acids and composition of human aortic plaques. *Lancet* 1994; 344: 1195-1196.
30. Mozaffarian D, et al. Dietary fats, carbohydrate, and progression of coronary atherosclerosis in postmenopausal women. *Am J Clin Nutr* 2004; 80: 1175-1184.
31. Knopp RH, Retzlaff BM. Saturated fat prevents coronary artery disease? An American paradox. *Am J Clin Nutr* 2004; 80: 1102-1103.
32. Richard JL. Coronary risk factors. The French paradox. *Arch Mal Coeur Vaiss* 1987; 80 Spec No: 17-21.
33. Renauld S, DeLorgeril M. Wine, alcohol, platelets, and the French paradox for heart disease. *Lancet* 1992; 339:1523-1526.
34. Hauswirth CB, et al. High ω-3 fatty acid content in alpine cheese: The basis for an alpine paradox. *Circulation* 2004; 109: 103-107.
35. Ulbright TLV, Southgate DAT. Coronary heart disease: seven dietary factors. *Lancet* 1991; 338: 985-992.
36. Serra-Majem L, et al. How could changes in diet explain changes in coronary heart disease mortality in Spain? The Spanish paradox. *Am J Clin Nutr* 1995; 61(6 Suppl): 1351S-1359S.
37. Grimes DS, et al. Respiratory infection and coronary heart disease: progression of a paradigm. *QJM* 2000; 93: 375-383.
38. Romagnoli E, et al. Hypovitaminosis D in an Italian population of healthy subjects and hospitalized patients. *Br J Nutr* 1999; 81: 133-137.
39. Gjonca A, Bobak M. Albanian paradox, another example of protective effect of Mediterranean lifestyle? *Lancet* 1997; 350: 1815-1817.

40. Evans AE, et al. Autres pays, autres coeurs? Dietary patterns, risk factors and ischaemic heart disease in Belfast and Toulouse. *QJM* 1995; 88: 469-477.

41. Yarnell JW. The PRIME study: classical risk factors do not explain the several-fold differences in risk of coronary heart disease between France and Northern Ireland. Prospective Epidemiological Study of Myocardial Infarction *QJM* 1998; 91: 667-676.

42. Marmot MG, et al. Changes in heart disease mortality in England and Wales and other countries. *Hlth Trends* 1981; 13: 33-42.

43. Yam D, et al. Diet and disease – the Israeli paradox: possible dangers of a high omega-6 polyunsaturated fatty acid diet. *Isr J Med Sci* 1996; 32: 1134-1143.

44. Malhotra SL. Serum lipids, dietary factors and ischemic heart disease. *Am J Clin Nutr* 1967; 20: 462-475.

45. (No authors listed.) Ghee, cholesterol, and heart disease. *Lancet* 1987; 2: 1144-1145.

46. Singh RB, et al. Low fat intake and coronary artery disease in a population with higher prevalence of coronary artery disease: The Indian paradox. *J Am Coll Nutr* 1998; 17: 342-350.

47. Rose GA, et al. Corn oil in treatment of ischaemic heart disease. *BMJ* 1965; 1: 1531-1533.

48. Hulley S. Editorial: Conference on low blood cholesterol. *Circulation* 1992; 86: 1026-1029.

49. Forette B, et al. Cholesterol as a risk factor for mortality in elderly women. *Lancet* 1989; i: 868-870.

50. Superko HR, et al. Small LDL and its clinical importance as a new CAD risk factor: a female case study. *Prog Cardiovasc Nurs* 2002; 17: 167-173.

51. Barnes BO. A practical diet for weight reduction. *Fed Proc* 1965; 24: 314.

52. Nicholls SJ, et al. Relationship between cardiovascular risk factors and atherosclerotic disease burden measured by intravascular ultrasound. *J Am Coll Cardiol* 2006; 47:1967-1975.

53. Liu J, et al. Non-high-density lipoprotein and very-low-density lipoprotein cholesterol and their risk predictive values in coronary heart disease. *Am J Cardiol* 2006; 98: 1363-1368.

54. Corsetti JP, et al. Elevated HDL is a risk factor for recurrent coronary events in a subgroup of non-diabetic postinfarction patients with hypercholesterolemia and inflammation. *Atherosclerosis* 2006; 187: 191–197.

55. Fonarow GC, et al. Lipid levels in patients hospitalized with coronary artery disease: an analysis of 136,905 hospitalizations in GWTG-CAD. http://astute. cardiosource.com/ 2007/vposters/pdf/275_Fonarow.pdf.

56. Rapaport E. Update in Cardiology. *Ann Intern Med* 2006; 145: 618-625.

57. Hayward RA, et al. Narrative review: lack of evidence for recommended low-density lipoprotein treatment targets: a solvable problem. *Ann Intern Med* 2006; 145: 520-530.

58. Hickie JB. The prevention of coronary heart disease. *Med J Aust* 1968; 1: 159-166.

59. Oliver MF. Should we not forget about mass control of coronary risk factors? *Lancet* 1983; ii: 37-38.

60. Grundy SM, et al. Rationale of the diet heart statement of the American Heart As-

sociation, report of the Nutrition Committee. *Circulation* 1982; 65: 839A-854A.

61. National Advisory Committee on Nutrition Education. *A Discussion Paper on Proposals for Nutritional Guidelines for Health Education in Britain.* HEC, 1983.

62. Committee on Medical Aspects of Food. *Diet and Cardiovascular Disease.* DHSS, 1984.

Chapter Four: Learning from history

1. Price WA. Nutrition and Physical Degeneration: A Comparison of Primitive and Modern Diets and Their Effects. Paul B. Hoeber, Inc, New York, 1939.

2. Grant GM. *Ocean to Ocean.* Toronto, 1873.

3. Peary RE. *Secrets of Polar Travel.* New York: Century Co, 1917.

4. Stefansson V. *The Fat of the Land.* New York: Macmillan Press, 1957.

5. Hanson EP. *Journey to Manaos.* New York: Reynal & Hitchcock. 1938.

6. Weinberg SL. The diet–heart hypothesis: A critique. *J Am Coll Cardiol* 2004; 43: 731-733.

Chapter Five: Fats – from tonic to toxic

1. Solomons NW, Bulux J. Plant sources of provitamin A and human nutriture. *Nutr Rev* 1993; 51: 199-204.

2. Fraps GS, Kemmerer AR. *Texas Agricultural Bulletin*, Feb 1938, No 560.

3. Volek JS, et al. Modification of lipoproteins by very low-carbohydrate diets. *J Nutr* 2005; 135: 1339-1342.

4. German JB, Dillard CJ. Saturated fats: what dietary intake? *Am J Clin Nutr* 2004; 80: 550-559.

5. Ravnskov U. The questionable role of saturated and polyunsaturated fatty acids in cardiovascular disease. *J Clin Epidemiol* 1998; 51: 443-460.

6. Grundy SM. Influence of stearic acid on cholesterol metabolism relative to other long-chain fatty acids. *Am J Clin Nutr* 1994; 60: 986S-990S.

7. French MA, et al. Cholesterolaemic effect of palmitic acid in relation to other dietary fatty acids. *Asia Pac J Clin Nutr* 2002; 11 Suppl 7: S401-S407.

8. Mozaffarian D, et al. Dietary fats, carbohydrate, and progression of coronary atherosclerosis in postmenopausal women. *Am J Clin Nutr* 2004; 80: 1175-1184.

9. Katan MB, et al. Dietary oils, serum lipoproteins, and coronary heart disease. *Am J Clin Nutr* 1995; 61: 1368S-1373S.

10. Berglund L, et al. HDL-subpopulation patterns in response to reductions in dietary total and saturated fat intakes in healthy subjects. *Am J Clin Nutr* 1999; 70: 992-1000.

11. Hays JH, et al. Effect of a high saturated fat and no-starch diet on serum lipid subfractions in patients with documented atherosclerotic cardiovascular disease. *Mayo Clin Proc* 2003; 78: 1331-1336.

12. Seshadri P, et al. A randomized study comparing the effects of a low-carbohydrate diet and a conventional diet on lipoprotein subfractions and C-reactive protein levels in patients with severe obesity. *Am J Med* 2004; 117: 398-405.

13. Wolf RB. Effect of temperature on soybean seed constituents. *J Am Oil Chem Soc* 1982; 59: 230-232.

14. Wolfe R. Chemistry of nutrients and world food. *Univ of Oregon Chem.* October 16, 1986; 121.

15. Paul AA, Southgate DAT. *McCance & Widdowson's The Composition of Foods.* Fourth revised extended edition of MRC Special Report, No 297. London: HMSO, 1979.

16. McHenry EW, Cornett ML. The role of vitamins in anabolism of fats. *Vit Horm* 1944; 2: 1-27.

17. Lambelet P, et al. Formation of modified fatty acids and oxyphytosterols during refining of low erucic acid rapeseed oil. *J Agric Food Chem* 2003; 51: 4284-4290.

18. Rausch HP, et al. The influence of calorie restriction and of dietary fat on the tumor formation with ultraviolet light. *Cancer Res* 1945; 5: 431.

19. Hannan D. Atherosclerosis: possible ill-effects of the use of highly unsaturated fats to lower serum cholesterol levels. *Lancet* 1957 II: 1116, 1957.

20. Ershoff BH. Effects of diet on fish oil toxicity in the rat. *J Nutr* 1960; 71: 45.

21. Norkin SA. Experimental nutritional cirrhosis in the rat. *Arch Pathol* 1967; 83:31.

22. Carroll KK, et al. Dietary fat and mammary cancer. *Can Med Assn J* 1968; 98: 590.

23. Ritchie JH, et al. Edema and hemolytic anemia in premature infants. *N Engl J Med* 1968; 279: 1185.

24. Pearce ML, Dayton S. Incidence of cancer in men on a diet high in polyunsaturated fat. *Lancet* 1971; i: 464.

25. Lawrence F (ed). *Additives: your complete survival guide.* Century, London, 1986.

26. Newsholme EA. Mechanism for starvation suppression and refeeding activity of infection. *Lancet* 1977; i: 654.

27. Miller JHD, et al. Double blind trial of linoleate supplementation in the diet in multiple sclerosis. *BMJ* 1973; i: 765-768.

28. Uldall PR, et al. Unsaturated fatty acids and renal transplantation. *Lancet* 1974; ii: 514.

29. *American Heart Association Monograph, No 25.* 1969.

30. Nauts HC. *Cancer Research Institute Monograph No 18.* 1984: 91.

31. Mackie BS. Do polyunsaturated fats predispose to malignant melanoma? *Med J Austr* 1974; 1: 810.

32. Karnauchow PN. Melanoma and sun exposure. *Lancet* 1995; 346: 915.

33. Kearney R. Promotion and prevention of tumour growth – effects of endotoxin, inflammation and dietary lipids. *Int Clin Nutr Rev* 1987; 7: 157.

34. Carroll KK. Dietary fats and cancer. *Am J Clin Nutr* 1991; 53: 1064S.

35. France T, Brown P. Test-tube cancers raise doubts over fats. *New Scientist*, 7 December 1991, p 12.

36. Franceschi S, et al. Intake of macronutrients and risk of breast cancer. *Lancet* 1996; 347: 1351-1356.

37. Hunter DJ, et al. Cohort studies of fat intake and the risk of breast cancer – a pooled analysis. *N Engl J Med* 1996; 334: 356-361.

38. Wolk A, et al. A prospective study of association of monounsaturated fat and other types of fat with risk of breast cancer. *Arch Intern Med* 1998; 158: 41-45.

39. Wirfält E, et al. Postmenopausal breast cancer is associated with high intakes of omega-6 fatty acids (Sweden). *Cancer Causes Control* 2002; 13: 883-93.
40. Cho E, et al. Premenopausal fat intake and risk of breast cancer. *J Natl Cancer Inst* 2003; 95: 1079-1085.
41. Holmes MD, et al. Meat, fish and egg intake and risk of breast cancer. *Int J Cancer* 2003; 104: 221-227.
42. Bingham SA, et al. Are imprecise methods obscuring a relation between fat and breast cancer? *Lancet* 2003; 362: 212-214
43. Ip C, et al. Conjugated linoleic acid: A powerful anticarcinogen from animal fat sources. *Cancer* 1994; 74(3 Suppl): 1050-1054.
44. Shultz TD, et al. Inhibitory effect of conjugated dienoic derivatives of linoleic acid and beta-carotene on the in vitro growth of human cancer cells. *Cancer Letters* 1992; 63: 125-133.
45. Lin H, et al. Survey of the conjugated linoleic acid contents of dairy products. *J Dairy Sci* 1995; 78: 2358-2365.
46. Cohen LA, et al. Dietary fat and mammary cancer. II. Modulation of serum and tumor lipid composition and tumor prostaglandins by different dietary fats: Association with tumor incidence patterns. *J Nat Cancer Inst* 1986; 77: 43.
47. Cox BD, Whichelow MJ. Frequent consumption of red meat is not a risk factor for cancer. *BMJ* 1997; 315: 1018.
48. Burr GO, Burr MM. A new deficiency disease produced by the rigid exclusion of fat from the diet. *J Biol Chem* 1929; 82: 345-367.
49. Deuel HJ, Reiser R. Physiology and biochemistry of the essential fatty acids. *Vit Horm* 1955; 13: 1-70.
50. Frost L, Vestergaard P. n–3 Fatty acids consumed from fish and risk of atrial fibrillation or flutter: the Danish Diet, Cancer, and Health Study. *Am J Clin Nutr* 2005; 81: 50-54.
51. Stender S, et al. High levels of industrially produced trans fat in popular fast foods. *N Engl J Med* 2006; 354: 1650-1652.
52. Mozaffrian D, et al. Trans fatty acids and cardiovascular disease. *N Engl J Med* 2006; 354: 1601-1613.
53. Astrup A. The trans fatty acid story in Denmark. *Atheroscler Suppl* 2006; 7: 43-46.
54. Sundram K, et al. Stearic acid-rich interesterified fat and trans-rich fat raise the LDL/HDL ratio and plasma glucose relative to palm olein in humans. *Nutr Metab* 2007; 4: 3.
55. Stare FJ (referee), Rathman DM, et al. Dynamic utilization of recent nutritional findings: diet and cardiovascular disease. *CRC Critical Reviews in Food Technology* 1970; 1: 331.

Chapter Six: The seeds of ill health

1. Stoskopf NC. *Cereal Grain Crops*. Reston: Reston Publishing Company, 1985.
2. Cordain L. *Cereal Grains: Humanity's Double-Edged Sword*. In: Simopoulos AP (ed): Evolutionary aspects of nutrition and health, diet, exercise, genetics and chronic disease. *World Rev Nutr Diet*. 1999; 84: 19-73.
3. Mangelsdorf PC. Genetic potentials for increasing yields of food crops and animals. *Proc Natl Acad Sci* 1966; 56: 370-375.

4. Cavalli-Sforza LL, et al. Demic expansions and human evolution. *Science* 1993; 259: 639-646.
5. Harlan JR. *Crops and Man.* American Society of Agronomy Inc. Madison, Wisconsin, 1992.
6. Zohary D. The progenitors of wheat and barley in relation to domestication and agricultural dispersal in the old world. In: Ucko PJ, Dimbleby GW (eds.) *The Domestication and Exploitation of Plants and Animals.* Chicago: Aldine Publishing Co, 1969 pp. 46-66.
7. Hawkes K, O'Connell JF. Optimal foraging models and the case of the !Kung. *Am Anthropologist* 1985; 87: 401-405.
8. Sinclair AJ, O'Dea K. Fats in human diets through history: Is the western diet out of step? In Wood JD, Fisher AV (eds): *Reducing Fat in Meat Animals.* London: Elsevier Applied Science, 1990, pp. 1-47.
9. E-Siong T. Carotenoids and retinoids in human nutrition. *Crit Rev Food Sci Nutr* 1992; 31: 103-163.
10. Rahmathullah L, et al. Reduced mortality among children in southern India receiving a small weekly dose of vitamin A. *N Engl J Med* 1990; 323: 929-935.
11. Lie C, et al. Impact of large-dose vitamin A supplementation on childhood diarrhoea, respiratory disease and growth. *Eur J Clin Nutr* 1992; 47: 88-96.
12. Hussey GD, Klein M. A randomized, controlled trial of vitamin A in children with severe measles. *N Engl J Med* 1990; 323: 160-164.
13. Glasziou PP, Mackerras DEM. Vitamin A supplementation in infectious diseases: Meta-analysis. *BMJ* 1993; 306: 360-367.
14. Jukes TH. Historical perspectives: The prevention and conquest of scurvy, beriberi, and pellagra. *Prevent Med* 1989; 18: 877-883.
15. Bollet AJ. Politics and pellagra: The epidemic of pellagra in the US in the early twentieth century. *Yale J Biol Med* 1992; 65: 211-221.
16. Roe DA. *A Plague of Corn, the Social History of Pellagra.* Ithaca: Cornell University Press, 1973.
17. Malfait P, et al. An outbreak of pellagra related to changes in dietary niacin among Mozambican refugees in Malawi. *Int J Epidemiol* 1993; 22: 504-511.
18. Nachbar MS, Oppenheim JD. Lectins in the United States diet: a survey of lectins in commonly consumed foods and a review of the literature. *Am J Clin Nutr* 1980; 33: 2338-2345.
19. Pusztai A. Review: Dietary lectins are metabolic signals for the gut and modulate immune and hormone functions. *Eur J Clin Nutr* 1993; 47: 691-699.
20. Reynolds RD. Bioavailability of vitamin B-6 from plant foods. *Am J Clin Nutr* 1988; 48: 863-867.
21. Bamji MS, Sarma KV. Relationship between biochemical and clinical indices of B-vitamin deficiency. A study of rural school boys. *Br J Nutr* 1979; 41: 431-441.
22. Natarajan VS, et al. Assessment of nutrient intake and associated factors in an Indian elderly population. *Age Ageing* 1993; 22: 103-108.
23. Kopinksi JS, et al. Biotin studies in pigs: Biotin availability in feedstuffs for pigs and chickens. *Brit J Nutr* 1989; 62: 773-780.
24. Herbert V. Vitamin B-12: Plant sources, requirements, and assay. *Am J Clin Nutr* 1988; 48: 852-858.

25. Chanarin I, et al. Megaloblastic anaemia in a vegetarian Hindu community. *Lancet* 1985; ii: 1168-1172.
26. Allen LH, et al. Vitamin B-12 deficiency and malabsorption are highly prevalent in rural Mexican communities. *Am J Clin Nutr* 1995; 62: 1013-1019.
27. Sly MR, et al. Exacerbation of rickets and osteomalacia by maize: A study of bone histomorphometry and composition in young baboons. *Calcif Tissue Int* 1984; 36: 370-379.
28. Hunt SP, et al. Vitamin D status in different subgroups of British Asians. *BMJ* 1976; ii: 1351-1354.
29. Brooke OG, et al. Observations of the vitamin D state of pregnant Asian women in London. *Br J Obstet Gynaecol* 1981; 88: 18-26.
30. Batchelor AJ, Compston JE. Reduced plasma half-life of radio-labelled 25-hydroxyvitamin D3 in subjects receiving a high-fibre diet. *Br J Nutr* 1983; 49: 213-216.
31. Torre M, et al. Effects of dietary fiber and phytic acid on mineral availability. *Crit Rev Food Sci Nutr* 1991; 1: 1-22.
32. Calvo MS. Dietary phosphorus, calcium metabolism and bone. *J Nutr* 1993; 123: 1627-1633.
33. Norman DA, et al. Jejunal and ileal adaptation to alterations in dietary calcium. *J Clin Invest* 1981; 67: 1599-1603.
34. Ford JA, et al. Biochemical response of late rickets and osteomalacia to a chupatty-free diet. *BMJ* 1972; ii: 446-447.
35. Berlyne GM, et al. Bedouin osteomalacia due to calcium deprivation caused by high phytic acid content of unleavened bread. *Am J Clin Nutr* 1973; 26: 910-911.
36. Robertson I, et al. The role of cereals in the aetiology of nutritional rickets: the lesson of the Irish national nutritional survey 1943-8. *Br J Nutr* 1981; 45: 17-22.
37. WHO-UNICEF: Indicators and strategies for iron deficiency and anaemia programs: World Health Organization Technical Report Series. New York, WHO-UNICEF, 1993.
38. Viteri FE. The consequences of iron deficiency and anemia in pregnancy on maternal health, the foetus and the infant. *Sci News* 1994; 11: 14-17.
39. International Nutritional Anemia Consultive Groups (INACG). *The effect of cereals and legumes on iron availability.* Washington, Nutrition Foundation, 1982.
40. Sandstrom B, et al. Zinc absorption in humans from meals based on rye, barley, oatmeal, triticale and whole wheat. *J Nutr* 1987; 117: 1898-1902.
41. Halsted JA, et al. Zinc deficiency in man, the Shiraz experiment. *Am J Med* 1972; 53: 277-284.
42. Reinhold JG. High phytate content of rural Iranian bread: a possible cause of human zinc deficiency. *Am J Clin Nutr* 1971; 24: 1204-1206
43. Lasztity R, Lasztity L. Phytic acid in cereal technology. In Pomeranz Y (ed): *Adv Cereal Tech* 1990; 10: 309-371.
44. Herms DA, Mattson WJ. The dilemma of plants: to grow or defend. *Quart Rev Biol* 1992; 67: 283-335.
45. Milton K. Primate diets and gut morphology: Implications for hominid evolution. In: Harris M, Ross EB (eds), *Food and Evolution*. Philadelphia: Temple University Press, 1987, pp. 93-115.

46. Brand-Miller JC, Colagiuri S. The carnivore connection: dietary carbohydrate in the evolution of NIDDM. *Diabetologia* 1994; 37: 1280-1286.
47. Greco L. *Why So Many Intolerant To Gluten?* Department of Pediatrics, University of Naples. 30 June 1995.

Chapter Seven: Climb off the bran wagon

1. Arbuthnot Lane W. *New Health for Everyman.* London: Geoffry Bles, 1932: 127.
2. Burkitt DP, et al. Some geographical variations in disease patterns in East and Central Africa. *E Afr Med J* 1963; 40: 1.
3. Lyon JL, et al. Low cancer incidence and mortality in Utah. *Cancer* 1977; 39: 2608.
4. Smith J. Nutrition and The Media. In: MR Turner, ed. *Preventative Nutrition and Society.* Academic Press, 1981.
5. Yudkin J. Food for thought. *BMJ* 1980; 281: 1563.
6. Trowell HC. Fibre and irritable bowels. *BMJ* 1974; 3: 44.
7. Kritchevsky D. Fibre and cancer. In: Vahouny GV and Kritchevsky D (eds). *Dietary Fibre: Basic And Clinical Aspects* Plenum, NY; 1986: 427.
8. Dietary studies of cancer of the large bowel in the animal model. In Vahouny GV, Kritchevsky D (eds). Op cit. p 469.
9. *Complex Carbohydrates in Foods: the Report of the British Nutrition Foundation's Task Force.* The British Nutrition Foundation. Chapman & Hall, 1990.
10. *Cancer of the Colon and Rectum: the Seventh King's Fund Forum.* London: King's Fund Centre, 1990.
11. Inoue M, et al. Subsite-specific risk factors for colorectal cancer: a hospital-based case-control study in Japan. *Cancer Causes Control* 1995; 6: 14-22.
12. Wasan HS, Goodlad RA. Fibre-supplemented foods may damage your health. *Lancet* 1996; 348: 319-320.
13. Various. Fibre and colorectal cancer. *Lancet* 1996; 348: 956-959.
14. Fuchs CS, et al. Dietary fiber and the risk of colorectal cancer and adenoma in women. *N Engl J Med* 1999; 340: 169-176, 223-224.
15. Park Y, et al. Dietary fiber intake and risk of colorectal cancer: a pooled analysis of prospective cohort studies. *JAMA* 2005; 294: 2849-2857.
16. Park Y, et al. Dietary fibre, ischaemic heart disease and diabetes mellitus. *Proc Nutr Soc* 1973; 32: 151.
17. Van Horn LV, et al. Serum lipid response to oat product intake with a fat-modified diet. *J Am Diet Assoc* 1986; 86: 759-764.
18. Connor WE. Dietary fiber – nostrum or critical nutrient? *N Engl J Med* 1990; 322: 193.
19. Swain JF, et al. Comparison of the effects of oat bran and low-fiber wheat on serum lipoprotein levels and blood pressure. *N Engl J Med* 1990; 322: 147.
20. Leadbetter J, et al. Effects of increasing quantities of oat bran in hypercholesterolemic people. *Am J Clin Nutr* 1991; 54: 841-845.
21. Marshall E. Diet advice, with a grain of salt and a large helping of pepper. *Science* 1986; 231: 537.

22. Sandström B, et al. The effects of vegetables and beet fibre on the absorption of zinc in humans from composite meals. *Br J Nutr* 1987; 58: 49.
23. Kelsay JL. A review of research on effect of fibre intake on man. *Am J Clin Nutr* 1978; 31: 142.
24. Sandstead HH. Fiber, phytates, and mineral nutrition. *Nutr Rev* 1992; 50: 30-31.
25. Hallberg L, et al. Phytates and the inhibitory effect of bran on iron absorption in man. *Am J Clin Nutr* 1987; 45: 988.
26. Turnlund JR, et al. A stable isotope study of zinc absorption in young men: effects of phytate and alpha-cellulose. *Am J Clin Nutr* 1984; 40: 1071.
27. Stevens J, et al. Effect of psyllium gum and wheat bran on spontaneous energy intake. *Am J Clin Nutr* 1987; 46: 812.
28. Balasubraminian R, et al. Effect of wheat bran on bowel function and fecal calcium in older adults. *J Am Coll Nutr* 1987; 6: 199.
29. Hallfisch J, et al. Mineral balances of men and women consuming high fibre diets with complex or simple carbohydrate. *J Nutr* 1987; 117: 403.
30. Kesaniemi YA, et al. Low vs high dietary fiber and serum, biliary, and fecal lipids in middle-aged men. *Am J Clin Nutr* 1990; 51: 1007.
31. Moynahan EJ. Nutritional hazards of high-fibre diet. *Lancet* 1977; i: 654-655.
32. Steinkraus KH, ed, *Handbook of Indigenous Fermented Foods*, New York: Marcel Dekker, Inc., 189-198.
33. Cassidy MM, et al. Effect of chronic intake of dietary fibers on the ultrastructual topography of rat jejunum and colon: a scanning electron microscopy study. *Am J Clin Nutr* 1981; 34: 218-228.
34. Ausman LM. Fiber and colon cancer: does the current evidence justify a preventive policy? *Nutrition Reviews*, 51(2), pp. 57-63.
35. Shelly E, Dean G. Multiple sclerosis. Western diseases: their emergence and prevention. *Nutrition Reviews*, 51(2), pp. 7-12.
36. Southgate DAT. Minerals, trace elements and potential hazards. *Am J Clin Nutr* 1987; 45: 1256.
37. BMA. *The Slimmers' Guide*. Family Doctor Publications, 1988. Latimer Trench & Co Ltd. Plymouth.
38. Miyake K, et al. Disruption-induced mucus secretion: repair and protection. *PLoS Biol* 2006; 4: e276.
39. Wayne Martin. Personal communication. 2001.

Chapter Eight: Why 'five portions'?

1. http://www.5aday.com/html/consumers/serving.php.
2. http://www.dh.gov.uk/PolicyAndGuidance/HealthAndSocialCareTopics/FiveADay/FiveADayFAQ/fs/en?CONTENT_ID=4039413&chk=hlJWRW.
3. Panagiotakos DB, et al. Consumption of fruits and vegetables in relation to the risk of developing acute coronary syndromes; the CARDIO2000 case-control study. *Nutr J* 2003; 2: 2.
4. Three fruit and veg are still healthy. *Daily Mail*, 2 September 2003, p. 8.
5. Hung H-C, et al. Fruit and vegetable intake and risk of major chronic disease. *J Nat Canc Inst* 2004; 96: 1577-1584.
6. Smith-Warner SA, et al. Intake of fruits and vegetables and risk of breast

cancer: a pooled analysis of cohort studies. *JAMA* 2001; 285: 769-776.
7. Geddes L. Watch out for the wrong kind of sugar. *New Scientist* 2008; 2662: 9.
8. Johnson RJ, et al. Potential role of sugar (fructose) in the epidemic of hypertension, obesity and the metabolic syndrome, diabetes, kidney disease, and cardiovascular disease. *Am J Clin Nutr* 2007; 86: 899-906.
9. Edwards HT, et al. Human respiratory quotients in relation to alveolar carbon
   dioxide and blood lactic acid after ingestion of glucose, fructose, or galactose. *J
   Nutr* 1944; 27: 241-251.
10. Brown CM, et al. Fructose ingestion acutely elevates blood pressure in healthy
    young humans. *Am J Physiol Regul Integr Comp Physiol* 2008; 294: R730-737.
11. Nothlings U, et al. Dietary glycemic load, added sugars, and carbohydrates as
    risk factors for pancreatic cancer: the Multiethnic Cohort Study. *Am J Clin Nutr*
    2007; 86: 1495-1501.
12. Beard J. *The Enzyme Treatment of Cancer and Its Scientific Basis*. London:
    Chatto & Windus, 1911; Chap VI.
13. Hoffer A. Editorial. *J Orthomolec Med* 2005; 20: 67.
14. Rene Dubos. *Mirage of Health*. Harper, 1959.
15. Kijak E, et al. Relationship of blood sugar level and leukocytic phagacytosis.
    South Calif Dent Assn 1964; 32: 349-351.
16. Sanchez A, et al. Role of sugars in human neutrophilic phagocytosis. *Am J Clin
    Nutr* 1973; 26: 1180-1184.
17. Hallfrisch J. Metabolic effects of dietary fructose. *FASEB J* 1990; 4: 2652-2660.
18. Spiro DM, et al. Wait-and-see prescription for the treatment of acute otitis media:
    a randomized controlled trial. *JAMA* 2006; 296: 1235-1241.
19. Pichichero ME, Casey JR. Emergence of a multiresistant serotype 19A pneumo-
    coccal strain not included in the 7-valent conjugate vaccine as an otopathogen in
    children. *JAMA* 2007; 298: 1772-1778.
20. Klevens RM, et al. Invasive methicillin-resistant *Staphylococcus aureus* infec-
    tions in the United States. *JAMA* 2007; 298: 1763-1771.
21. Dayan GH, et al. Recent resurgence of mumps in the United States. *N Engl J
    Med* 2008; 358: 1580-1589.
22. Given HDC. *A New Angle on Health*. London: John Bale, Sons & Danielsson
    Ltd. 1935.
23. Richardson R. Measurement of phagocytic activity in diabetes mellitus. *Am J
    Med Sci* 1942; 204: 29.
24. Bybee JD, Rodgers DE. The phagocytic activity of polymorphonuclear leukocytes
    obtained from patients with diabetes mellitus. *J Lab Clin Med* 1964; 64: 1.
25. Parkin DM. The global health burden of infection-associated cancers in the year
    2002. *Int J Cancer* 2006; 118: 3030-3044.
26. Oparil S. Baylor College of Medicine, *Lectures on Atherosclerosis*. 2001.
27. Patel P, et al. Association of Helicobacter pylori and Chlamydia pneumoniae
    infections with coronary heart disease and cardiovascular risk factors. *BMJ* 1995;
    311: 711-714.
28. Namuzaki K, Chiba S. Chlamydia pneumoniae infection and coronary heart dis-
    ease. *BMJ* 1997; 315: 1538-1539.
29. Madjid M, et al. Systemic infections cause exaggerated local inflammation in
    atherosclerotic coronary arteries: clues to the triggering effect of acute infections

on acute coronary syndromes. *Tex Heart Inst J* 2007; 34: 11-18.

30. Svilaas A, et al. Intakes of antioxidants in coffee, wine, and vegetables are correlated with plasma carotenoids in humans. *J Nutr* 2004; 134: 562-567.
31. Joshipura KJ, et al. The effect of fruit and vegetable intake on risk for coronary heart disease. *Ann Intern Med* 2001; 134: 1106-1114.
32. MRC/BHF Heart Protection Study of antioxidant vitamin supplementation in 20 536 high-risk individuals: a randomised placebo-controlled trial. *Lancet* 2002; 360: 23-33.
33. Azzi A, et al. Free radical biology – terminology and critical thinking. *FEBS Letters* 2004; 558: 3-6.
34. Stefansson V. *The Fat of the Land*. New York: Macmillan Press, 1957.
35. Ratliff JC, et al. Eggs modulate the inflammatory response to carbohydrate restricted diets in overweight men. *Nutr & Metab* 2008; 5:6doi:10.1186/ 1743-7075-5-6.

Chapter Nine: The phoney war on salt

1. Spitzer S, et al. The influence of social situations on ambulatory blood pressure. *Psychosom Med* 1992; 54: 71.
2. Singer AJ, Hollander JE. Blood pressure – assessment of interarm differences. *Arch Int Med* 1996; 156: 2005-2008
3. Stallones RA. The rise and fall of ischaemic heart disease. *Sci Am* 1980; 24: 43-49.
4. Nakatsuka H, et al. Effectiveness of attention to reduce salt in diet, as evidenced by reduced urinary excretion of salt. *Ecol Food Nutr* 1991; 26: 323-332.
5. Gothberg G, et al. Response to slow graded bleeding in salt depleted rats. *J Hypertens* 1983; 1(Suppl 2): 24.
6. Wassertheil-Smoller S, et al. Effect of antihypertensives on sexual function and quality of life: the TAIM Study. *Ann Intern Med* 1991; 114: 613-620.
7. Medical Research Council Working Party: MRC trial of treatment of mild hypertension: principal results. *BMJ* 1985; 291: 97-104.
8. Medical Research Council Working Party. Adverse reactions to bendrofluazide and propranolol. *Lancet* 1981; ii: 632.
9. Editorial. More on hypertension labelling. *Lancet* 1985; i: 1138.
10. Milne BJ, et al. Alteration in health perception and life-style in treated hypertensives. *J Chronic Dis* 1985; 38: 37.
11. Brown JJ, et al. Salt and hypertension. *Lancet* 1984; ii: 456.
12. Swales J. *Salt and high blood pressure: a study in education, persuasion and naïveté. a diet of reason.* London: Social Affairs Unit, 1986.
13. Shimamoto T, et al. Trends for coronary heart disease and stroke and their risk factors in Japan. *Circulation* 1989; 3: 503.
14. Gillman MW, et al. Inverse association of dietary fat with development of ischemic stroke in men. *JAMA* 1997; 278: 2145.
15. Barker DJP, et al. The relation of fetal length, ponderal index and head circumference to blood pressure and the risk of hypertension in later life. *Paed Perinat Epidem* 1992; 6: 35.

16. Doyle W, et al. Maternal nutrient intake and birthweight. *J Hum Nutr Dietet* 1989; 2: 451-422.
17. Alderman MN, et al. Dietary sodium intake and mortality: the National Health and Nutrition Examination Survey (NHANES I). *Lancet* 1998; 351: 781-785.
18. Whalley H. Salt and Hypertension: consensus or controversy? *Lancet* 1997; 350: 1686.
19. Graudal NA, et al. Effects of sodium restriction on blood pressure, renin, aldosterone, catecholamines, cholesterols, and triglyceride: a meta-analysis. *JAMA* 1998; 279: 1383-1391.
20. Elliott P, et al. Intersalt: an international study of electrolyte excretion and blood pressure. Results for 24-hour urinary sodium and potassium excretion. *BMJ* 1988; 297: 319-328.
21. Folkow B. Salt and blood pressure – centenarian bone of contention. *Läkartidningen* 2003; 100: 3142-3147.
22. Merlo J, et al. Incidence of myocardial infarction in elderly men being treated with antihypertensive drugs: population based cohort study. *BMJ* 1996; 313: 457-461.
23. Cohen JS. *Overdose: the Case Against the Drug Companies.* New York, N.Y.: Tarcher/Putnam, 2001; 109.
24. Kaufmann JM. *Malignant Medical Myths.* Infinity Publishing, West Conshohocken, PA. 2006, p. 126.
25. Tunstall-Pedoe H, et al. Pattern of declining blood pressure across replicate population surveys of the WHO MONICA project, mid-1980s to mid-1990s, and the role of medication. *BMJ* 2006; 332: 629-632.
26. Herrick WW. Hypertension and hyperglycaemia. *JAMA* 1923; 81:1942-1944.
27. Reaven PD, et al. Abnormal glucose tolerance and hypertension. *Diabetes Care* 1990; 13: 119-125.
28. Bloom W L. Inhibition of salt excretion by carbohydrate. *Arch Int Med* 1962; 109: 26-32.
29. Friedman GD, et al. Precursors of essential hypertension: body weight, alcohol and salt use, and parental history of hypertension. *Prev Med* 1988; 17: 387-400.
30. The sixth report of the Joint National Committee on Prevention, Detection, Evaluation, and Treatment of High Blood Pressure. *Arch Intern Med* 1997; 157: 2413-2446.
31. Dwyer JH, et al. Dietary calcium, calcium supplementation, and blood pressure in African American adolescents. *Am J Clin Nutr* 1998; 68: 648-655.
32. Appel LJ, et al. A clinical trial of the effects of dietary patterns on blood pressure. *N Engl J Med* 1997; 336: 1117-1124.
33. McCarron DA, et al. Blood pressure and nutrient intake in the United States: an analysis of the Health and Nutrition Examination Survey I. *Science* 1984; 224: 1392-1398.
34. McCarron DA, et al. Dietary calcium in human hypertension. *Science* 1982; 217: 267-269.
35. Le Fanu J. Cross cultural studies such as Intersalt study cannot be used to infer causality. *BMJ* 1997; 315: 484.
36. Alderman M. Data linking sodium intake to subsequent morbid and fatal outcomes must be studied. *BMJ* 1997; 315: 484-485.

Chapter Ten: Soy, fluoride and the thyroid

1. Malysheva LV. Tissue respiration rate in certain organs in experimental hyper-cholesterolemia and atherosclerosis. *Fed Proc* 1964; 23: T562.

2. Barnes BO, Barnes CW. *Heart Attack Rareness in Thyroid-Treated Patients.* Springfield, Illinois: Charles C. Thomas, Publisher, 1972.

3. Katz SH. Food and biocultural evolution: a model for the investigation of modern nutritional problems. In: *Nutritional Anthropology.* New York: Alan R. Liss Inc., 1987, p. 50.

4. Rackis JJ, et al. The USDA trypsin inhibitor study. I: Background, objectives and procedural details. In: *Qualification of Plant Foods in Human Nutrition*, 1985; vol. 35.

5. Final Rule Re Food Labeling: Health Claims; Soy Protein And Heart Disease. FDA, October 19, 1999.

6. El Tiney AH. Proximate composition and mineral and phytate contents of legumes grown in Sudan. *J Food Compos Analysis* 1989; 2: 6778.

7. Ologhobo AD, et al. Distribution of phosphorus and phytate in some Nigerian varieties of legumes and some effects of processing. *J Food Sci* 1984; 49: 199-201.

8. Sandstrom B, et al. Effect of protein level and protein source on zinc absorption in humans. *J Nutr* 1989; 119: 48-53.

9. Tait S, et al. The availability of minerals in food, with particular reference to iron. *J Res Soc Health* 1983; 103: 74-77.

10. Leviton R. *Tofu, Tempeh, Miso and Other Soyfoods: The 'Food of the Future' – How to Enjoy its Spectacular Health Benefits.* New Canaan, CT: Keats Publishing, Inc., 1982.

11. Yassa R, et al. Plasma magnesium in chronic schizophrenia. A preliminary report. *Int Pharmacopsychiatry* 1979; 14: 57-64.

12. White LR, et al. Brain aging and midlife tofu consumption. *J Am Coll Nutr* 2000; 19: 242-255.

13. Ishizuki Y, et al. The effects on the thyroid gland of soybeans administered experimentally in healthy subjects. *Nippon Naibunpi Gakkai Zasshi* 1991; 767: 622-629.

14. Divi RL, et al. Anti-thyroid isoflavones from the soybean. *Biochem Pharm* 1997; 54: 1087-1096.

15. IEH Assessment on Phytoestrogens in the Human Diet. Final Report to the Ministry of Agriculture, Fisheries and Food, UK, November 1997, p. 11.

16. Bakery says new loaf can help reduce hot flushes. Reuters, 15 September 1997.

17. Cassidy A, et al. Biological effects of a diet of soy protein rich in isoflavones on the menstrual cycle of premenopausal women. *Am J Clin Nutr* 1994; 60: 333-340.

18. Bulletin de L'Office Fédéral de la Santé Publique, No. 28, 20 July 1992.

19. Matrone G, et al. Effect of genistein on growth and development of the male mouse. *J Nutr* 1956; 235-240.

20. Keung WM. Dietary oestrogenic isoflavones are potent inhibitors of B-hydroxysteroid dehydrogenase of P. testosteronii. *Biochemical and Biophysical Research Committee* 1995; 215: 1137-1144.

21. Makela SI, et al. Estrogen-specific 12 B-hydroxysteroid oxidoreductase type 1

(E.C. 1.1.1.62) as a possible target for the action of phytoestrogens. *PSEBM* 1995; 208: 51-59.

22. Setchell KD, et al. Dietary oestrogens – a probable cause of infertility and liver disease in captive cheetahs. *Gastroenterol* 1987; 93: 225-233.

23. Leopald AS. Phytoestrogens: Adverse effects on reproduction in California Quail. *Science* 1976; 191: 98-100.

24. Drane HM, et al. Oestrogenic activity of soy-bean products. *Food, Cosmetics and Technology* 1980; 18: 425-427.

25. Kimura S, et al. Development of malignant goiter by defatted soybean with iodine-free diet in rats. *Gann* 1976; 67: 763-765.

26. Pelissero C, et al. Oestrogenic effect of dietary soybean meal on vitellogenesis in cultured Siberian Sturgeon Acipenser baeri. *Gen Comp End* 1991; 83: 447-457.

27. Braden, et al. The oestrogenic activity and metabolism of certain isoflavones in sheep. *Aust J Agric Res* 1967; 18: 335-348.

28. Setchell KD, et al. Isoflavone content of infant formulas and the metabolic fate of these early phytoestrogens in early life. *Am J Clin Nutr* 1998; Supplement: 1453S-1461S.

29. Irvine C, et al. The potential adverse effects of soybean phytoestrogens in infant feeding. *NZ Med J* 1995; May 24: 318

30. Herman-Giddens ME, et al. Secondary sexual characteristics and menses in young girls seen in office practice: a study from the pediatric research in office settings network. *Pediatrics* 1997; 99: 505-512.

31. Hagger C, Bachevalier J. Visual habit formation in 3-month-old monkeys (Macaca mulatta): reversal of sex difference following neonatal manipulations of androgen. *Behav Brain Res* 1991; 45: 57-63

32. Doerge D. Goitrogenic and estrogenic activity of soy isoflavones. *Environ Health Perspect* 2002; 110, Suppl 3: 349-353.

33. Coward L, et al. Genistein, daidzen and their betaglycoside conjugates: Antitumor isoflavones in soybean food from American and Asian diets. *J Agric Food Chem* 1993; 41: 1961-1967.

34. Trock BJ, et al. Meta-analysis of soy intake and breast cancer risk. *JNCI* 2006; 98: 459-471.

35. Jefferson W, et al. Neonatal genistein treatment alters ovarian differentiation in the mouse: inhibition of oocyte nest breakdown and increased oocyte survival. *Biol Reprod* 2006; 74: 161-168.

36. Fraser LR, et al. Effects of estrogenic xenobiotics on human and mouse spermatozoa. *Hum Reprod* 2006; 21: 1184-1193.

37. Adeoya-Osiguwa SA, et al. 17 beta-Estradiol and environmental estrogens significantly affect mammalian sperm function. *Hum Reprod* 2003; 18: 100-107.

38. Amsterdam A, et al. Persistent sexual arousal syndrome associated with increased soy intake. *J Sex Med* 2005; 2: 338-340.

39. Wallace GM. Studies on the processing and properties of soymilk. *J Sci Food Agric* 1971; 22: 526-535.

40. http://vm.cfsan.fda.gov/%7Edjw/pltx.cgi?QUERY=soy.

41. von Mundy G. Influence of fluoride and iodine on the metabolism, especially on the thyroid gland. *Münch Med Wochenschrift* 1963; 105: 234-247.

42. Ruiz-Payan A, et al. Chronic effects of fluoride on growth, blood chemistry, and

thyroid hormones in adolescents residing in northern Mexico. *Fluoride* 2005; 38: 46.

43. Pesić M, et al. Cardiovascular risk factors in patients with subclinical hypothyroidism. *Vojnosanit Pregl* 2007; 64: 749-752.
44. Ito M, et al. Effect of levo-thyroxine replacement on non-high-density lipoprotein cholesterol in hypothyroid patients. *J Clin Endocrinol Metab* 2007; 92: 608-611.
45. Tennakone K, Wickramanayake S. Aluminium leaching from cooking utensils. *Nature* 1987; 325: 202.
46. Jansen I, Thomson HM. Heart deaths and fluoridation. *Fluoride* 1974; 7: 52-56.

Chapter Eleven: Our irrational fear of sunlight

1. American Cancer Society. *Cancer facts and figures 1998*. Atlanta: The Society, 1998.
2. MacLennan R, et al. Increasing incidence of cutaneous melanoma in Queensland, Australia. *J Natl Cancer Inst* 1992; 84: 1427-1432.
3. Potten CS, et al. DNA damage in UV-irradiated human skin in vivo: automated direct measurement by image analysis (thymine dimers) compared with indirect measurement (unscheduled DNA synthesis) and protection by 5-methoxypsoralen. *Int J Radiat Biol* 1993; 63: 313-324.
4. Diffey BL, et al. Melanin, melanocytes and melanoma. *Lancet* 1995; 346: 1713.
5. Council on Scientific Affairs. Harmful effects of ultraviolet radiation. *JAMA* 1989; 262: 380-384.
6. Hacker SM, Flowers FP. Squamous cell carcinoma of the skin. *Postgrad Med* 1993; 93: 115-126.
7. Lee JAH. The relationship between malignant melanoma of skin and exposure to sunlight. *Photochem Photobiol* 1989; 50: 493-496.
8. Malignant melanoma – Report of a meeting of physicians and scientists, University College, London Medical School. *Lancet* 1992; 340: 948-951.
9. *Canadian Cancer Statistics*. Statistics Canada, 1991.
10. Reynolds T. Sun plays havoc with light skin down under. *J Natl Cancer Inst* 1992; 84: 1392-1394.
11. Fitzpatrick TB, Haynes HA. Photosensitivity and other reactions to light. In: *Harrison's Principles of Internal Medicine*. 7th ed, New York: McGraw-Hill, 1974; 281-284.
12. Marks R, Whiteman D. Sunburn and melanoma: how strong is the evidence? *BMJ* 1994; 308: 75-76.
13. Karnauchow PN. Melanoma and sun exposure. *Lancet* 1995; 346: 915.
14. Shuster S. Melanoma and sun exposure. *Lancet* 1995; 346: 1224.
15. Kricker A, et al. Sun exposure and non-melanocytic skin cancer. *Cancer Causes and Controls* 1994; 5: 367-392.
16. Garland CF, et al. Could sunscreens increase melanoma risk? *Am J Publ Hlth* 1992; 82: 614-615.
17. Garland CF, et al. Effect of sunscreens on UV radiation-induced enhancement of melanoma growth in mice. *J Natl Cancer Inst* 1994; 86: 798-801
18. Kirk-Othmer. *Encyclopedia of Chemical Technology*. 1981; 13: 367-368.
19. Stern RS, Laid N. The carcinogenic risk of treatments for severe psoriasis. *Cancer* 1994; 73: 2759-2764.

20. Autier P, et al. Melanoma and use of sunscreens: an EORTC case-control study in Germany, Belgium and France. *Int J Cancer* 1995; 61: 749-755.
21. Fackelmann K. Melanoma madness. The scientific flap over sunscreens and skin cancer. *Science News* June 6, 1998; 153 (23): 360.
22. Dover JS, Arndt KA. Dermatology. *JAMA* 1994; 271: 1662-1663.
23. Alberts D, et al. Safety and Efficacy of Dose-Intensive Oral Vitamin A in Subjects with Sun-Damaged Skin. *Clin Cancer Res* 2004; 10: 1875-1880.
24. Ball P. Nanoparticles in sun creams can stress brain cells. *NatureNews* 2006; doi:10.1038/news060612-14.
25. Mackie BS, Mackie LE. Dietary polyunsaturated fats. *Med J Aust* 1988; 149: 449.
26. Holborow P. Melanoma and fatty acids. *NZ J Med* 1991; 104: 19.
27. Rees J L. The melanoma epidemic: reality or artefact. *BMJ* 1996; 312: 137-138.
28. Allen S. BU advocate of sunlight draws ire. *Boston Globe*, April 13, 2004.
29. Bauer HH. Science in the 21st century: knowledge monopolies and research cartels. *JSE* 2004; 18: 643-660.
30. Apperly FL. The relation of solar radiation to cancer mortality in North America. *Cancer Res* 1941; 1: 191-195.
31. Garland FC, et al. Geographic variation in breast cancer mortality in the United States: a hypothesis involving exposure to solar radiation. *Prev Med* 1990; 19: 614-622.
32. Gorham ED, et al. Sunlight and breast cancer incidence in the USSR. *Int J Epidemiol* 1990; 19: 820-824.
33. Martinez ME, Willett WC. Calcium, vitamin D, and colorectal cancer: a review of the epidemiologic evidence. *Cancer Epidemiol Biomarkers Prev* 1998; 7: 163-168.
34. Skinner HG, et al. Vitamin D Intake and the Risk for Pancreatic Cancer in Two Cohort Studies. *Cancer Epidemiol Biomarkers Prev* 2006; 15: 1688-1695.
35. Ainsleigh HG. Beneficial effects of sun exposure on cancer mortality. *Prev Med* 1993; 22: 132-140.
36. Freedman DM, et al. Prospective study of serum vitamin D and cancer mortality in the United States. *J Natl Cancer Inst* 2007; 99: 1594-1602.
37. *WHO World Cancer Report* 2003. WHO, Geneva, 3 April 2003.
38. Grant W. An estimate of premature cancer mortality in the U.S. due to inadequate doses of solar ultraviolet-B radiation. *Cancer* 2002; 94: 1867-1875.
39. Garland CF. More on preventing skin cancer: sun avoidance will increase incidence of cancers overall. *BMJ* 2003; 327: 1228.
40. Freedman DM, et al. Sunlight and mortality from breast, ovarian, colon, prostate, and non-melanoma skin cancer: a composite death certificate based case-control study. *Occup Environ Med* 2002; 59: 257-262.
41. Hughes AM, et al. Sun exposure may protect against non-Hodgkin lymphoma: a case-control study. *Int J Cancer* 2004; 112: 865-871.
42. Smedby KE, et al. Ultraviolet radiation exposure and risk of malignant lymphomas. *J Natl Cancer Inst* 2005; 97: 199-209.
43. John EM, et al. Residential sunlight exposure is associated with a decreased risk of prostate cancer. *J Steroid Biochem Mol Biol* 2004; 89-90: 549-552.
44. Robsahm TE, et al. Vitamin D3 from sunlight may improve the prognosis of breast-, colon- and prostate cancer (Norway). *Cancer Causes Control.* 2004; 15: 149-158.

45. Moan J, et al. Solar radiation, vitamin D and survival rate of colon cancer in Norway. *J Photochem Photobiol B* 2005; 78: 189-193.

46. Zhou W, et al. Vitamin D predicts overall survival in early stage non-small cell lung cancer patients. *Am. Assoc. Cancer Res. Annual Meeting, Abstract LB-231.* 2005.

47. Grant WB. Insufficient sunlight may kill 45,000 Americans each year from internal cancer. *J Cos Dermatol* 2004; 3: 176-178.

48. Webb AR, et al. Influence of season and latitude on the cutaneous synthesis of vitamin D3: exposure to winter sunlight in Boston and Edmonton will not promote vitamin D3 synthesis in human skin. *J Clin Endocrinol Metab* 1988; 67: 373-378.

49. Roth DE, et al. Are national vitamin D guidelines sufficient to maintain adequate blood levels in children? *Can J Public Health* 2005; 96: 443-449.

50. Jablonski NG, Chaplin G. The evolution of human skin coloration. *J Hum Evol* 2000; 39: 57-106.

51. Holick MF. Sunlight and vitamin D for bone health and prevention of autoimmune diseases, cancers, and cardiovascular disease. *Am J Clin Nutr* 2004; 80: 1678S-1688S.

52. Marshall TG. Vitamin D discovery outpaces FDA decision making. *BioEssays* 2008; 30: 173-182.

53. Romagnoli E, et al. Hypovitaminosis D in an Italian population of healthy subjects and hospitalized patients. *Br J Nutr* 1999; 81: 133-137.

54. Chapuy MC, et al. Prevalence of vitamin D insufficiency in an adult normal population. *Osteoporos Int* 1997; 7: 439-443.

55. Evans AE, et al. Autres pays, autres coeurs? Dietary patterns, risk factors and ischaemic heart disease in Belfast and Toulouse. *QJM* 1995; 88: 469-477.

56. Yam D, et al. Diet and disease – the Israeli paradox: possible dangers of a high omega-6 polyunsaturated fatty acid diet. *Isr J Med Sci* 1996; 32: 1134-1143.

57. Mukamel MN, et al. Vitamin D deficiency and insufficiency in Orthodox and non-Orthodox Jewish mothers in Israel. *Isr Med Assoc J* 2001; 3: 419-421.

58. Hochwald O, et al. Hypovitaminosis D among inpatients in a sunny country. *Isr Med Assoc J* 2004; 6: 82-87.

59. Gannage-Yared MH, et al. Hypovitaminosis D in a sunny country: relation to lifestyle and bone markers. *J Bone Miner Res* 2000; 15: 1856-1862.

60. Bouillon R, et al. Polyunsaturated fatty acids decrease the apparent affinity of vitamin D metabolites for human vitamin D-binding protein. *J Steroid Biochem Mol Biol* 1992; 42: 855-861.

61. Grimes DS, et al. Sunlight, cholesterol and coronary heart disease. *QJM* 1996; 89: 579-589.

62. Voors AW, Johnson WD. Altitude and arteriosclerotic heart disease mortality in white residents of 99 of the 100 largest cities in the United States. *J Chronic Dis* 1979; 32: 157-162.

63. Leaf A. Getting old. *Sci Am* 1973; 229: 44-52.

64. Scragg R. Seasonality of cardiovascular disease mortality and the possible protective effect of ultra-violet radiation. *Int J Epidemiol* 1981; 10: 337-341.

65. Zittermann A, et al. Putting cardiovascular disease and vitamin D insufficiency into perspective. *Br J Nutr* 2005; 94: 483-492.

66. Zittermann A, et al. Low vitamin D status: a contributing factor in the

pathogenesis of congestive heart failure? *J Am Coll Cardiol* 2003; 41: 105-112.
67. Rostand SG. Ultraviolet light may contribute to geographic and racial blood pressure differences. *Hypertension* 1997; 30: 150-156.
68. Fiori G, et al. Relationships between blood pressure, anthropometric characteristics and blood lipids in high- and low-altitude populations from Central Asia. *Ann Hum Biol* 2000; 27: 19-28.
69. Santos JL, et al. Low prevalence of type 2 diabetes despite a high average body mass index in the Aymara natives from Chile. *Nutrition* 2001; 17: 305-309.
70. Garancini P, et al. Incidence and prevalence rates of diabetes mellitus in Italy from routine data: a methodological assessment. *Eur J Epidemiol* 1991; 7: 55-63.
71. Lora-Gomez RE, et al. Incidence of Type 1 diabetes in children in Caceres, Spain, during 1988-1999. *Diabetes Res Clin Pract* 2005; 69: 169-174.
72. Suarez L, Barrett-Connor E. Seasonal variation in fasting plasma glucose levels in man. *Diabetologia* 1982; 22: 250-23.
73. Tseng CL, et al. Seasonal patterns in monthly hemoglobin A1c values. *Am J Epidemiol* 2005; 161: 565-574.
74. Kohn MA, et al. Three summertime outbreaks of influenza type A. *J Infect Dis* 1995; 172: 246-249.
75. Curwen M. Excess winter mortality in England and Wales with special reference to the effects of temperature and influenza. In: Charlton J, Murphy M, (eds). *The Health of Adult Britain 1841–1994*. London: The Stationery Office, 1997, pp. 205-216.
76. Hope-Simpson RE. The role of season in the epidemiology of influenza. *J Hyg* 1981; 86: 35-47.
77. Cannell JJ, et al. Epidemic influenza and vitamin D. *Epidemiol Infect* 2006; 134: 1129-1140.
78. Jefferson T, et al. Efficacy and effectiveness of influenza vaccines in elderly people: a systematic review. *Lancet* 2005; 366: 1165-1174.
79. Groll DL, Thomson DJ. Incidence of influenza in Ontario following the Universal Influenza Immunization Campaign. *Vaccine* 2006; 24: 5245-5250.
80. Rizzoa C, et al. Influenza-related mortality in the Italian elderly: No decline associated with increasing vaccination coverage. *Vaccine* 2006; 24: 6468-6475.
81. Jefferson T. Influenza vaccination: policy versus evidence. *BMJ* 2006; 333: 912-915.
82. Kilbourne E. *Influenza.* New York: Plenum Press, 1987. p. 291.
83. Munger KL, et al. Serum 25-hydroxyvitamin D levels and risk of multiple sclerosis. *JAMA* 2006; 296: 2832-2838.
84. Hochberg Z, et al. Consensus development for the supplementation of vitamin D in childhood and adolescence. *Horm Res* 2002; 58: 39-51.
85. Hess AF, Unger LJ. The cure of infantile rickets by sunlight. *JAMA* 1921; 77: 39.
86. Park EA. The therapy of rickets. *JAMA* 1940; 115: 370-379.
87. Welch TR, et al. Vitamin D-deficient rickets: The re-emergence of a once-conquered disease. *J Pediatr* 2000; 137: 143-145.
88. Kreiter SR, et al. Nutritional rickets in African American breast-fed infants. *J Pediatr* 2000; 137: 153-157.
89. Joiner TA, et al. The many faces of vitamin D deficiency rickets. *Pediatr Rev* 2000; 21: 296-302.

90. Wharton BA. Low plasma vitamin D in Asian toddlers in Britain. *BMJ* 1999; 318: 2-3.
91. Kruger DM, et al. Vitamin D deficiency rickets: report on three cases. *Clin Orthop* 1987; 224: 277-283.
92. Al-Jurayyan NA, et al. Nutritional rickets and osteomalacia in school children and adolescents. *Saudi Med J* 2002; 23: 182-185.
93. Zlotkin S. Limited vitamin D intake and use of sunscreens may lead to rickets. *BMJ* 1999; 318: 1417.
94. El-Hajj Fuleihan G, et al. Hypovitaminosis D in healthy schoolchildren. *Pediatrics* 2001; 107: E53.
95. Chalmers J. Vitamin D deficiency in elderly people. *BMJ* 1991; 303: 314-315.
96. LeBoff MS, et al. Occult vitamin D deficiency in postmenopausal US women with acute hip fracture. *JAMA* 1999; 281: 1505-1511.
97. Dobnig H, et al. Independent association of low serum 25-hydroxyvitamin D and 1,25-dihydroxyvitamin D levels with all-cause and cardiovascular mortality. *Arch Intern Med* 2008; 168: 1340-1349.
98. Grant WB. Solar ultraviolet irradiance and cancer incidence and mortality. *Adv Exp Med Biol* 2008; 624: 16-30.

Chapter Twelve: Exercise care

1. Prentice AM, Jebb SA. Obesity in Britain: gluttony or sloth? *BMJ* 1995; 311: 437-439.
2. Björntorp P, et al. Physical training in human hyperplasic obesity. IV: Effects on hormonal status. *Metab* 1977; 26: 319.
3. Krotkiewski M, et al. Effects of long-term physical training on body fat, metabolism, and blood pressure in obesity. *Metab* 1979; 28: 650.
4. Yale J-F, et al. Metabolic responses to intense exercise in lean and obese subjects. *J Clin Endocrin Metab* 1989; 68: 438-445.
5. Oomura Y, et al. eds. *Progress in Obesity Research*. London: John Libby, 1990; p 563.
6. Voorrips LE, et al. History of body weight and physical activity of elderly women differing in current physical activity. *Int J Obes* 1992; 16: 199.
7. Votruba SB. The role of exercise in the treatment of obesity. *Nutrition* 2000; 16: 179-188.
8. Reilly JJ, et al. Physical activity to prevent obesity in young children: cluster randomised controlled trial. *BMJ* 2006; doi:10.1136/bmj.38979.623773.55.
9. Swinburn BA, et al. Estimating the effects of energy imbalance on changes in body weight in children. *Am J Clin Nutr* 2006; 83: 859-863.
10. Roberts SB. High-glycemic index foods, hunger, and obesity: is there a connection? *Nutr Rev* 2000; 58: 163-169.
11. Zelasko C. Exercise for weight loss: What are the facts? *J Am Diet Assoc* 1995; 95: 1414-1417.
12. Yudkin J. Diet and coronary thrombosis. Hypothesis and fact. *Lancet* 1957; ii: 155.
13. Solomon HA. *The Exercise Myth*. Orlando, FL: Harcourt Brace Jovanovich, 2004.

14. Morris JN, et al. Vigorous exercise in leisure time and the incidence of coronary heart disease. *Lancet* 1973; i: 333.

15. Hambrecht R, et al. Various intensities of leisure time physical activity in patients with coronary artery disease: effects on cardiorespiratory fitness and progression of coronary atherosclerotic lesions. *J Am Coll Cardiol* 1993; 22: 468-477.

16. Rose G, et al. UK Heart Disease Prevention Project: Incidence and mortality results. *Lancet* 1983; iv: 1062.

17. Stern MP. The recent decline in ischaemic heart disease mortality. *Ann Intern Med* 1979; 91: 630.

18. Bürger M. *Altern und Krankheit als Problem der Biomorphose*. 3rd ed, Leipzig: Georg Thieme, 1957.

19. Dargie H, Grant S. The Health of the Nation: The BMJ View. *BMJ* 1992; 305: 156.

20. Schwartz B, et al. Exercise associated amenorrhea: a distinct entity? *Am J Obstet Gynecol* 1981; 141: 662.

21. Cumming DC, et al. Exercise and reproductive function in women. *Prog Clin Biol Res* 1983; 117: 113.

22. Reid RL, van Vugt DA. Weight-related changes in reproductive function. *Fertil Steril* 1987; 48: 905.

23. Editorial. Reduced testosterone and prolactin in male distance runners. *JAMA* 1984; 252: 514.

24. Coplan NL, et al. Exercise and sudden cardiac death. *Am Heart J* 1988; 115: 207-212.

25. Hillis WS, et al. Sudden death in sport. *BMJ* 1994; 309: 657-661.

26. Weinstein CE. Exercise-induced allergic syndromes on the increase. *Cleveland Clin J Med* 1989; 56: 665-666.

27. Tikkanen HO, Helenius I. Asthma in runners. *BMJ* 1994; 309: 1087.

28. Ketelhut R, et al. Is a decrease in arterial pressure during long-term exercise caused by a fall in cardiac pump function? *Am Heart J* 1994; 127: 567-571.

29. Sholter DE, Armstrong PW. Adverse effects of corticosteroids on the cardiovascular system. *Can J Cardiol* 2000; 16: 505-511.

30. Sawrey WL, Weisz JD. An experimental method of producing gastric ulcers. *J Comp Physio Psychol* 1956; 49: 269.

31. Selye H. *The stress of life*. McGraw-Hill, New York, 1956.

32. Solomon GF. Psychophysiological aspects of rheumatoid arthritis and autoimmune disease. In: Hill OW (ed). *Modern Trends in Psychosomatic Medicine – 2*. London: Butterworths, 1970.

33. Axt P, Axt-Gadermann M. *The joy of laziness: how to slow down and live longer*. London: Bloomsbury, 2005.

Chapter Thirteen: Homo carnivorous

1. Abrams HL Jr. The Relevance of Paleolithic Diet in Determining Contemporary Nutritional Needs. *J Applied Nutr* 1979; 31: 43-59.

2. Abrams HL Jr Vegetarianism: an anthropological/nutritional evaluation. *J Applied Nutr* 1980; 32: 53-87.

3. Chapman CA, Chapman LJ. Dietary variability in primate populations. *Primates* 1990; 31: 121-128.

4. Goodall J. *Miss Goodall and the Wild Chimpanzees*. A documentary film of Jane Goodall's studies of wild chimpanzees in their natural habitat in a rain forest in Tanzania, Africa. *National Geographic*, 1966.
5. *Search For the Great Apes*. A documentary film on the ethological research on gorillas by Dian Fossey and the ethological research of orang-utans by Birute Galdikas-Brindamour. *National Geographic*, 1975.
6. Perry R. *Life in Forest and Jungle*. New York: Taplinger Publishing Co; 1976, 165-185.
7. Campbell S. Noah's Ark in Tomorrow's zoo: animals are a-comin', two-by-two. *Smithsonian* 1978; 8: 42-50.
8. Eaton SB, et al. An evolutionary perspective enhances understanding of human nutritional requirements. *J Nutr* 1996; 126: 1732-1740.
9. Hawkes JG. The hunting hypothesis. In: Ardrey R, (ed). *The Hunting Hypothesis*. Collins, London; 1976.
10. Bryant VM, Williams-Dean G. The coprolites of man. *Sci Am*, January 1975.
11. Crawford M, Crawford S. *The Food We Eat Today*. Spearman, London; 1972.
12. Leopold AC, Ardrey R. Toxic substances in plants and food habits of early Man. *Science* 1972; 176: 512-514.
13. McHenry HM. How big were early hominids? *Evol Anthropol* 1992; 1: 15-20.
14. Stefansson V. *The Fat of The Land*. MacMillan, New York, 1960; 15-39.
15. Sinclair AJ. Long-chain polyunsaturated fatty acids in mammalian brain. *Proc Nutr Soc* 1975; 34: 287-291.
16. Crawford MA, et al. A new theory of evolution: quantum theory. In: Sinclair A, Gibson R, eds. *Essential fatty acids and eicosanoids*. Champlaign, Ill.: American Oil Chemists Society, 1992. 87-95.
17. Leonard WR, Robertson ML. Evolutionary perspectives on human nutrition: the influence of brain and body size on diet and metabolism. *Am J Human Biol* 1994; 6: 77-88.
18. Aiello LC, Wheeler P. The expensive tissue hypothesis: the brain and the digestive system in human and primate evolution. *Current Anthropology* 1995; 36: 199-221.
19. Milton K. Primate diets and gut morphology: implications for hominid evolution. In: Harris M, Ross EB (eds). *Food and Evolution: Toward a Theory of Food Habit*. Philadelphia: Temple University Press, 1987; 93-115.
20. Martin RD, et al. Gastrointestinal allometry in primates and other mammals. In: Jungers WL (ed). *Size and Scaling in Primate Biology*. New York: Plenum Press, 1985; 61-89.
21. Ruff CB, et al. Body mass and encephalization in Pleistocene Homo. *Nature* 1997; 387: 173-176.
22. Eaton SB, et al. *Evolution, diet and health*. Presented in association with the scientific session, Origins and Evolution of Human Diet. 14th International Congress of Anthropological and Ethnological Sciences, Williamsburg, Virginia; 1998.
23. Callender ST, Spray GH. Latent pernicious anaemia. *Br J Haematol* 1962; 8: 230.
24. Halstead JA, et al. Serum and tissue concentration of vitamin B 12 in certain pathologic states. *N Engl J Med* 1959; 260: 575.
25. Herbert V. Vitamin B-12: plant sources, requirements and assay. *Am J Clin Nutr* 1988; 48: 852.

26. Miller DR, et al. Vitamin B-12 status in a macrobiotic community. *Am J Clin Nutr* 1991; 53: 524-529.
27. Chanarin I, et al. Megaloblastic anaemia in a vegetarian Indian community. *Lancet* 1985; 2: 1168-1172.
28. Stefansson V. *The Fat of The Land.* New York: Macmillan Press, 1957.
29. Wilkins GH. *Undiscovered Australia.* London: G. P. Putnam & Sons, 1928.
30. Beeton, Mrs Isabella. *Beeton's Book of Household Management.* London: S. O. Beeton, 1861; p 279.
31. Eaton SB, et al. Stoneagers in the fast lane: chronic degenerative diseases in evolutionary perspective. *Am J Med* 1988; 84: 739-749.

Chapter Fourteen: The metabolic syndrome and the glycaemic index

1. Alberts B. *Molecular Biology of the Cell*, 4th edn. Garland Science, New York; 2002, p. 93.
2. McLaughlin T, et al. Prevalence of insulin resistance and associated cardiovascular disease risk factors among normal weight, overweight, and obese individuals. *Metabolism* 2004; 53: 495-499.
3. Kahn CR, et al. The syndromes of insulin resistance and acanthosis nigricans: insulin receptor disorders in man. *N Engl J Med* 1976; 294: 739-745.
4. Krook A, O'Rahilly S. Mutant insulin receptors in syndromes of insulin resistance. *Bailliers Clin Endocrinol Metab* 1996; 10: 97-122.
5. Brand-Miller JC, Colagiuri S. The carnivore connection: dietary carbohydrate in the evolution of NIDDM. *Diabetologia* 1994; 37: 1280-1286.
6. Despres JP, et al. Hyperinsulinemia as an independent risk factor for ischemic heart disease. *N Engl J Med* 1996; 334: 952-957.
7. Cordain L. Syndrome X: Just the tip of the hyperinsulinemia iceberg. *Medikament* 2001; 6: 46-51.
8. Szathmary EJE, et al. Dietary changes and plasma glucose levels in an Amerindian population undergoing cultural transition. *Soc Sci Med* 1987; 24: 791-804.
9. Schraer CD, et al. Prevalence of diabetes in Alaskan Eskimos, Indians and Aleuts. *Diabetes Care* 1988; 11: 693-700.
10. Brand JC, et al. Plasma glucose and insulin responses to traditional Pima Indian meals. *Am J Clin Nutr* 1990; 51: 416-420.
11. Gustavsson J, et al. Insulin-stimulated glucose uptake involves the transition of glucose transporters to a caveolae-rich fraction within the plasma cell membrane: implications for type II diabetes. *Molec Med* 1996; 2: 367-372.
12. Ganong WF. *Review of Medical Physiology*, 19th edition 1999; 9: 26-33.
13. Pan DA, et al. Skeletal muscle membrane lipid composition is related to adiposity and insulin action. *J Clin Invest* 1995; 96: 2802-2808.
14. Lillioja S, et al. Insulin resistance and insulin secretory dysfunction as precursors of non-insulin-dependent diabetes mellitus: Prospective studies of Pima Indians. *N Engl J Med* 1993; 329: 1988-1992.
15. Haffner SM, et al. Decreased insulin secretion and increased insulin resistance are independently related to the 7-year risk of NIDDM in Mexican Americans. *Diabetes* 1995; 44: 1386-1391.
16. Sicree RA, et al. Plasma insulin responses among Nauruans: Prediction of

deterioration in glucose tolerance over 6 years. *Diabetes* 1987; 36: 179-186.

17. Wise PH, et al. Diabetes and associated variables in the South Australian Aborigines. *Aust NZ Med* 1976; 6: 191-196.

18. Putnam JJ, Allshouse JE. Food consumption, prices and expenditures, 1970-97. Economic Research Service, US Department of Agriculture. *Stat Bull* 1999; 965: 24.

19. Sorensen T. The genetics of obesity. *Metabolism* 1995; 44: 4-6.

20. Ganrot PO. Insulin resistance syndrome: possible key role of blood flow in resting muscle. *Diabetologia* 1993; 36: 876-879.

21. Nakagawa T, et al. Hypothesis: fructose-induced hyperuricemia as a causal mechanism for the epidemic of the metabolic syndrome. *Nat Clin Pract Nephrol* 2005; 1: 80-86.

22. Brand-Miller JC. Glycemic load and chronic disease. *Nutr Rev* 2003; 61: S49-55.

23. Ludwig DS, et al. High glycaemic index foods, overeating, and obesity. *Pediatrics* 1999; 103: E26-E32.

24. Parilo M, et al. Effect of a low fat diet on carbohydrate metabolism in patients with hypertension. *Hypertension* 1988; 22: 244-248.

25. Liu S, et al. A prospective study of dietary glycemic load, carbohydrate intake, and risk of coronary heart disease in US women. *Am J Clin Nutr* 2000; 71: 1455-1461.

26. Salmeron J, et al: Dietary fibre, glycemic load, and risk of NIDDM in men. *Diabetes Care* 1997; 20: 545-550.

27. Gannon MC, et al. The serum insulin and plasma glucose response to milk and fruit products in type 2 (non-insulin-dependent) diabetic patients. *Diabetologia* 1986; 29: 784-791.

28. Pelletier X, et al. Glycaemic and insulinaemic responses in healthy volunteers upon ingestion of maltitol and hydrogenated glucose syrups. *Diabetes Metab*1994; 20: 291-296.

29. Schenk S, et al. Different glycemic indexes of breakfast cereals are not due to glucose entry into blood but to glucose removal by tissue. *Am J Clin Nutr* 2003; 78: 742-748.

30. Chan EM, et al. Postprandial glucose response to Chinese foods in patients with type 2 diabetes. *J Am Diet Assoc* 2004; 104: 1854-1858.

31. Chiu CJ, et al. Carbohydrate intake and glycemic index in relation to the odds of early cortical and nuclear lens opacities. *Am J Clin Nutr* 2005; 81: 1411-1416.

32. Mayer-Davis, et al. Towards understanding of glycaemic index and glycaemic load in habitual diet: associations with measures of glycaemia in the Insulin Resistance Atherosclerosis Study. *Br J Nutr* 2006; 95: 397-405.

33. Elliott SS, et al. Fructose, weight gain, and the insulin resistance syndrome. *Am J Clin Nutr* 2002; 76: 911-922.

34. Gannon MC, et al. An increase in dietary protein improves the blood glucose response in persons with type 2 diabetes. *Am J Clin Nutr* 2003; 78: 734-741.

35. Collier G, et al. Effect of co-ingestion of fat on the metabolic responses to slowly and rapidly absorbed carbohydrates. *Diabetologia* 1984; 26: 50-54.

36. Gannon MC, et al. The effect of fat and carbohydrate on plasma glucose, insulin, C-peptide, and triglycerides in normal male subjects. *J Am Coll Nutr* 1993; 12: 36-41.

37. Holt SHA, et al. An insulin index of foods: The insulin demand generated by 1,000-kJ portions of common foods. *Am J Clin Nutr* 1997; 66: 1264-1276.

Chapter Fifteen: Unhealthy dogma means unhealthy food

1. Rohrmann S, et al. Meat and dairy consumption and subsequent risk of prostate cancer in a US cohort study. *Cancer Causes Control* 2007; 18: 41-50.
2. Mitrou PN, et al. A prospective study of dietary calcium, dairy products and prostate cancer risk (Finland). *Int J Cancer* 2007; 120: 2466-2473.
3. Willett WC. Nutrition and cancer. *Salud Publica Mex* 1997; 39: 298-309.
4. Chan JM, et al. Dairy products, calcium, and prostate cancer risk in the Physicians' Health Study. *Am J Clin Nutr* 2001; 74: 549-554.
5. Tseng M, et al. Dairy, calcium, and vitamin D intakes and prostate cancer risk in the National Health and Nutrition Examination Epidemiologic Follow-up Study cohort. *Am J Clin Nutr* 2005; 81: 1147-1154.
6. Veierod MB, et al. Dietary fat intake and risk of prostate cancer: a prospective study of 25,708 Norwegian men. *Int J Cancer* 1997; 73: 634-638.
7. Grant WB. An ecologic study of dietary links to prostate cancer. *Altern Med Rev* 1999; 4: 162-169.
8. Kushi LH, et al. Prospective study of diet and ovarian cancer. *Am J Epidemiol* 1999; 149: 21-31.
9. Fairfield KM, et al. A prospective study of dietary lactose and ovarian cancer. *Int J Cancer* 2004; 110: 271-277.
10. Schwartz GG, Hulka BS. Is vitamin D deficiency a risk factor for prostate cancer? (Hypothesis). *Anticancer Res* 1990; 10: 1307-1311.
11. Miller A, et al. Conjugated linoleic acid (CLA)-enriched milk fat inhibits growth and modulates CLA-responsive biomarkers in MCF-7 and SW480 human cancer cell lines. *Br J Nutr* 2003; 90: 877-885.
12. O'Shea M, et al. Milk fat conjugated linoleic acid (CLA) inhibits growth of human mammary MCF-7 cancer cells. *Anticancer Res* 2000; 20: 3591-3601.
13. Larsson SC, et al. High-fat dairy food and conjugated linoleic acid intakes in relation to colorectal cancer incidence in the Swedish Mammography Cohort. *Am J Clin Nutr* 2005; 82: 894-900.
14. Chavarro JE, et al. A prospective study of dairy foods intake and anovulatory infertility. *Hum Reprod* 2007; 22: 1340-1347.
15. Adebamowo CA, et al. High school dietary dairy intake and teenage acne. *J Am Acad Dermatol* 2005; 52: 207-14.
16. Grant WB. Milk and other dietary influences on coronary heart disease. *Altern Med Rev* 1998; 3: 281-94.
17. Riedler J, et al. Exposure to farming in early life and development of asthma and allergy: a cross-sectional survey *Lancet* 2001; 358: 1129-1133.
18. Mikolon AB, et al. Risk factors for brucellosis seropositivity of goat herds in the Mexicali Valley of Baja California, Mexico. *Prev Vet Med* 1998; 37: 185-195.
19. Kanis JA, et al. A meta-analysis of milk intake and fracture risk: low utility for case finding. *Osteoporos Int* 2005; 16: 799-804.

Chapter Sixteen: So what should we eat?

1. Livesy G. A perspective on food energy standards for nutrition labelling. *Br J Nutr* 2001; 85: 271-287.
2. Ershoff BH. Beneficial effect of liver feeding on swimming capacity of rats in cold water. *Proc Soc Exp Biol Med* 1951; 77: 488-491.
3. Macrae F. Junk diet is causing famine symptoms. *Daily Mail*, 6 May 2007.
4. Hickman M. Caution: Some soft drinks may seriously harm your health: Expert links additive to cell damage. *The Independent on Sunday*, 27 May 2007
5. Susiarjo M, et al. Bisphenol A exposure in utero disrupts early oogenesis in the mouse. *PLoS Genet* 2007; 3(1): e5, doi:10.1371/journal.pgen.0030005.
6. Humphries P, et al. Direct and indirect cellular effects of aspartame on the brain. *Eur J Clin Nutr* 2008; 62: 451-462.
7. O'Driscoll C. Skimmed milk straight from the cow. *Chem & Ind* 2007; 10: 11.
8. Hayashi K, et al. Laughter lowered the increase in postprandial blood glucose. *Diabetes Care* 2003; 26: 1651-1652.
9. Waldhaus WK, et al. Effect of stress hormones on splanchnic substrate and insulin disposal after glucose ingestion in healthy humans. *Diabetes* 1987; 36: 127-135.

Chapter Seventeen: Why low-carb diets must be high-fat, not high-protein

1. Cahill GF. Survival in starvation. *Am J Clin Nutr* 1998; 68: 1-2.
2. Exton JH. Gluconeogenesis. *Metabolism* 1972; 21: 945-990.
3. Volek JS, et al. Body composition and hormonal responses to a carbohydrate-restricted diet. *Metabolism* 2002; 51: 864-870
4. Cox M, Nelson DL. *Lehninger Principles of Biochemistry*. London: Palgrave Macmillan, 2004.
5. Vazquez JA, Kazi U. Lipolysis and gluconeogenesis from glycerol during weight reduction with very low calorie diets. *Metabolism* 1994; 43: 1293-1299.
6. Phinney SD, et al. The human metabolic response to chronic ketosis without caloric restriction: physical and biochemical adaptation. *Metabolism* 1983; 32: 757-768.
7. Bisshop PH, et al. The effects of carbohydrate variation in isocaloric diets on glycogenolysis and gluconeogenesis in healthy men. *J Clin Endocrinol Metab* 2000; 85: 1963-1967.
8. Cahill GF Jr. Starvation in man. *N Engl J Med* 1970; 19: 668-675.
9. Klein S, Wolfe RR. Carbohydrate restriction regulates the adaptive response to fasting. *Am J Physiol* 1992; 262: E631-E636.
10. Sherwin RS, et al. Effect of ketone infusions on amino acid and nitrogen metabolism in man. *J Clin Invest* 1975; 55: 1382-1390.
11. Neely JR, Morgan HE. Relationship between carbohydrate and lipid metabolism and the energy balance of heart muscle. *Annu Rev Physiol* 1974; 36: 413-459.
12. Speth JD, Spielmann KA. Energy source, protein metabolism, and hunter-gatherer subsistence strategies. *J Anthropol Archaeol* 1982; 2: 1-31.

13. Noli D, Avery G. Protein poisoning and coastal subsistence. *J Archaeol Sci* 1988; 15: 395-401.
14. McClelland WS, du Bois EF. Clinical Calorimetry. XLV, XLVI, XLVII Prolonged meat diets with a study of kidney function and ketosis. *J Biol Chem* 1930-1931; 87: 651-658; 87: 669; and 93: 419.
15. Dulloo AG, et al. Differential effects of high-fat diets varying in fatty acid composition on the efficiency of lean and fat tissue deposition during weight recovery after low food intake. *Metabolism* 1995; 44: 273-279.
16. Bang HO, et al. Plasma lipid and lipoprotein pattern in Greenlandic West-Coast Eskimos. *Lancet* 1971; i: 1143-1146.
17. Feldman SA, et al. Lipid and cholesterol metabolism in Alaskan arctic Eskimos. *Arch Pathol* 1972; 94: 42-58.
18. Bjerregaard P, Dyerberg J. Mortality from ischaemic heart disease and cerebrovascular disease in Greenland. *Int J Epidem* 1988; 17: 514-519.
19. Sagild U, et al. Epidemiological studies in Greenland 1962-1964. I. Diabetes mellitus in Eskimos. *Acta Med Scand* 1966; 179: 29-39.
20. Stefansson V. *The Fat of The Land.* New York: Macmillan Press, 1957.
21. Sinclair HM. The diet of Canadian Indians and Eskimos. *Proc Nutr Soc* 1952; 12: 69-82.

Chapter Eighteen: Prevention is better

1. Barker DJP, et al. Weight in infancy and death from ischaemic heart disease. *Lancet* 1989; ii: 579.
2. Barker DJP. The intrauterine origins of cardiovascular and obstructive lung disease in adult life. *J R Coll Phys* 1991; 25: 129.
3. Barker DJP, et al. The relation of fetal length, ponderal index and head circumference to blood pressure and the risk of hypertension in later life. *Paed Perinat Epidem* 1992; 6: 35.
4. Davies A. *Let's Have Healthy Children.* London: Unwin Paperbacks, 1981.
5. Doyle W, et al. Maternal nutrient intake and birthweight. *J Hum Nutr & Dietet* 1989; 2: 415.
6. Menon RK, et al. Transplacental passage of insulin in pregnant women with insulin dependent diabetes mellitus: its role in fetal macrosomia. *N Engl J Med* 1990; 323: 309-315.
7. Chavarro JE, et al. Dietary fatty acid intakes and the risk of ovulatory infertility. *Am J Clin Nutr* 2007; 85: 231-237.
8. Chavarro JE, et al. Iron intake and risk of ovulatory infertility. *Obstet Gynecol* 2006; 108: 1145-1152.
9. Barton M, Weisner BP. The role of special diets in the treatment of female infecunditis. *BMJ* 1948; 2: 847-851.
10. Smith C A. The effect of wartime starvation upon pregnancy and its produce. *Am J Obstet Gynecol* 1947; 53: 599-608.
11. Sunshine could boost chances of fatherhood. *Daily Mail*, 19 October 2004.
12. Godfrey K, et al. Maternal nutrition in early and late pregnancy in relation to placental and fetal growth. *BMJ* 1996; 312: 410-414.
13. Hanson LA. Breast-feeding provides passive and likely long-lasting active

immunity. *Ann Allergy Asthma Immunol* 1998, 81: 523-533.

14. Oddy WH, et al. Breast feeding and respiratory morbidity in infancy: a birth cohort study. *Arch Dis Child* 2003; 88: 224-228.

15. Kalliomaki M, et al. Transforming growth factor-beta in breast milk: a potential regulator of atopic disease at an early age. *J Allergy Clin Immunol* 1999; 104: 1251-1257.

16. Shu XO, et al. Breast-feeding and risk of childhood acute leukemia. *J Nat Cancer Inst* 1999; 91: 1765-1772.

17. Singhal A, et al. Breastmilk feeding and lipoprotein profile in adolescents born preterm: follow-up of a prospective randomised study. *Lancet* 2004; 363: 1571-1578.

18. Uauy R, Peirano P. Breast is best: human milk is the optimal food for brain development. *Am J Clin Nutr* 1999; 70: 433-4.

19. Dewey KG, et al. Breast-fed infants are leaner than formula-fed infants at 1 y of age: The DARLING Study. *Am J Clin Nutr* 1993; 57: 140-145.

20. Arenz S, et al. Breast-feeding and childhood obesity – a systematic review. *Int J Obes Relat Metab Disord* 2004; 28:1247-1256.

21. Bonbiot G. Don't listen to what the rich world's leaders say – look at what they do. *The Guardian*, 5 June 2007.

22. Dewey KG, et al. Maternal weight-loss patterns during prolonged lactation. *Am J Clin Nutr* 1993; 58: 162-166.

23. Janney C, et al. Lactation and weight retention. *Am J Clin Nutr* 1997; 66: 1116-1124.

24. Fomon S. *Infant Nutrition.* 2nd ed. Philadelphia, USA: W. B. Saunders, 1974. p. 455.

25. Durie P.R. Inherited causes of exocrine pancreatic dysfunction. *Can J Gastroenterol* 1997; 11: 145-152.

26. Simopoulos AP, Salem N Jr. Egg yolk as a source of long-chain polyunsaturated fatty acids in infant feeding; *Am J Clin Nutr* 1992; 55: 411-414.

27. Makrides M, et al. Nutritional effect of including egg yolk in the weaning diet of breast-fed and formula-fed infants: a randomized controlled trial. *Am J Clin Nutr* 2002; 75: 1084-1092.

28. Carvalho NF, et al. Severe nutritional deficiencies in toddlers resulting from health food milk alternatives. *Pediatrics* 2001; 107: E46.

29. Etcheverry P, et al. Effect of beef and soy proteins on the absorption of non-heme iron and inorganic zinc in children. *J Am Coll Nutr* 2006; 25: 34-40.

30. Garemo M H. *Nutrition and health in 4-year-olds in a Swedish well-educated urban community.* PhD Dissertation 14, December 2006, Department of Paediatrics, Göteborg, published by the Swedish Research Council.

31. Makrides M, et al. Are long-chain polyunsaturated fatty acids essential nutrients in infancy? *Lancet* 1995; 345: 1463-1468.

32. Richards J, et al. Quality of drinking water. *BMJ* 1992; 304: 571.

33. Groves, BA. *Fluoride: drinking ourselves to death?* Dublin: Newleaf, 2001.

34. Schwartz MB, et al. Examining the nutritional quality of breakfast cereals marketed to children. *JADA* 2008; 108: 702-705.

Chapter Nineteen: 'Healthy eating' is fattening

1. Mokdad AH, et al: The continuing epidemic of obesity in the United States. *JAMA* 2000; 184: 1650-1651.
2. Wooley SC, Garner DM. Dietary treatments for obesity are ineffective. *BMJ* 1994; 309: 655.
3. Garrow JS. Should obesity be treated? *BMJ* 1994; 309: 654.
4. Willett W. Is dietary fat a major determinant of body fat? *Am J Clin Nutr* 1998; 67(3 Suppl): 556S-562S.
5. Sheppard L, et al. Weight loss in women participating in a randomized trial of low-fat diets. *Am J Clin Nutr* 1991; 54: 821-828.
6. Heini AF, Weinsier RL. Divergent trends in obesity and fat intake patterns: the American paradox. *Am J Med* 1997; 102: 259-264.
7. Bruning JC, et al. Role of brain insulin receptor in control of body weight and reproduction. *Science* 2000; 289: 2122-2125.
8. Odeleye OE, et al. Fasting hyperinsulinemia is a predictor of increased body weight gain and obesity in Pima Indian children. *Diabetes* 1997; 46: 1341-1345.
9. Sigal RJ, et al. Acute postchallenge hyperinsulinemia predicts weight gain: a prospective study. *Diabetes* 1997; 46: 1025-1029.
10. Braun T, et al. Factor in human urine inhibiting lipid metabolism. *Experientia* 1963; 19: 319-320.
11. Kekwick A, Pawan GLS. The effects of high fat and high carbohydrate diets on rates of weight loss in mice. *Metabolism* 1964; 13: 87-97.
12. Li CH. Lipotropin: A new active peptide from pituitary glands. *Nature* 1964; 201: 924.
13. Kanarek RB, Hirsch E. Dietary-induced overeating in experimental animals. *Fed Proc* 1977; 36: 154-158.
14. Kreitzman SN. Factors influencing body composition during very-low-calorie diets. *Am J Clin Nutr* 1992; 56: 217S-223S.
15. Somogyi M. Studies of arteriovenous differences in blood sugar; II. Effect of hypoglycemia on the rate of extrahepatic glucose assimilation. *J Biolog Chem* 1948; 174: 597-604.
16. Feinman RD, Fine EJ. Thermodynamics and metabolic advantage of weight loss diets. *Metab Synd Rel Dis* 2003; 1: 209-219.
17. Young C. Weight loss on 1800 kcal diets varying in carbohydrate content. *Am J Clin Nutr* 1971; 290-296.
18. Lyon DM, Dunlop DM. The treatment of obesity: a comparison of the effects of diet and of thyroid extract. *Quart J Med* 1932; 1: 331.
19. Yancy WS. New research examines effectiveness and weight loss maintenance of the low carbohydrate diet. *NAASO 2000* – Annual Scientific Meeting, Long Beach, California. 30 October 2000.
20. Flegal KM, et al. Excess deaths associated with underweight, overweight, and obesity. *JAMA* 2005; 293: 1861-1867.
21. Kim D-J, et al. Visceral adiposity and subclinical coronary artery disease in elderly adults: Rancho Bernardo Study. *Obesity* 2008; 16: 853-858.
22. Gordon ES, et al. A new concept in the treatment of obesity. *JAMA* 1963; 186: 50-60.

Chapter Twenty: Diabetes deceit

1. Mitka M. Diabetes management remains suboptimal: even academic centers neglect curbing risk factors. *JAMA* 2005; 293: 1845-1846

2. Yudkin J. Evolutionary and historical changes in dietary carbohydrates. *Am J Clin Nutr* 1967; 20: 108 115.

3. Mouratoff GJ, et al. Diabetes mellitus in Eskimos. *JAMA* 1967; 199: 107-112.

4. Menon RK, et al. Transplacental passage of insulin in pregnant women with insulin dependent diabetes mellitus: its role in fetal macrosomia. *N Engl J Med* 1990; 323: 309-315.

5. MacFarlane AJ, et al. A type 1 diabetes-related protein from wheat (Triticum aestivum): cDNA clone of a wheat storage globulin, Glb1, linked to islet damage. *J Biol Chem* 2003; 278: 54-63.

6. Ziegler A-G, et al. Early infant feeding and risk of developing type 1 diabetes-associated autoantibodies. *JAMA* 2003; 290: 1721-1728.

7. Harris MI. Epidemiologic studies on the pathogenesis of non-insulin-dependent diabetes mellitus (NIDDM). *Clin Invest Med* 1995; 18: 231-239.

8. Manson JE, Spelsberg A. Primary prevention of non-insulin dependent diabetes mellitus. *Am J Prev Med* 1994; 10: 172-184.

9. Gohdes D, et al. Diabetes in American Indians: an overview. *Diabetes Care* 1993; 16: 239-243.

10. Hodge AM, et al. Dramatic increase in the prevalence of obesity in Western Samoa over the 13 year period 1978-1991. *Int J Obes Relat Metab Disord* 1994; 18: 419-428.

11. United Kingdom Prospective Diabetes Study (UKPDS) IV. Characteristics of newly diagnosed type 2 diabetic patients and their association with different clinical and biochemical risk factors. *Diabetes Res* 1990; 13: 1-11.

12. UK Prospective Diabetes Study Group. UK Prospective Diabetes Study (UKPDS) VIII. Study design, progress and performance. *Diabetologia* 1991; 34: 877-890.

13. Murray CJL, Lopez AD. *The Global Burden of Disease.* Geneva: WHO, 1996.

14. Rayner M, Petersen S. *European Cardiovascular Disease Statistics.* London: British Heart Foundation, 2000; Table 2.2.

15. Diabetes Control and Complications Trial Research Group. The effect of intensive treatment of diabetes on the development and progression of long-term complications in insulin-dependent diabetes mellitus. *N Engl J Med* 1993; 329: 977-986.

16. Sánchez CD, et al. Diabetes-related knowledge, atherosclerotic risk factor control, and outcomes in acute coronary syndromes. *Am J Cardiol* 2005; 95: 1290-1294.

17. Meier JJ, et al. Sustained beta cell apoptosis in patients with long-standing type 1 diabetes: indirect evidence for islet regeneration? *Diabetologia* 2005; 48: 2221-2228.

18. Robertson MD, et al. Extended effects of evening meal carbohydrate-to-fat ratio on fasting and postprandial substrate metabolism. *Am J Clin Nutr* 2002; 75: 505-510.

19. Gannon MC, et al. An increase in dietary protein improves the blood glucose response in persons with type 2 diabetes. *Am J Clin Nutr* 2003; 78: 734-741.
20. Jenkins DJ, et al. Effect of wheat bran on glycemic control and risk factors for cardiovascular disease in type 2 diabetes. *Diabetes Care* 2002; 25: 1522-1528.
21. Bunn HF, Higgins PJ. Reaction of monosaccharides with proteins: possible evolutionary significance. *Science* 1981; 213: 222-229.
22. Bierman EL. George Lyman Duff Memorial Lecture. Atherogenesis in diabetes. *Arterioscler Thromb* 1992; 12: 647-656.
23. Swanson JE, et al. Metabolic effects of dietary fructose in healthy subjects. *Am J Clin Nutr* 1992; 55: 851-856.
24. Rohatgi A, McGuire DK. Effects of the thiazolidinedione medications on micro- and macrovascular complications in patients with diabetes – update 2008. *Cardiovasc Drugs Ther* 2008 Mar 29. [Epub ahead of print]
25. Meigs JB, et al. Hyperinsulinemia, hyperglyceima, and impaired hemostasis. The Framingham offspring study. *JAMA* 2000; 283: 221-229.
26. DeFronzo RA, Eleuterio F. Insulin resistance: a multifaceted syndrome responsible for NIDDM, obesity, hypertension, dyslipidemia, and atherosclerotic cardiovascular disease. *Diabetes Care* 1991; 14: 173-191.
27. Rosen Q. Serum insulin-like growth factors and insulin-like growth factor-binding proteins: clinical implications. *Clin Chem* 1999; 45: 1384-1390.
28. Goodwin PJ, et al. Fasting insulin and outcome in early-stage breast cancer: results of a prospective cohort study. *J Clin Oncol* 2002; 20: 42-51.
29. Amowitz LL, Sobel BE. Cardiovascular consequences of polycystic ovary syndrome. *Endocrinol Metab Clin North Am* 1999; 28: 438-458.
30. Ciampelli M, et al. Insulin in obstetrics: a main parameter in the management of pregnancy. *Hum Reprod Update* 1998; 4: 904-914.
31. Joslin EP. Arteriosclerosis in Diabetes. *Ann Intern Med* 1930; 4: 54-66.
32. Chen YD, et al. Why do low-fat, high-carbohydrate diets accentuate postprandial lipemia in patients with NIDDM? *Diabetes Care* 1995; 18: 10-16.
33. Gaist D, et al. Statins and risk of polyneuropathy: A case-control study. *Neurology* 2002; 58: 1333-1337.
34. Vaughan TB, Bell DS. Statin neuropathy masquerading as diabetic autoimmune polyneuropathy. *Diabetes Care* 2005; 28: 2082.

Chapter Twenty-One: Diseases of the heart and blood vessels

1. VACABSCSG. Eleven year survival in the veterans administration randomized trial of coronary bypass surgery for stable angina. *N Engl J Med* 1984 311; 1333-1339.
2. Willis GC. An experimental study of the intimal hemorrhages and in the precipitation of coronary thrombi. *Can Med Assoc J* 1953; 69:17-22.
3. Brown MS, et al. 1985 Nobel laureates in medicine. *J Invest Med* 1996; 44: 14-23.
4. Saul GD. Arterial stress from intraluminal pressure modified by tissue pressure offers a complete explanation for the distribution of atherosclerosis. *Med Hyp* 1999; 52: 349-351.
5. Michalodimitrakis M, et al. Lessons learnt from the autopsies of 445 cases of

sudden cardiac death in adults. *Coron Art Dis* 2005; 16: 385-389.
6. Boushey CJ, et al. A quantitative assessment of plasma homocysteine as a risk for vascular disease. Probable benefits of raising folic acid intakes. *JAMA* 1995; 274: 1049-1057.
7. De Bree A, et al. Homocysteine determinants and the evidence to what extent homocysteine determines risk of coronary heart disease. *Pharmacol Rev* 2002; 54: 599-618.
8. Newbold HL. Reducing the serum cholesterol level with a diet high in animal fat. *South Med J* 1988; 81: 61-3
9. Lackland DT, Wheeler FC. The need for accurate nutrition survey methodology: The South Carolina experience. *J Nutr* 1990; 120: 11S: 1433-6.
10. Castelli WP. Concerning the possibility of a nut . . . *Arch Int Med* 1992; 152: 1371-1372.
11. Ravnskov, Uffe. *The Cholesterol Myths*. Washington, DC: New Trends Publishing Inc, 2000. p. 109.
12. Djoussé L, Gaziano MJ. Egg consumption and risk of heart failure in the Physicians' Health Study. *Circulation* 2008; 117: 512-516.
13. Mann GV (ed). *Coronary Heart Disease: The dietary sense and nonsense*. London: Veritas Society, 1993.
14. Henriques de Gouveia R, et al. Sudden unexpected death in young adults. *Eur Heart J* 2002; 23: 1433-1440.
15. de Lorgeril M, Salen P. Cholesterol lowering and mortality: time for a new paradigm? *Nutr Metab Cardiovasc Dis* 2006; 16: 387-390.
16. Plat J, et al. Oxidized plant sterols in human serum and lipid infusions as measured by combined gas-liquid chromatography-mass spectrometry. *J Lipid Res* 2001; 42: 2030-2038.
17. Weingärtner O, et al. Plant sterols as dietary supplements for the prevention of cardiovascular diseases. *Dtsch Med Wochenschr* 2008; 133: 1201-4.
18. Enig M. *Know Your Fats: the complete primer on fats and cholesterol*. Maryland: Bethesda Press, 2000, 76-81.
19. Smith R, Pinckney E. *Diet, Blood Cholesterol, And Coronary Heart Disease: a critical review of the literature*. California; Vector Enterprises, 1991.
20. Cherubini A, et al. The VASA Study Group. High vitamin E plasma levels and low low-density lipoprotein oxidation are associated with the absence of atherosclerosis in octogenarians. *J Am Geriatr Soc* 2001; 49: 651-654.
21. Silaste M-L, et al. Changes in dietary fat intake alter plasma levels of oxidized low-density lipoprotein and lipoprotein(a). *Arterioscler Thromb Vasc Biol* 2004; 24: 498-503.
22. McGee DL, et al. Ten-year incidence of coronary heart disease in Honolulu Heart Programme – Relationship to nutrient intake. *Am J Epidemiol* 1984; 119: 667-676.
23. Halton TL, et al. Low-carbohydrate-diet score and the risk of coronary heart disease in women. *N Engl J Med* 2006; 355: 1991-2002.
24. Selvin E, et al. Glycemic control, atherosclerosis, and risk factors for cardiovascular disease in individuals with diabetes: the atherosclerosis risk in communities study. *Diabetes Care* 2005; 28: 1965-1973.
25. West J, et al. Risk of vascular disease in adults with diagnosed coeliac disease: a

population-based study. *Aliment Pharmacol Ther* 2004; 20: 73-79.

26. Nemetz PN, et al. Recent trends in the prevalence of coronary disease: A population-based autopsy study of nonnatural deaths. *Arch Intern Med.* 2008; 168: 264-270.

27. Chen YD, et al. Why do low-fat, high-carbohydrate diets accentuate postprandial lipemia in patients with NIDDM? *Diabetes Care* 1995; 18: 10-16.

28. Selvin E, et al. Glycemic control and coronary heart disease risk in persons with and without diabetes: the atherosclerosis risk in communities study. *Arch Intern Med* 2005; 165: 1910-1916.

29. Jeppeson J, et al. Effects of low-fat, high-carbohydrate diets on risk factors for ischemic heart disease in postmenopausal women. *Am J Clin Nutr* 1997; 65: 1027-1033.

30. Bürger M. *Altern und Krankheit als Problem der Biomorphose.* 3rd ed, Leipzig: Georg Thieme, 1957.

31. Abbasi F, et al. High carbohydrate diets, triglyceride-rich lipoproteins and coronary heart disease risk. *Am J Cardiol* 2000; 85: 45-48.

32. Norhammar A, et al. Glucose metabolism in patients with acute myocardial infarction and no previous diagnosis of diabetes mellitus: a prospective study. *Lancet* 2002; 359: 2140-2144.

33. Sharman MJ, et al. A ketogenic diet favorably affects serum biomarkers for cardiovascular disease in normal-weight men. *J Nutr* 2002; 132: 1879-1885.

34. Westman EC, et al. Effect of 6-month adherence to a very low carbohydrate diet program. *Am J Med* 2002; 113: 30-36.

35. Editorial. Prevention of coronary heart disease. *BMJ* 1968; 2: 689-690.

36. Lucas FL, et al. Temporal trends in the utilization of diagnostic testing and treatments for cardiovascular disease in the United States, 1993-2001. *Circulation* 2006; 113: 374-379.

37. Barzilay JI, et al. The association of fasting glucose levels with congestive heart failure in diabetic adults ≥65 years: the Cardiovascular Health Study. *J Am Coll Cardiol* 2004; 43: 2236-2241.

38. Rauchhaus M, et al. The relationship between cholesterol and survival in patients with chronic heart failure. *J Am Coll Cardiol* 2003; 42:1933-1940.

39. Wattanakit K, et al. Risk factors for peripheral arterial disease incidence in persons with diabetes: the Atherosclerosis Risk in Communities (ARIC) Study. *Atherosclerosis* 2005; 180: 389-397.

40. Gaede P, et al. Multifactorial intervention and cardiovascular disease in patients with type 2 diabetes. *N Engl J Med* 2003; 348: 383-393.

41. Vermeer SE, et al. Impaired glucose tolerance increases stroke risk in nondiabetic patients with transient ischemic attack or minor ischemic stroke. *Stroke* 2006; 37: 1413-1417.

42. Jern S. Effects of acute carbohydrate administration on central and peripheral hemodynamic responses to mental stress. *Hypertension* 1991; 18: 790-797.

43. Pyorala M, et al. Hyperinsulinemia and the risk of stroke in healthy middle-aged men: the 22-year follow-up results of the Helsinki Policemen Study. *Stroke* 1998; 29: 1860-1866.

44. Kamide K, et al, Insulin resistance is related to silent cerebral infarction in patients with essential hypertension. *Am J Hypertens* 1997; 10: 1245-1249.

45. Biessels GJ. Cerebral complications of diabetes: clinical findings and pathogenic mechanisms. *Neth J Med* 1999; 54: 35-45.
46. Hsueh WA, et al. Insulin resistance and the endothelium. *Am J Med* 2004; 117: 109-117.
47. Selvin E, et al. Glycaemia (haemoglobin A1c) and incident ischaemic stroke: the Atherosclerosis Risk in Communities (ARIC) Study. *Lancet Neurol* 2005; 4: 821-826.
48. Hur C, et al. Analysis of aspirin-associated risks in healthy individuals. *Ann Pharmacotherapy* 2005; 39: 51-57.
49. US Dep't of Labor, Bureau of Labor statistics. Census of fatal occupational injuries. http:// www.bis.gov/mirappendix.pdf, Table 5.
50. Cohen JT, Graham JD. A revised economic analysis of restrictions on the use of cell phones whilst driving. *Risk Analysis* 2003; 23: 5-17.

Chapter Twenty-Two: The dangers of low blood cholesterol

1. Anderson KM, et al. Cholesterol and mortality. 30 years of follow-up from the Framingham Study. *JAMA* 1987; 257: 2176-2180.
2. Rauchhaus M, et al. The relationship between cholesterol and survival in patients with chronic heart failure. *J Am Coll Cardiol* 2003; 42: 1933-1940.
3. Kame C, et al. Estimation of effect of lipid lowering treatment on total mortality rate and its cost-effectiveness determined by intervention study of hypercholesterolemia. *Nippon Eiseigaku Zasshi* 2007; 62: 39-46.
4. Horwich, et al. Low serum total cholesterol is associated with marked increase in mortality in advanced heart failure. *J Cardiac Fail* 2002; 4: 216-224.
5. Steffens DC, et al. Cholesterol-lowering medication and relapse of depression. *Psychopharmacology Bull* 2003; 37: 92-98.
6. Adachi H, Hino A. Trends in nutritional intake and serum cholesterol levels over 40 years in Tanushimaru, Japanese men. *J Epidemiol* 2005; 15: 85-89.
7. Liu L, et al. Changes in stroke mortality rates for 1950 to 1997. A great slowdown of decline trend in Japan. *Stroke* 2001; 32: 1745.
8. Shimamoto T, et al. Trends for coronary heart disease and stroke and their risk factors in Japan. *Circulation*. 1989; 3: 503-515.
9. Iso H, et al. Trends of cardiovascular risk factors and diseases in Japan: implications for primordial prevention. *Prev Med* 1999; 29: S102-S105.
10. Sauvaget C, et al. Animal protein, animal fat, and cholesterol intakes and risk of cerebral infarction mortality in the Adult Health Study. *Stroke* 2004; 35: 1351.
11. Gillman MW, et al. Inverse association of dietary fat with development of ischemic stroke in men. *JAMA* 1997; 278: 2145-2150.
12. Atkins D, et al. Cholesterol reduction and the risk of stroke in men. A meta-analysis of randomized, controlled trials. *Ann Int Med* 1993; 119: 136-145.
13. Dyker AG, et al. Influence of cholesterol on survival after stroke: retrospective study. *BMJ* 1997; 314: 1584.
14. Ruiz-Sandoval JL, et al. Intracerebral hemorrhage in young people: analysis of risk factors, location, causes, and prognosis. *Stroke* 1999; 30: 537-541.
15. He K, et al. Dietary fat intake and risk of stroke in male US healthcare professionals: 14-year prospective cohort study. *BMJ* 2003; 327: 777-782.

16. Isles CG, et al. Plasma cholesterol, coronary heart disease, and cancer in the Renfrew and Paisley survey. *BMJ* 1989; 298: 920-924.

17. Oliver MF. Low cholesterol and increased risk. *Lancet* 1989; ii: 163.

18. Muller CP, et al. The prognostic significance of total serum cholesterol in patients with Hodgkin's disease. *Cancer* 1992; 69: 1042-1046.

19. Winawer SJ, et al. Declining serum cholesterol prior to diagnosis of colon cancer. *JAMA* 1990; 263: 2083-2085.

20. Siemianowicz K, et al. Serum total cholesterol and triglycerides levels in patients with lung cancer. *Int J Mol Med.* 2000; 5: 201-205.

21. Okamura T, et al. What cause of mortality can we predict by cholesterol screening in the Japanese general population? *J Intern Med* 2003; 253: 169-180.

22. Scolozzi R, et al. Hypocholesterolemia in multiple myeloma. Inverse relation to the component M and the clinical stage. *Minerva Med* 1983; 74: 2359-2364.

23. Nakagawa T, et al. Marked hypocholesterolemia in a case with adrenal adenoma-enhanced catabolism of low density lipoprotein (LDL) via the LDL receptors of tumor cells. *J Clin Endocrinol Metab* 1995; 80: 3391-3392.

24. Aixala M, et al. Hypocholesterolemia in hematologic neoplasms. *Sangre* (Barc) 1997; 42: 7-10.

25. Pandolfino J, et al. Hypocholesterolemia in hairy cell leukemia: a marker for proliferative activity. *Am J Hematol* 1997; 55: 129-133.

26. Grieb P, et al. Serum cholesterol in cerebral malignancies. *J Neurooncol* 1999; 41: 175-180.

27. Tomiki Y, et al. Reduced low-density-lipoprotein cholesterol causing low serum cholesterol levels in gastrointestinal cancer: a case control study. *J Exp Clin Cancer Res* 2004; 23: 233-240.

28. Mazza A, et al. Predictors of cancer mortality in elderly subjects. *Eur J Epidemiol* 1999; 15: 421-427.

29. Wannamethee G, et al. Low serum total cholesterol concentrations and mortality in middle aged British men. *BMJ* 1995; 311: 409-413.

30. Newman TB, Hulley SB. Carcinogenicity of lipid-lowering drugs. *JAMA* 1996; 275: 55-60.

31. Muldoon MF, et al. Immune system differences in men with hypo- or hypercholesterolemia. *Clin Immunol Immunopathol* 1997; 84: 145-149.

32. Perez-Guzman C, et al. A cholesterol-rich diet accelerates bacteriologic sterilization in pulmonary tuberculosis. *Chest* 2005; 127: 643-651.

33. Leardi S, et al. Blood levels of cholesterol and postoperative septic complications. *Ann Ital Chir* 2000; 71: 233-237.

34. Crook MA, et al. Hypocholesterolaemia in a hospital population. *Ann Clin Biochem* 1999; 36: 613-616.

35. Bonville DA, et al. The relationships of hypo-cholesterolemia to cytokine concentrations and mortality in critically ill patients with systemic inflammatory response syndrome. *Surg Infect* 2004; 5: 39-49.

36. Pacelli F, et al. Prognosis in intra-abdominal infections. Multivariate analysis on 604 patients. *Arch Surg* 1996; 131: 641-645.

37. Ravnskov U. High cholesterol may protect against infections and atherosclerosis. *Quart J Med* 2003; 96: 927-934.

38. Dursun SM, et al. Low serum cholesterol and depression. *BMJ* 1994; 309: 273-274.

References 469

39. Ryman A. Cholesterol, violent death, and mental disorder. *BMJ* 1994; 309: 421-422.
40. Glueck CJ, et al. Hypocholesterolemia and affective disorders. *Am J Med Sci* 1994; 308: 218-225.
41. Law M. Having too much evidence (depression, suicide and low serum cholesterol). *BMJ* 1996; 313: 651-652.
42. Zureik M, et al. Serum cholesterol concentration and death from suicide in men: Paris Prospective Study I. *BMJ* 1996; 313: 649-651.
43. Engleberg H. Low serum cholesterol and suicide. *Lancet* 1992; 339: 727-729.
44. Buydens-Branchey L, Branchey M. Association between low plasma levels of cholesterol and relapse in cocaine addicts. *Psychosom Med* 2003; 65: 86-91.
45. Zhang J, et al. Association of serum cholesterol and history of school suspension among school-age children and adolescents in the United States. *Am J Epidemiol* 2005; 161: 691-699.
46. Bürger M. *Altern und Krankheit als Problem der Biomorphose.* 3rd dd, Leipzig: Georg Thieme, 1957.
47. Corrigan FM, et al. Dietary supplementation with zinc sulphate, sodium selenite and fatty acids in early dementia of Alzheimer's Type II: Effects on lipids. *J Nutr Med* 1991; 2: 265-271.
48. Elias PK, et al. Serum cholesterol and cognitive performance in the Framingham Heart Study. *Psychosom Med* 2005; 67: 24-30.
49. de Lau LML, et al. Serum cholesterol levels and the risk of Parkinson's disease. *Am J Epidemiol* 2006; 164: 998-1002.
50. Franzblau A, Criqui MH. Characteristics of persons with marked hypocholesterolemia. A population-based study. *J Chronic Dis* 1984; 37: 387-395.
51. Obialo CI, et al. Role of hypoalbuminemia and hypocholesterolemia as copredictors of mortality in acute renal failure. *Kidney Int.* 1999; 56: 1058-1063.
52. Kalantar-Zadeh K, et al. Reverse epidemiology of cardiovascular risk factors in maintenance dialysis patients. *Kidney Int* 2003; 63: 793-808.
53. Levy E, et al. Altered lipid profile, lipoprotein composition, and oxidant and antioxidant status in pediatric Crohn disease. *Am J Clin Nutr* 2000; 71: 807-815.
54. VanderJagt DJ, et al. Hypocholesterolemia in Nigerian children with sickle cell disease. *J Trop Pediatr* 2002; 48: 156-161.
55. Child mortality under age 5 per 1,000. *1992 Britannia Book of the Year.* Chicago, US: Encyclopaedia Britannica.
56. Weverling-Rijnsburger AWE, et al. Total cholesterol and risk of mortality in the oldest old. *Lancet* 1997; 350: 1119-1123.
57. Jonsson A, et al. Total cholesterol and mortality after age 80 years. *Lancet* 1997; 350: 1778-1779.
58. Hu P, et al. Does inflammation or undernutrition explain the low cholesterol-mortality association in high-functioning older persons? MacArthur studies of successful aging. *J Am Geriatr Soc* 2003; 51: 80-84.
59. Shibata H, et al. Nutrition for the Japanese elderly. *Nutr Health* 1992; 8: 165-175.
60. Stehbens WE. *The Lipid Hypothesis of Atherogenesis.* Austin, Texas: R. G. Landes Co, 1993.
61. Schatz IJ, et al. Cholesterol and all-cause mortality in elderly people from the Honolulu Heart Program: a cohort study. *Lancet* 2001; 358: 351-355.

62. Garasto S, et al. Low cholesterol trait linked to shorter life span. *BMC Medical Genetics* 2004; 5: 3.
63. Dunnigan MG. The problem with cholesterol: No light at the end of this tunnel? *BMJ* 1993; 306: 1355-1356.
64. Ravnskov U. Cholesterol lowering trials in coronary heart disease: frequency of citation and outcome. *BMJ* 1992; 305: 15-19.
65. Kassirer, JP. Why should we swallow what these studies say? *The Washington Post.* 1 August 2004; B03.
66. Dugdale AE. Serum cholesterol and mortality rates. *Lancet* 1987; i: 155-156.

Chapter Twenty-Three – Cancer – disease of civilization

1. From Cancer Research UK's Memorandum and Articles of Association, 2001.
2. Mortality statistics: cause, England and Wales, 2005. Series DH2 no.32, London: HMSO, 2006.
3. Jones HB. A Report on Cancer. Speech delivered to the American Cancer Society's 11th Annual Science Writers' Conference, New Orleans, Louisiana, 7 March 1969, published in *The Choice*, May 1977.
4. Simone CB, II, et al. Cancer, lifestyle modification and glucarate. *J Orthomol Med* 2001; 16: 83.
5. Pert, CB. *Molecules of Emotion.* Scribner, New York, NY, 1997.
6. Hutton SK. *Health Conditions and Disease Incidence among the Eskimos of Labrador.* Poole, England: Wessex Press 1925.
7. Amundsen R. *The Northwest Passage.* London: Archibald Constable, 1908.
8. Schweitzer A. In: Berglas A. *Cancer: Nature, Cause and Cure.* Paris: Institute Pasteur, 1957.
9. Hoffman FL. *The Mortality from Cancer Throughout the World.* Newark, NJ: The Prudential Press, 1915.
10. Cope, J. *Cancer: Civilization and Degeneration.* London: 1932.
11. Berglas A. *Cancer: Nature, Cause and Cure.* Paris: Institute Pasteur, 1957.
12. McCarrison R. *Studies in Deficiency Disease.* Cornell University Library, 1921.
13. Jenness D. *The Copper Eskimos. Vol. XII,* Report of the Canadian Arctic Expedition, 1913-18. Ottawa: The King's Printer, 1923.
14. Quoted in: Stefansson V. *Cancer: Disease Of Civilization?* American Book-Stratford Press, Inc. 1960, Chapter 14.
15. Clemmesen J. The Danish Cancer Registry. *Dan Med Bull* 1955; 2: 124-128.
16. Warburg O. On the origin of cancer cells. *Science* 1956; 123: 309-314.
17. Shim H, et al. A Unique Glucose-Dependent Apoptotic Pathway Induced by c-Myc. *Proc Natl Acad Sci US* 1998; 95: 1511-1516.
18. Rossi-Fanelli F, et al. Abnormal substrate metabolism and nutritional strategies in cancer management. *J Parenter Enteral Nutr* 1991; 15: 680-683.
19. Grant JP. Proper use and recognized role of TPN in the cancer patient. *Nutr* 1990; 6 (4 Suppl): 6S-7S, 10S.
20. Pedersen PL. Tumor mitochondria and the bioenergetics of cancer cells. *Prog Exp Tumor Res* 1978, 22:190-274.
21. Tanchou S. Recherches sur la fréquence du cancer. *Gaz d hop Par* 1843; 2: 313.
22. West J, et al. Malignancy and mortality in people with coeliac disease:

population based cohort study. *BMJ* 2004; 329: 716-719.

23. Seeley S. Diet and breast cancer: the possible connection with sugar consumption. *Med Hyp* 1983; 11: 319-327.
24. Moerman CJ, et al. Dietary sugar intake in the aetiology of biliary tract cancer. *Int J Epidemiol* 1993; 22: 207-214.
25. Yam D, et al. Hyperinsulinemia in colon, stomach and breast cancer patients. *Cancer Lett* 1996; 104: 129-132.
26. Takenaka T, et al. Fatty acids as an energy source for the operation of axoplasmic transport. *Brain Res* 2003; 972, 1-2: 38-43.
27. Hockerts T, Hingerty D. *Medizinische* 1937; 289. Cited by Werner E. Adenosinetriphosphate in the blood of children. *Monatsschr Kinderheilk* 1960; 108: 5-8.
28. Roslin M, et al. Baseline levels of glucose metabolites, glutamate and glycerol in malignant glioma assessed by stereotactic microdialysis. *J Neurooncol* 2003; 61: 151-160.
29. Oudard S, et al. Gliomas are driven by glycolysis: putative roles of hexokinase, oxidative phosphorylation and mitochondrial ultrastructure. *Anticancer Res* 1997; 17: 1903-1911.
30. Nagamatsu S, et al. Rat C6 glioma cell growth is related to glucose transport and metabolism. *Biochem J* 1996; 319: 477-482.
31. Mies G, et al. Relationship between of blood flow, glucose metabolism, protein synthesis, glucose and ATP content in experimentally-induced glioma (RG1 2.2) of rat brain. *J Neurooncol* 1990; 9: 17-28.
32. Floridi A, et al. Modulation of glycolysis in neuroepithelial tumors. *J Neurosurg Sci* 1989; 33: 55-64.
33. Galarraga J, et al. Glucose metabolism in human gliomas: correspondence of in situ and in vitro metabolic rates and altered energy metabolism. *Metab Brain Dis* 1986; 1: 279-291.
34. Rhodes CG, et al. In vivo disturbance of the oxidative metabolism of glucose in human cerebral gliomas. *Ann Neurol* 1983; 14: 614-626.
35. Patel MS, et al. Ketone-body metabolism in glioma and neuroblastoma cells. *Proc Natl Acad Sci US* 1981; 78: 7214-7218.
36. Roeder LM, et al. Utilization of ketone bodies and glucose by established neural cell lines. *J Neurosci Res* 1982; 8: 671-682.
37. Seyfried TN, Mukherjee P. Targeting energy metabolism in brain cancer: review and hypothesis. *Nutr Metab* 2005; 2: 30.
38. Hoehn SK, et al. Complex versus simple carbohydrates and mammary tumors in mice. *Nutr Cancer* 1979; 1: 27.
39. Nimptsch K, et al. Dietary intake of vitamin K and risk of prostate cancer in the Heidelberg cohort of the European Prospective Investigation into Cancer and Nutrition (EPIC-Heidelberg). *Am J Clin Nutr* 2008; 87: 985-992.

Chapter Twenty-Four: Gut reaction

1. Talley NJ, et al. Association of upper and lower gastrointestinal tract symptoms with body mass index in an Australian cohort. *Neurogastroenterol Motil* 2004; 16: 413-419.
2. Aro P, et al. Body mass index and chronic unexplained gastrointestinal

symptoms: an adult endoscopic population-based study. *Gut* 2005: 54: 377-383.
3. Lutz W. *Dismantling a Myth*. Munich, Germany: Selecta-Verlag Dr Ildar Idris GmbH & Co, KG, 1986; 125-180.
4. Nanji AA, French SW. Dietary linoleic acid is required for development of experimentally induced alcoholic liver-injury. *Life Sciences* 1989; 44: 223-301.
5. Laitinen M, et al. Effects of dietary cholesterol feeding on the membranes of liver cells and on the cholesterol metabolism in the rat. *Int J Biochem* 1982; 14: 239-241.
6. Sargin M, et al. Association of nonalcoholic fatty liver disease with insulin resistance: is OGTT indicated in nonalcoholic fatty liver disease? *J Clin Gastroenterol* 2003; 37: 399-402.
7. Schwimmer JB, et al. Obesity, insulin resistance, and other clinicopathological correlates of pediatric nonalcoholic fatty liver disease. *J Pediatr* 2003; 143: 500-505.
8. Diet for obese patient tied to liver inflammation. Reuters Health, 27 October 2003. http://www.reuters.co.uk/newsArticle.jhtml?type=healthNews&storyID=3698408 &section=news, accessed 28 October 2003.
9. Nanji AA, et al. Medium chain triglycerides and vitamin E reduce the severity of established experimental alcoholic liver disease. *J Pharmacol Exp Ther* 1996; 277: 1694-1700.
10. Liddle RA, et al. Gallstone formation during weight-reduction dieting. *Arch Intern Med* 1989; 149: 1750-1753.
11. Heaton KW. Breakfast – do we need it? Report of a meeting of the Forum on Food and Health, 16 June 1989. *J R Soc Med* 1989; 82: 770-771.
12. Tsai C-J, et al. Prospective study of abdominal adiposity and gallstone disease in US men. *Am J Clin Nutr* 2004; 80: 38-44.
13. Dayton S, et al. A controlled clinical trial of a diet high in unsaturated fat in preventing complications of atherosclerosis. *Circulation* 1969; 40 (Suppl 2): 1-63.
14. Thom JA, et al. The influence of refined carbohydrate on urinary calcium excretion. *Br J Urol* 1978; 50:7, 459-464.
15. http://www.niddk.nih.gov/health/kidney/pubs/stonadul/stonadul.htm, accessed 21 August 2003.
16. http://www.kidney.org/general/atoz/content/kstones.html, accessed 21 August 2003.
17. Poortmans JR, Dellalieux O. Do regular high protein diets have potential health risks on kidney function in athletes? *Int J Sport Nutr Exercise Metab* 2000; 10: 28-38.
18. Blum M, et al. Protein intake and kidney function in humans: its effect on normal aging. *Arch Int Med* 1989; 149: 211-212.
19. Skov AR, et al. Changes in renal function during weight loss induced by high vs low-protein low-fat diets in overweight subjects. *Int J Obes* 1999; 23: 1170-1177.
20. Wrone EM, et al. Association of dietary protein intake and microalbuminuria in healthy adults: Third National Health and Nutrition Examination Survey. *Am J Kidney Dis* 2003; 41: 580-587.
21. Knight EL, et al. The impact of protein intake on renal function decline in women with normal renal function or mild renal insufficiency. *Ann Int Med* 2003; 138: 460-467.
22. Facchini FS, Saylor KL. A low-iron-available, polyphenol-enriched,

carbohydrate-restricted diet to slow progression of diabetic nephropathy. *Diabetes* 2003; 52: 1204-1209.

23. Nielsen JV, et al. A low-carbohydrate diet may prevent end-stage renal failure in type 2 diabetes. A case report. *Nutr Metab* 2006; 3: 23.
24. Catassi C, et al. The coeliac iceberg in Italy: a multicentre antigliadin antibodies screening for coeliac disease in school-age subjects. *Acta Paediatr Suppl* 1996; 412: 29-35.
25. Fasano A, et al. Prevalence of celiac disease in at-risk and not-at-risk groups in the United States: a large multicenter study. *Arch Intern Med* 2003; 163: 286-292.
26. West J, et al. Malignancy and mortality in people with coeliac disease: population based cohort study. *BMJ* 2004; 329: 716-719.
27. Burkitt DP, et al. Effect of dietary fibre on stools and transit times, and its role in the causation of disease. *Lancet* 1972; ii: 1408-1411.
28. Lucey MR, et al. Is bran efficacious in irritable bowel syndrome? A double-blind placebo controlled cross-over study. *Gut* 1987; 28: 221-225.
29. Francis CY, Whorwell PJ. Bran and irritable bowel syndrome: time for reappraisal. *Lancet* 1994; 344: 39-40.
30. Editorial. The bran wagon. *Lancet*. 1987; i: 782-783.
31. Choi K, et al. Fructose intolerance: an under-recognized problem. *Am J Gastroenterol* 2003; 98: 1348-1353.
32. Janes SEJ, et al. Management of diverticulitis. *BMJ* 2006; 332: 271-275.
33. Inoue M, et al. Subsite-specific risk factors for colorectal cancer: a hospital-based case-control study in Japan. *Cancer Causes & Control* 1995; 6: 14-22.
34. Guller R, Reber M. Mechanical obstruction of the large intestine by wheat bran. *Schweiz Med Wochenschr* 1980; 110: 89-91.
35. Dukes HH. *The Physiology of Domestic Animals.* Ithaca, NY: Comstock Publishing Company, 1955.
36. Voegtlin WL. *The Stone Age Diet.* New York, NY: Vantage Press Inc, 1975.
37. *JAMA* 9 May 1966 and *Medical World News* 20 May 1966. Quoted in Voegtlin, 1975.
38. Tran TT, et al. Hyperinsulinemia, but not other factors associated with insulin resistance, acutely enhances colorectal epithelial proliferation in vivo. *Endocrinology* 2006; 147: 1830-1837.
39. Larsson SC, et al. High-fat dairy food and conjugated linoleic acid intakes in relation to colorectal cancer incidence in the Swedish Mammography Cohort. *Am J Clin Nutr* 2005; 82: 894-900.
40. Lakhani K, et al. Polycystic ovary syndrome, diabetes and cardiovascular disease: risks and risk factors. *J Obstet Gynaecol* 2004; 24: 613-621.

Chapter Twenty-Five: Deficiency diseases

1. *Fractured neck of femur: prevention and management.* A report of the Royal College of Physicians, London. 1989.
2. Bengner U. Changes in the incidence of fracture of the upper humerus during a 30-year period: a study of 2125 fractures. *Clin Orthop* 1988; 231: 179-182.
3. Love S. *Dr Susan Love's Hormone Book.* New York: Random House, 1997; p. 85.

4. Frost H. The pathomechanics of osteoporosis. *Clin Orthop* 1985; 200: 198-225.
5. Consensus Development Conference. Prophylaxis and treatment of osteoporosis. Conference Report. *Am J Med* 1991: 107-110.
6. Brown S. *Better Bones, Better Body.* Connecticut, US: Keats Publishing, 1996, 38.
7. Kerstetter JE, et al. Low protein intake: The impact on calcium and bone homeostasis in humans. *J Nutr* 2003; 133: 855S-861S.
8. Fehily AM. Dietary determinants of bone mass and fracture risk: a review. *J Hum Nutr and Diet* 1989; 2: 299.
9. Spencer H, Kramer L. Factors contributing to osteoporosis. *J Nutr* 1986; 116: 316-319.
10. Hunt J, et al. High- versus low-meat diets: Effects on zinc absorption, iron status, and calcium, copper, iron, magnesium, manganese, nitrogen, phosphorus, and zinc balance in postmenopausal women. *Amer J Clin Nutr* 1995; 62: 621-632.
11. Spencer H, et al. Do protein and phosphorus cause calcium loss? *J Nutr* 1988; 118: 657-660.
12. Cooper C, et al. Dietary protein and bone mass in women. *Calcif Tiss Int* 1996; 58: 320-325.
13. Munger RG, et al. Prospective study of dietary protein intake and risk of hip fracture in postmenopausal women. *Amer J Clin Nutr* 1999; 69: 147-152.
14. Hannan MT, et al. Effect of dietary protein on bone loss in elderly men and women: the Framingham Osteoporosis Study. *J Bone & Min Res* 2000; 15: 2504-2512.
15. Dawson-Hughes B, Harris SS. Calcium intake influences the association of protein intake with rates of bone loss in elderly men and women. *Am J Clin Nutr* 2002; 75: 773-779.
16. Fallon S, Enig M. Dem bones – do high protein diets cause osteoporosis? *Wise Traditions* 2000; 1: 4: 38-41.
17. Watkins BA, et al. Importance of vitamin E in bone formation and in chondrocyte function. *American Oil Chemists Society Proceedings* 1996, at Purdue University.
18. Watkins BA, Saifert MF. Food lipids and bone health. In: McDonald RE, Min DB, (eds). *Food Lipids and Health.* NY: Marcel Dekker Co. 1996.
19. Dhonukshe-Rutten RA, et al. Homocysteine and vitamin B12 status relate to bone turnover markers, broadband ultrasound attenuation, and fractures in healthy elderly people. *J Bone Miner Res* 2005; 20: 921-929.
20. Chiu JF, et al. Long-term vegetarian diet and bone mineral density in postmenopausal Taiwanese women. *Calcif Tissue Int* 1997; 60: 245-249.
21. Lau EM, et al. Bone mineral density in Chinese elderly female vegetarians, vegans, lacto-vegetarians and omnivores. *Eur J Clin Nutr* 1998; 52: 60-64.
22. Kocjan T, et al. Vitamin d status in patients with osteopenia or osteoporosis – an audit of an endocrine clinic. *Int J Vitam Nutr Res* 2006; 76: 307-313.
23. Abramson J. *Overdo$ed America*, Harper Collins, 2004.
24. Darlington LG, et al. Placebo-controlled, blind study of dietary manipulation therapy in rheumatoid arthritis. *Lancet* 1986; i: 236-238.
25. Karvonen RL, et al. Periarticular osteoporosis in osteoarthritis of the knee. *J Rheumatol* 1998; 25: 2187-2194.
26. National Institutes of Health. *Clinical guidelines on the identification, evaluation,*

and treatment of overweight and obesity in adults: the Evidence Report. Bethesda, MD: US Department of Health and Human Services, 1998.

27. *Medical World News.* December 18, 1964.
28. Morbidity and Mortality Weekly Report: Prevalence of Arthritis – United States, 1997. *MMWR* 2001; 50: 334-336.
29. Price WA. *Nutrition and Physical Degeneration.* New York & London: Paul B. Hoeber, Inc, 1939: Chap 6.
30. Ibid: Chap 15.
31. Lepore L, et al. Prevalence of celiac disease in patients with juvenile arthritis. *J Pediatr* 1996; 129: 311-313.
32. O'Farrelly C, et al. Association between villous atrophy in rheumatoid arthritis and a rheumatoid factor and gliadin-specific IgG. *Lancet* 1988; ii: 819-822.
33. Lepore L, et al. Anti-alpha-gliadin antibodies are not predictive of celiac disease in juvenile chronic arthritis. *Acta Paediatr* 1993; 82: 569-573.
34. Shatin R. Preliminary report of the treatment of rheumatoid arthritis with high protein gluten-free diet and supplements. *Med J Aust* 1964; 2: 169-172.
35. Williams R. Rheumatoid arthritis and food: A case study. *BMJ* 1981; 283: 563.
36. Beri D, et al. Effect of dietary restrictions on disease activity in rheumatoid arthritis. *Ann Rheum Dis* 1988; 47: 69-77.
37. Lunardi C, et al. Food allergy and rheumatoid arthritis. *Clin Exp Rheumatol* 1988; 6: 423-426.
38. Hagfors L, et al. Fat intake and composition of fatty acids in serum phospholipids in a randomized, controlled, Mediterranean dietary intervention study on patients with rheumatoid arthritis. *Nutr Metab* 2005; 2: 26.
39. Gerli R, Goodson NJ. Cardiovascular involvement in rheumatoid arthritis. *Lupus* 2005; 14: 679-682.
40. Stefansson V. *Discovery: The autobiography of Vilhjalmur Stefansson.* New York: McGraw-Hill Book Co., 1964.
41. Ebringer A, Wilson C. The use of a low starch diet in the treatment of patients suffering from ankylosing spondylitis. *Clin Rheumatol* 1996; 15, Suppl 1: 62-66.
42. Welch TR, et al. Vitamin D-deficient rickets: the re-emergence of a once-conquered disease. *J Pediatr* 2000; 137: 143-145.
43. Wargovitch MJ, Baer AR. Basic and clinical investigations of dietary calcium in the prevention of colorectal cancer. *Prev Med* 1989; 18: 672.
44. BBC. *Horizon: The Poison That Waits.* BBC2 broadcast 16 Jan. 1989.
45. Addy D. Happiness is: iron. *BMJ* 1986; 292: 969
46. Bryce-Smith D, Simpson R. Anorexia, depression and zinc deficiency. *Lancet* 1984; ii: 1162.
47. Meadows N, et al. Zinc and small babies. *Lancet* 1981; ii: 1135.
48. Lifshitz F, et al. Nutritional dwarfing in adolescents. *Semin Adolesc Med* 1987; 3: 255-266.
49. Lozoff B, et al. Long-term developmental outcome of infants with iron deficiency. *N Engl J Med* 1991; 325: 687-694.
50. Hughes RE, Johns E. Apparent relation between dietary fibre and reproductive function in the female. *Ann Hum Biol.* 1985; 12: 325.
51. Hughes RE. A new look at dietary fibre. *Hum Nutr Clin Nutr* 1986; 40c: 81.

52. Lloyd T, et al. Inter-relationships of diet, athletic activity, menstrual status and bone density in collegiate women. *Am J Clin Nutr* 1987; 46: 681.

Chapter Twenty-Six: Diet and the brain

1. Goldman J, et al. Behavioral effects of sucrose on preschool children. *J Abnormal Child Psych* 1986; 14: 565-577.
2. Behar D, et al. Sugar testing with children considered behaviorally sugar reactive. *Nutritional Behavior* 1984; 1: 277-288.
3. Schauss A. *Diet, Crime and Delinquency.* Berkeley, CA: Parker House, 1981.
4. Christensen L. The role of caffeine and sugar in depression. *The Nutrition Report* 1991; 9 (3): 17-24.
5. Hadjivassiliou M, et al. Does cryptic gluten sensitivity play a part in neurological illness? *Lancet* 1996; 347: 369-371.
6. Levitt Katz LE, et al. Neuropsychiatric disorders at the presentation of type 2 diabetes mellitus in children. *Pediatr Diabetes* 2005; 6: 84-89.
7. Benton D, et al. The delivery rate of dietary carbohydrates affects cognitive performance in both rats and humans. *Psychopharmacology* 2003; 166: 86-90.
8. Reichelt KL, et al. Gluten, milk proteins and autism: Dietary intervention effects on behavior and peptide secretion. *J Appl Nutr* 1990; 42: 1-11.
9. Sponheim E. Gluten-free diet in infantile autism: A therapeutic trial. *Tidsskr Norsk Laegeforen* 1991; 111: 704-707.
10. Baughman, FA Jr., Hovey C. *The ADHD Fraud: How Psychiatry Makes "Patients" Out of Normal Children.* Victoria, BC, Canada: Trafford Publishing, 2007.
11. Egger J, et al. Controlled trial of oligoantigenic treatment in the hyper kinetic syndrome. *Lancet* 1985; 1: 540-545.
12. Stevens LJ, et al. Essential fatty acid metabolism in boys with attention deficit hyperactivity disorder. *Am J Clin Nutr* 1995; 62: 761-768.
13. Swanson JM, et al. Effects of stimulant medication on growth rates across 3 years in the MTA Follow-up. *JAACAP* 2007; 46 1015-1027.
14. Murray, CJL, Lopez, AD (eds). *The Global Burden of Disease.* Cambridge, Mass.: Harvard University Press, 1996.
15. Moreno C, et al. National trends in the outpatient diagnosis and treatment of bipolar disorder in youth. *Arch Gen Psychiatry* 2007; 64: 1032-1039.
16. Zureik M, et al. Serum cholesterol concentration and death from suicide in men: Paris Prospective Study I. *BMJ* 1996; 313: 649-651.
17. Dunnigan M G. The problem with cholesterol: No light at the end of this tunnel? *BMJ* 1993; 306: 1355-1356.
18. Ellison LF, Morrison HI. Low serum cholesterol concentration and risk of suicide. *Epidemiology* 2001; 12: 168-172.
19. Vevera J, et al. Cholesterol concentrations in violent and non-violent women suicide attempters. *Eur Psychiatry* 2003; 18: 23-27.
20. Lalovic A, et al. Cholesterol content in brains of suicide completers. *Int J Neuropsychopharmacol* 2007; 10: 159-166.
21. Sublette ME, et al. Omega-3 polyunsaturated essential fatty acid status as a predictor of future suicide risk. *Am J Psychiatry* 2006; 163: 1100-1102.

22. Hibbeln JR, et al. Increasing homicide rates and linoleic acid consumption among five Western countries, 1961-2000. *Lipids* 2004; 39: 1207-1213.
23. Barker DJP, et al. Low weight gain and suicide in later life. *BMJ* 1995; 311: 1203.
24. Wells AS, et al. Alterations in mood after changing to a low-fat diet. *Br J Nutr* 1998; 79: 23-30
25. Harris G. Psychiatrists top list in drug maker gifts. *New York Times*, 27 June 2007.
26. Hammad TA, et al. Suicidality in pediatric patients treated with antidepressant drugs. *Arch Gen Psychiatry* 2006; 63: 332-339.
27. http://www.neuro.jhmi.edu/epilepsy/keto.html. Accessed February 2002.
28. Lefevre F, Aronson N. Ketogenic diet for the treatment of refractory epilepsy in children: a systematic review of efficacy. *Pediatrics* 2000; 105: e46.
29. The diet that can treat epilepsy. *The Guardian* 15 April 2008.
30. Sirven J, et al. The ketogenic diet for intractable epilepsy in adults: preliminary results. *Epilepsia* 1999; 40: 1721-1726.
31. American Academy of Neurology. *Lower IQ found in children of women who took epilepsy drug.* AAN Press Release, Newswise, Wed 11-Apr-2007. http://www. newswise.com/articles/view/528880/?sc=dwhn.
32. Qin P, et al. Risk for schizophrenia and schizophrenia-like psychosis among patients with epilepsy: population based cohort study. *BMJ* 2005; 331: 23.
33. Dohan FC, Grasberger JC. Relapsed schizophrenics: earlier discharge from the hospital after cereal-free, milk-free diet. *Am J Psychiatry* 1973; 130: 685-688.
34. Lorenz K. Cereals and schizophrenia. *Adv Cereal Sci Technol* 1990; 10: 435-469.
35. Dohan FC, et al. Relapsed schizophrenics: More rapid improvement on a milk and cereal free diet. *Br J Psychiatry* 1969; 115: 595-596.
36. Singh MM, Kay SR. Wheat gluten as a pathogenic factor in schizophrenia. *Science* 1976; 191: 401-402.
37. Laugharne JD, et al. Fatty acids and schizophrenia. *Lipids*, 1996; 31 Suppl: S163-165.
38. Price WA. *Nutrition and Physical Degeneration.* New York: Paul B. Hoeber, Inc, 1939, Chap 19.
39. Thorndike EL. Big Chief's G. G. *Time*, 1937; 30: 25.
40. Gesch CB, et al. Influence of supplementary vitamins, minerals and essential fatty acids on the antisocial behaviour of young adult prisoners. Randomised, placebo-controlled trial. *Br J Psych* 2002; 181 22-28.
41. Zhang J, et al. Association of serum cholesterol and history of school suspension among school-age children and adolescents in the United States. *Am J Epidemiol* 2005; 161: 691-699.
42. Wilder J. Nutrition and mental deficiency. *Nervous Child* 1944; 3: 174.
43. Goldman JA, et al. Behavioral effects of sucrose on preschool children. *J Abnorm Child Psychol* 1986; 14: 565-577.
44. Leibson CL, et al. Risk of dementia among persons with diabetes mellitus: a population-based cohort study. *Am J Epidemiol* 1997; 145: 301-308.
45. Stolk RP, et al. Insulin and cognitive function in an elderly population. The Rotterdam Study. *Diabetes Care* 1997; 20, 792-795.

46. Henderson ST. High carbohydrate diets and Alzheimer's disease. *Med Hyp* 2004; 62: 689-700.
47. Rosedale R. Insulin and Its Metabolic Effects, Presented at Designs for Health Institute's BoulderFest, August 1999 Seminar. http://www.mercola.com/2001/jul/14/insulin2.htm. Accessed 8 December 2005.
48. Arvanitakis Z, et al. Diabetes mellitus and risk of Alzheimer disease and decline in cognitive function. *Arch Neurol* 2004; 61: 661-666.
49. Strachan, MWJ. Insulin and cognitive function. *Lancet* 2003; 362: 1253.
50. Zhao WQ, et al. Amyloid beta oligomers induce impairment of neuronal insulin receptors. *FASEB J* 2008; 22: 246-260.
51. Rönnemaa E, et al. Impaired insulin secretion increases the risk of Alzheimer disease. *Neurology* 2008, Apr 9. [Epub ahead of print]
52. Bertram L, et al. Alzheimer Research Forum. http://www.alzgene.org.
53. Lane RM, Farlow MR. Lipid homeostasis and apolipoprotein E in the development and progression of Alzheimer's disease. *J Lipid Res* 2005; 46: 949-968.
54. Van der Auwera I, et al. A ketogenic diet reduces amyloid beta 40 and 42 in a mouse model of Alzheimer's disease. *Nutr Metab* 2005; 2: 28.
55. Newmark HL, Newmark J. Vitamin D and Parkinson's disease – A hypothesis. *Movement Disorders* 2007; 22: 461-468.
56. Ebert D, et al. Energy contribution of octanoate to intact rat brain metabolism measured by 13C nuclear magnetic resonance spectroscopy. *J Neurosci* 2003; 23: 5928-5935.
57. Takenaka T, et al. Fatty acids as an energy source for the operation of axoplasmic transport. *Brain Res* 2003; 972: 38-43.
58. VanItallie TB, Nufert TH. Ketones: metabolism's ugly duckling. *Nutr Rev* 2003; 61: 327-341.
59. Kashiwaya Y, et al. D-b-Hydroxybutyrate protects neurons in models of Alzheimer's and Parkinson's disease. *PNAS* 2000: 97: 5440-5444.
60. Dupuis L, et al. Dyslipidemia is a protective factor in amyotrophic lateral sclerosis. *Neurology* 2008; 70: 1004-1009
61. Fergani A, et al. Increased peripheral lipid clearance in an animal model of amyotrophic lateral sclerosis. *J Lipid Res* 2007; 48: 1571-1580.
62. Dupuis L, et al. Evidence for defective energy homeostasis in amyotrophic lateral sclerosis: benefit of a high-energy diet in a transgenic mouse model. *Proc Natl Acad Sci USA* 2004; 101: 11159-11164.
63. Zoccolella S, et al. Elevated plasma homocysteine levels in patients with amyotrophic lateral sclerosis. *Neurology* 2008; 70: 222-225.

Chapter Twenty-Seven: Multiple sclerosis

1. van Oosten BW, et al. Multiple sclerosis therapy, a practical guide. *Drugs* 1995; 49: 200-212.
2. Ebers G, et al. A population-based study of MS twins. *N Engl J Med* 1986; 315: 1638-1642.
3. Mumford C, et al. The British Isles Survey of multiple sclerosis in twins. *Neurology* 1994; 44: 11-15.

4. Ebers GC. Genetic epidemiology of multiple sclerosis. *Curr Opin Neurol* 1996; 9: 155-158.
5. Kurtzke JF. Epidemiologic contributions to multiple sclerosis: an overview. *Neurology* 1980; 30: 61-79.
6. Poser CM. The epidemiology of multiple sclerosis: a general overview. *Ann Neurol* 1994; 36: S181-S193.
7. Kurtzke JF. Multiple sclerosis from an epidemiological point of view. In: Field EJ (ed). *Multiple Sclerosis: A critical conspectus.* Lancaster: MTP Press Inc; 1977; 83-142.
8. Alter M, et al. Multiple sclerosis among Orientals and Caucasians in Hawai'i. *Neurology* 1971; 21: 122-130.
9. Elian M, et al. Multiple sclerosis among the United Kingdom-born children of immigrants from the Indian subcontinent, Africa, and the West Indies. *J Neurol Neurosurg Psychiatry* 1990; 53: 906-911.
10. Poser C. The pathogenesis of multiple sclerosis: Additional considerations. *J Neuro Sci* 1993; 115 (suppl): S3-S15.
11. Munger KL, et al. Vitamin D intake and incidence of multiple sclerosis. *Neurology* 2004; 62: 60-65.
12. Munger KL, et al. Serum 25-hydroxyvitamin D levels and risk of multiple sclerosis. *JAMA* 2006; 296: 2832-2838.
13. Shatin R. Multiple Sclerosis and geography. *Neurology* 1964; 14: 338-344.
14. Agranoff BW, Goldberg D. Diet and the geographical distribution of multiple sclerosis. *Lancet* 1974; 2: 1061-1066.
15. Alter M, et al. Multiple sclerosis and nutrition. *Arch Neur* 1974; 31: 267-272.
16. Lauer K. The risk of multiple sclerosis in the US in relation to sociogeographic features: a factor analytic study. *J Clin Epidemiology* 1994; 47: 43-48.
17. Malosse D, et al. Correlation between milk and dairy product consumption and multiple sclerosis prevalence, a worldwide study. *Neuroepidemiol* 1992; 11: 304-312.
18. McGrath A. *One Man's Poison.* County Cork, Eire: Tower House; 1990.
19. Bürger M. *Altern und Krankheit als Problem der Biomorphose.* 3rd ed. Leipzig: Georg Thieme; 1957.
20. Eckel K, Lutz W. Über die Behandlung der Multiple Sklerose mittels Kohlenhydratentzuges. *Wien Klin Wschr* 1961; 493-495.

Chapter Twenty-Eight: The signs of 'healthy eating'

1. Cordain L, et al. Acne vulgaris: a disease of western civilization. *Arch Dermatol* 2002; 138: 1584-1590.
2. Dyer DG, et al. Accumulation of Maillard reaction products in skin collagen in diabetes and aging. *J Clin Invest* 1993; 91: 2463-2469.
3. Price WA. *Nutrition And Physical Degeneration: A Comparison Of Primitive And Modern Diets And Their Effects.* New York and London: Paul B. Hoeber, Inc, 1939.
4. Lingstrom P, Birkhed D. Plaque pH and oral retention after consumption of starchy snack products at normal and low salivary secretion rate. *Acta Odontol Scand* 1993; 51: 379-388.

5. Herod EL. The effect of cheese on dental caries: a review of the literature. *Aust Dent J* 1991; 36: 120-125.

6. Moynihan PJ, et al. The cariostatic potential of cheese: cooked cheese-containing meals increase plaque calcium concentration. *Br Dent J* 1999; 187: 664-667.

7. Kashket S, DePaola DP. Cheese consumption and the development and progression of dental caries. *Nutr Rev* 2002; 60: 97-103.

8. Distribution of Myopia by Region, Age, Gender and Ethnicity. *The Myopia Manual*. The University of Illinois at Chicago, 2006: Chap 3.1.

9. Nesse RM, Williams GC. *Why We Get Sick*. New York, US: Times Books, 1994; 91-106.

10. Holm S. The ocular refraction state of the Palae-Negroids in Gabon, French Equatorial Africa. *Acta Ophthalmol* 1937; Suppl 13: 1-29.

11. Skeller E. Anthropological and ophthalmological studies on the Angmagssalik Eskimos. *Meddr Gronland* 1954; 107: 167-211.

12. Young FA, et al. The transmission of refractive errors within Eskimo families. *Am J Optom Arch Am Acad Optom* 1969; 46: 676-685.

13. Stefansson V. *My Life with the Eskimo*. New York, US: MacMillan Co. 1919.

14. Cass E. Ocular conditions amongst the Canadian western arctic Eskimo. In: Weigelin E (ed.). *Proceedings of the XX International Congress of Ophthalmology*. New York, US: Excerpta Medica Foundation: 1966; 1041-1053.

15. Cordain L, et al. An evolutionary analysis of the etiology and pathogenesis of juvenile-onset myopia. *Acta Opthalmolgica* 2002; 80:125-135.

16. Fox D. Short-sightedness may be tied to refined diet. *New Scientist* http://www.newscientist.com/article.ns?id=dn2120 accessed 8 August 2008.

17. Cordain L. Cereal grains: humanity's double-edged sword. *World Rev Nutr Diet* 1999; 84: 19-73.

18. Mutti DO, et al. Naturally occurring vitreous chamber-based myopia in the Labrador retriever. *Invest Ophthalmol Vis Sci* 1999; 40: 1577-1584.

19. Thorburn AW, et al. Plasma glucose and insulin responses to starchy foods in Australian Aborigines: a population now at high risk of diabetes. *Am J Clin Nutr* 1987; 46: 282-285.

20. Lucidi EA. Cataracts, macular degeneration, blindness – Focus of eye research. *J Longev* 1998; 4: 24-26.

21. Vingerling JR, et al. Age-related macular degeneration is associated with atherosclerosis. *Am J Epidemiology* 1995; 142; 4: 404-409.

22. Seddon JM, et al. Dietary fat and risk for advanced age-related macular degeneration. *Arch Ophthalmol* 2001; 119: 1191-1199.

23. Cho E, et al. Prospective study of dietary fat and the risk of age-related macular degeneration. *Am J Clin Nutr* 2001; 73: 209-218.

24. Seddon JM, et al. Dietary carotenoids, vitamins A, C, and E, and advanced age-related macular degeneration. *JAMA* 1994; 272: 1413-1420.

25. http://seven.com.au/todaytonight/story/macular.

26. Moeller SM, et al. The potential role of dietary xanthophylls in cataract and age-related macular degeneration. *J Am Coll Nutr* 2000; 19 (5 Suppl): 522S-527S.

27. Gale CR, et al. Lutein and zeaxanthin status and risk of age-related macular degeneration. *Invest Ophthalmol Vis Sci* 2003; 44: 2461-2465.

28. Granado F, et al. Nutritional and clinical relevance of lutein in human health. *Br J Nutr* 2003; 90: 487-502.
29. Wang W, et al. Effect of dietary lutein and zeaxanthin on plasma carotenoids and their transport in lipoproteins in age-related macular degeneration. *Am J Clin Nutr* 2007; 85: 762-769.
30. Chiu C-J, et al. Dietary glycemic index and carbohydrate in relation to early age-related macular degeneration. *Am J Clin Nutr* 2006; 83: 880-886.
31. Schwartz G. *In Bad Taste: The MSG Syndrome.* Albuquerque, NM: Health Press; 1988.
32. Blaylock Russell L. *Excitotoxins: The Taste that Kills.* Albuquerque, NM: Health Press; 1995.
33. Lee L. *Radiation Protection Manual,* 3rd edition 1990.
34. Roberts HJ. Aspartame (NutraSweet®) addiction. *Townsend Ltr Doc & Patients* 2000; Jan: 52-57.
35. Harmful effects of ultraviolet radiation. *JAMA* 1989; 262: 380-384.
36. Ames BN, et al. Oxidants, antioxidants, and the degenerative diseases of aging. *Proc Natl Acad Sci US* 1993; 90:7915-7922.
37. Black HS, et al. Relation of antioxidants and level of dietary lipids to epidermal lipid peroxidation and ultraviolet carcinogenesis. *Cancer Res* 1985; 45: 6254-6259.
38. Leske MC, et al. Antioxidant vitamins and nuclear opacities. *Ophthalmology* 1998; 105: 18-36.
39. Das BN, et al. The prevalence of age related cataract in the Asian community in Leicester: a community based study. *Eye* 1990; 4: 723-726.
40. Rattan SIS, et al. Protein synthesis, post-translational modifications, and aging. *Ann NY Acad Sci* 1992; 663: 48-62.
41. Chiu C-J, et al. Carbohydrate intake and glycemic index in relation to the odds of early cortical and nuclear lens opacities. *Am J Clin Nutr* 2005; 81: 1411-1416.
42. Chiu C-J, et al. Dietary carbohydrate intake and glycemic index in relation to cortical and nuclear lens opacities in the Age-Related Eye Disease Study. *Am J Clin Nutr* 2006; 83: 1177-1184.
43. Mori M, et al. Lanosterol synthase mutations cause cholesterol deficiency-associated cataracts in the Shumiya cataract rat. *J Clin Invest* 2006; 116: 395-404.
44. Judd GP. Evidence against fluoride continues to mount. *Health Freedom News,* November/December 1994, p. 29.
45. Miljanovic B, et al. Relation between dietary n-3 and n-6 fatty acids and clinically diagnosed dry eye syndrome in women. *Am J Clin Nutr* 2005 82: 887-893.
46. Cruickshanks KJ, et al. The 5-year incidence and progression of hearing loss. *Arch Otolaryngol Head Neck Surg* 2003; 129:1041-1046.
47. Kakarlapudi V, et al. The effect of diabetes on sensorineural hearing loss. *Otol Neurotol* 2003; 24: 382-386.
48. Kashyap AS, Kashyap S. Increased prevalence of impaired hearing in patients with type 2 diabetes in western India. *Postgraduate Med J* 2000; 76: 38.
49. Rosen S, et al. Dietary prevention of hearing loss. *Acta Otolaryngol* 1970; 70: 242-247.
50. Fukushima H, et al. Cochlear changes in patients with type 1 diabetes mellitus. *Otolaryngol Head Neck Surg* 2005; 133: 100-106.

51. Dessein PH, et al. Beneficial effects of weight loss associated with moderate calorie/carbohydrate restriction, and increased proportional intake of protein and unsaturated fat on serum urate and lipoprotein levels in gout: a pilot study. *Ann Rheum Dis* 2000; 59: 539-543.
52. Johnson RJ, et al. Potential role of sugar (fructose) in the epidemic of hypertension, obesity and the metabolic syndrome, diabetes, kidney disease, and cardiovascular disease. *Am J Clin Nutr* 2007; 86: 899-906.
53. Choi HK, et al. Soft drinks, fructose consumption, and the risk of gout in men: prospective cohort study. *BMJ* 2008; 336: 309-312.

Chapter Twenty-Nine: And, finally . . .

1. Cleave TL. *The Saccharine Disease*. New Canaan, CT: Keats Publishers. 1974.
2. Schaeffer O. When the Eskimo comes to town. *Nutrition Today* 1971; Nov-Dec: 8-16.
3. Barclay AW, et al. Glycemic index, glycemic load, and chronic disease risk – a metaanalysis of observational studies. *Am J Clin Nutr* 2008; 87: 627-637.
4. Nemetz PN, et al. Recent trends in the prevalence of coronary disease: a population-based autopsy study of nonnatural deaths. *Arch Intern Med* 2008; 168: 264-270.
5. *FDA Science and Mission at Risk: Report of the Subcommittee on Science and Technology*. Prepared for the FDA Science Board, November 2007.
6. Miller K. Numbers of chronic patients soar as GPs are paid by the case. *The Sunday Telegraph*, 14 January 2007.
7. Kuhn TS. The structure of scientific revolutions. In Neurath O, ed. *International Encyclopedia of Unified Science*. Vol 2, No 2, University of Chicago Press, 1970.
8. Moynihan R. Who pays for the pizza? Redefining the relationships between doctors and drug companies. 2: Disentanglement. *BMJ* 2003; 326: 1193-1196.
9. Kishore S. Statins added to WHO model list of essential medicines! *ProCOR*, 7 June 2007.
10. Willman D. Scientist admits conflict of interest. *Los Angeles Times*, December 9, 2006, Part A, p. 21.
11. Toop L. *Report calls for ban on advertising prescription drugs*. University of Otago, Media Release, February 16, 2003.
12. Campbell EG, et al. Institutional academic-industry relationships. *JAMA* 2007; 298: 1779-1786.
13. Hardin G. The tragedy of the commons. *Science* 1968; 162: 1243-1248.
14. Weed LL. Medical records that guide and teach. *N Engl J Med* 1968; 278: 593-600.

Glossary

AIDS. Acquired immune deficiency syndrome or acquired immunodeficiency syndrome (AIDS or Aids) is a set of symptoms and infections resulting from the damage to the human immune system caused by the human immunodeficiency virus (HIV). AIDS progressively reduces the effectiveness of the immune system and leaves individuals susceptible to infections and tumours.

AMA. American Medical Association.

ATP. All living things, both plants and animals, require a continual supply of energy for all the processes which keep them alive. These include the metabolism of foods; the synthesis of important molecules such as proteins and DNA; and the transport of molecules and ions throughout the body. Other processes include muscle contraction and other cellular movements. Animals obtain their energy from foods. However, before the energy can be used, it is first transformed into a form which can be handled easily. This special carrier of energy is the molecule *adenosine triphosphate*, or ATP.

BDA. British Diabetic Association or British Dietetic Association.

Cals. (see kcals)

CDC. The Centers for Disease Control and Prevention (CDC) is an agency of the United States Department of Health and Human Services. It works to protect public health and safety by providing information to enhance health decisions, and it promotes health through partnerships with state health departments and other organizations. The CDC focuses national attention on developing and applying disease prevention and control, environmental health, health promotion, and education activities designed to improve the health of the people of the US.

CHD. Coronary heart disease, otherwise known as ischaemic heart disease, is a condition where the coronary arteries which supply blood to the heart muscle become blocked. The result is a heart attack.

CHF. Congestive heart failure or chronic heart failure. More deaths are attributed to CHF than to CHD.

CLA. Conjugated linoleic acid, a family of at least 13 isomers of linoleic acid found naturally, especially in the meat and dairy products derived from ruminant animals. CLA is a trans-fatty acid but, unlike other trans-fatty acids, it is beneficial, not harmful, having both antioxidant and anti-cancer properties.

COMA. The Committee on the Medical Aspects of Food and Nutrition Policy was an advisory committee of independent experts providing advice to UK government agencies. COMA was disbanded in March 2000 and replaced by a new committee, the Scientific Advisory Committee on Nutrition (SACN).

CRP. C-reactive protein is a marker for inflammatory processes occurring in the body and acute inflammation can cause as much as a 50,000-fold rise. Arterial damage is thought to result from inflammation due to chemical insults. For this reason CRP can be used as a very rough proxy for heart disease risk. Although many things can cause elevated CRP, and it is not a very specific prognostic indicator, nevertheless, it is a better indicator than cholesterol. A level above 2.4 mg/L has been associated with a doubled risk of a coronary event compared to levels below 1 mg/L.

CVD. Cardiovascular disease, an alternative acronym for CHD.

DHA. Docosahexaenoic acid (also known as cervonic acid) is an omega-3 fatty acid with 22-carbon atoms and and six double bonds. Fish oils are rich in DHA. Most animals make very little DHA through metabolism; however small amounts are manufactured internally through the consumption of alpha-linoleic acid, an omega-3 fatty acid found in chia, flax, and many other seeds and nuts. DHA is a major fatty acid in sperm and brain phospholipids, and in the retina.

EORTC. The European Organization for Research and Treatment of Cancer.

EPA. There are two meanings of EPA used in this book:
1. *The U.S. Environmental Protection Agency* is an agency of the federal government of the United States charged with protecting human health and with safeguarding the natural environment.
2. *Eicosapentaenoic acid* is an omega-3 fatty acid with five double bonds. It is particularly important for proper functioning of the brain. It is found in human breast milk. It is also obtained by eating oily fish

or fish oil. EPA can also be made in the body from the parent omega-3 alpha-linoleic acid.

FDA. The Food and Drug Administration (FDA) is an agency of the United States Department of Health and Human Services. It is responsible for the safety and regulation of most types of foods, dietary supplements, drugs, vaccines, biological medical products, blood products, medical devices, radiation-emitting devices, veterinary products, and cosmetics.

GI. The Glycaemic Index is an index of the amount by which blood glucose levels are raised by carbohydrate-containing foods

GL. The Glycaemic Load is a measure similar to the glycaemic index, except that this ranking system for carbohydrate content in food portions is based on both their glycemic index (GI) and the portion size combined.

GLA. *Gamma-linolenic acid* (GLA) is a non-essential omega-6 fatty acid found primarily in vegetable oils. The body can synthesize GLA from linoleic acid.

GP. General Practitioner, or family doctor.

GSK. Glaxo SmithKline is a UK-based pharmaceutical company. GSK is the world's second largest pharmaceutical company with a wide portfolio of pharmaceutical products.

HbA1c. (*Haemoglobin A1c, glycosylated* or *glycated* haemoglobin) is a form of haemoglobin used primarily to identify and measure the average blood glucose concentration over prolonged periods of time. In the normal 120-day life span of a red blood cell, glucose molecules join haemoglobin, forming glycosylated haemoglobin. Once a haemoglobin molecule is glycosylated, it remains that way. A buildup of glycosylated haemoglobin within the red cell reflects the average level of glucose to which the cell has been exposed during its life cycle. Measuring the HbA1c level tells average blood glucose concentration over the previous four weeks to three months.

HDL. Fats and cholesterol are not water-soluble. They cannot travel around the body on their own but have to be transported. High Density Lipoprotein (HDL) is one of the five major groups of lipoproteins which enable fats and cholesterol to move within the water based solution of the blood stream. About 30% of cholesterol in the bloodstream is carried by HDL.

Hg. The chemical symbol for mercury.

HPS. The Heart Protection Study was a large randomized controlled trial run by the Clinical Trial Service Unit, and funded by the Medical Research Council (MRC) and the British Heart Foundation (BHF) in the United Kingdom. It studied the use of simvastatin medication and vitamin supplementation in patients with cardiovascular disease. It is the largest study to investigate the use of statins in the prevention of cardiovascular disease.

IU. In medicine, the International Unit (IU) is a unit of measurement for the amount of a substance, based on measured biological activity or effect. The precise definition of one IU differs from substance to substance and is established by international agreement for each substance. There is no equivalence among different substances. So, one IU of vitamin A does not contain the same number of milligrams as one IU of vitamin E.

LDL. Low-density lipoprotein (LDL) is a lipoprotein that transports cholesterol and triglycerides from the liver to peripheral tissues. (see also HDL).

kcals. Calories are a unit of heat. One calorie is the amount of heat required to heat one gram of water by 1°C. This calorie is written with a small 'c'. A Calorie with a capital 'C' is the amount of heat required to heat a kilogramme of water through 1°C. It is this Calorie that is used when calorie counting for weight loss. However, as this is usually shortened to 'cals' with a small 'c', it can be confusing. The name now used is kilocalories (which means 1,000 calories), and that is usually shortened to kcals.

LI. Leukocytes, which are types of white blood cells, are cells of the immune system which defend the body against both infectious diseases and foreign materials. The Leukocytic Index (LI) is a measure of the effectiveness of leukocytes to mop up and kill bacteria and viruses.

MEP. A member of the European Parliament.

MMR. A combined vaccine against measles, mumps and rubella.

MRFIT. The Multiple Risk Factor Intervention Trial (MRFIT) sought to evaluate the effect of multiple risk factor intervention on mortality from coronary heart disease in high risk men. After 6-8 years of follow-up, risk factor levels declined in both treatment and control groups but slightly more in the special intervention group. Mortality from coronary heart disease and from all causes was not significantly different among the two groups.

MRSA. Methicillin-resistant *Staphylococcus aureus* (MRSA) is a bacterium responsible for difficult-to-treat infections in humans. It may also be referred to as multiple-resistant *Staphylococcus aureus*.

NACNE. The National Advisory Committee on Nutrition Education (NACNE) was an ad hoc working party that published a discussion paper on nutritional guidelines for the UK in 1983.

NCEP. The National Cholesterol Education Program, managed by the National Heart, Lung and Blood Institute, a division of the National Institutes of Health in the US, was set up in 1985. Its remit is to reduce increased cardiovascular disease rates in the US due to elevated cholesterol levels.

NCI. The National Cancer Institute (NCI) is part of the US government's National Institutes of Health. The NCI is one of eight agencies that compose the Public Health Service in the United States Department of Health and Human Services. The NCI coordinates the National Cancer Program.

NHANES. The National Health and Nutrition Examination Survey (NHANES) is a program of studies designed to assess the health and nutritional status of adults and children in the US. The survey is unique in that it combines interviews and physical examinations. It includes demographic, socioeconomic, dietary, and health-related questions. Medical, dental, and physiological measurements are also made. Data from the survey are used in epidemiological studies and health sciences research, which help develop sound public health policy, direct and design health programs and services, and expand knowledge about health.

NHLBI. The National Heart, Lung, and Blood Institute (NHLBI) is a division of the US National Institutes of Health. The NHLBI mission statement states it 'provides leadership for a national program in diseases of the heart, blood vessels, lung, and blood; blood resources; and sleep disorders'.

NHS. The term National Health Service (NHS) refers to the four publicly-funded healthcare systems of the United Kingdom. collectively, though technically it is only the health service in England that is called the NHS. It began operating on 5 July 1948.

NICE. The National Institute for Health and Clinical Excellence (NICE) was set up as the National Institute for Clinical Excellence in 1999 in an attempt to defuse the 'postcode lottery' system of healthcare in England and Wales, where treatments that were available depended upon the area in which the patient happened to live. In April 2005, it joined with the Health Development Agency to become the new National Institute for Health and Clinical Excellence. NICE publishes clinical appraisals of whether particular treatments should be considered worthwhile by the NHS. These appraisals are based primarily on cost-effectiveness.

PSA. Prostate specific antigen (PSA) is a protein produced by the cells of the prostate gland. It is present in small quantities in the blood of all healthy men. But PSA is often elevated in the presence of prostate cancer and in other prostate disorders. A blood test to measure PSA is used to detect prostate cancer. However, it is not a very accurate test as many benign conditions also raise PSA levels.

PUF. A polyunsaturated fatty acid (PUF) is any fatty acid with two or more double bonds.

QOF. Quality and Outcomes Frameworks (UK).

SARS. Severe acute respiratory syndrome (SARS) is a respiratory disease in humans which is caused by the SARS coronavirus, passed on to humans from birds. There has only been one epidemic so far. That was in China in 2002. Although there was a near panic by governments around the world, there were a mere 8,096 known infected cases and just 774 deaths.

UV. Light in the ultraviolet spectrum. There are three wavebands UVA, UVB and UVC.

WHO. The World Health Organization.

Appendix

Resources

References

Most of the medical references used in this book may be checked and verified online. Usually at least an abstract is available free; in some cases you may be able to read the whole paper. The website to use is at http://www.ncbi.nlm.nih.gov/entrez/query.fcgi.

Books

For more information on how to live a low-carb, high-fat lifestyle, Barry Groves' book, *Natural Health & Weight Loss*, gives detailed practical advice, recipes and menus.

Malignant Medical Myths, subtitled 'Why medical treatment causes 200,000 deaths in the USA each year, and how to protect yourself', by Professor Joel M. Kauffman, is worth its weight in gold as a resource.

Dr Malcolm Kendrick is a British GP with a special interest in heart disease. His book, *The Great Cholesterol Con*, is both informative and humorous. It also covers statins. There is a similarly titled book in the USA written by Anthony Colpo which is also worth reading.

Also in the USA, Dr Duane Graveline's books, *Statin Drugs Side Effects* and *Lipitor, Thief of Memory*, are available from www.spacedoc.net.

Websites

Barry Groves' websites

The author's websites contain more detail on the diseases highlighted in this book and more will be added as the evidence is published at www.second-opinions.co.uk, www.cholesterol-and-health.org.uk and www.diabetes-diet.org.uk. Barry Groves can be e-mailed via any of these websites.

Other websites

For more on disease mongering see *PLoS Medicine*, an open-access medical journal published by the nonprofit organisation, the Public Library of Science. http://collections.plos.org/diseasemongering-2006.php.

The International Network of Cholesterol Skeptics at www.thincs.org is a forum run by Dr Uffe Ravnskov in Sweden. Its membership is composed mostly of highly qualified medical professionals from all over the world.

The Weston A. Price Foundation at www.westonaprice.org has a copious amount of information on eating a natural diet.

www.factsmart.org provides information from reviewed and published medical journals concerning health maintenance and risk factors. It includes tutorials about terms and concepts that are used.

There are several websites that discuss baby-led weaning. One such is at www.babycentre.co.uk/referencedarticles/baby/babyledweaning/.

Read about the dark side of soy at: www.soyonlineservice.co.nz.

The Vitamin D Council website is a valuable source of information about sunlight, vitamin D and your health. www.vitamindcouncil.com.

The National Pure Water Association, the campaign for pure drinking water in the UK, is at www.npwa.org.uk. The international Fluoride Action Network's website is at www.fluoridealert.org.

The Medical Accountability Network provides resources on issues of integrity in medicine. www.medicalaccountability.net focuses on informed consent as the keystone to an ethical physician/patient relationship.

At www.numberwatch.co.uk find out about the scares, scams, junk, panics, and flummery cooked up by the media, politicians, bureaucrats, so-called scientists and others who try to confuse you with wrong numbers and statistics.

Index

About the author

Barry Groves, who lives with his wife, Monica, in the Oxfordshire Cotswolds, can rightfully claim to be Britain's leading exponent of the low-carb, high-fat way of life as he has lived on, researched, lectured and written about it for 46 years.

He and Monica were overweight from 1957 to 1962, when he discovered the low-carb, high-fat regime for weight loss. It worked. This started his questioning conventional diets and, in 1982, he took up a full-time research into the relationship between diet and 'diseases of civilization' such as obesity, diabetes, heart disease and cancer. As a result of his researches, he realised that the perceived wisdoms, both of low-calorie dieting for weight loss and 'healthy eating' for the control of heart disease, were seriously flawed.

In 2002 he won the Sophie Coe Prize at the Oxford Symposium on Food History and was awarded a doctorate in nutritional science. Now an international author, Barry has written both popular and more technical books which have been published in countries as far apart as Argentina and Russia, as well as all English-speaking countries. He currently divides his time between researching and writing books, and lecturing about the management and prevention of obesity, diabetes and associated conditions. He also gives less technical talks to Rotary, Women's Institute, Probus, and similar groups.

Barry Groves is a director of the Foundation for Thymic Cancer Research, (www.thymic.org), an honorary board member of the Weston A. Price Foundation (www.westonaprice.org), a founder member of The International Network of Cholesterol Sceptics (www.thincs.org), and a founder member of the Fluoride Action Network (www.fluoridealert.org). He also maintains three internationally respected health information websites.

Barry Groves does not confine himself to medical and dietary research. With a long-term interest in energy conservation, he and his wife, Monica, designed and built their own solar-heated house over three years from 1977 to 1980.

For relaxation, in 1982, Barry took up archery. He was a British Champion every year from 1987 to 2008 taking over 20 British Records in Target, Clout and Flight archery. He is also a six times World Champion with five World Records.

Barry Groves' other books

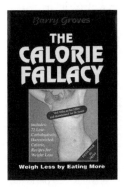

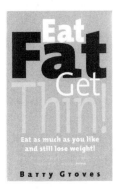

Eat Fat, Get Thin!
'Eat Fat, Get Thin! turns conventional weight loss wisdom on its head – and it works!' *Prima magazine*

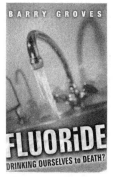

Fluoride: drinking ourselves to death?
'I commend this book to all active clinical practitioners as deserving a place in the practice library, and would go further and say it should be essential reading for all undergraduates.'

Dr Keith Marshall. *Dental Practice.*

'Writing primarily for the general reader, he nevertheless has assembled an impressive array of referenced information of interest to anyone who engaged in research concerning important biomedical and environmental aspects of fluoride and fluoridation.'

Professor Albert Burgstahler

Natural Health & Weight Loss
'the best non-technical book on diet I have ever seen.'
Professor Joel Kaufmann, University of the Sciences, Philadelphia

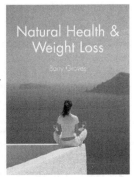

'For those unacquainted with the truth in matters of human nutrition, the contents of Natural Health & Weight Loss will raise some eyebrows . . . Yes, Groves is right, if there are any culprits to be found in our nutrients, macro- or micro-, it is the carbohydrates.'

Dr Herbert Nehrlich, Australia

'the best non-technical book on diet I have ever seen.'
Professor Joel Kauffman, University of the Sciences, Philadelphia

Natural Health & Weight Loss

the perfect companion to

Trick and Treat

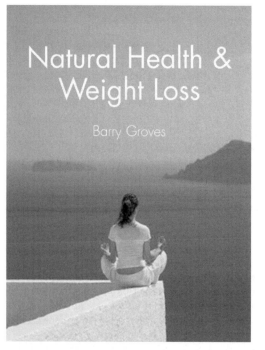

ISBN: 978-1905140-15-2

Based on years of research, and personal experience, this book tells us how to change our diets and what the benefits of doing so will be.

Practical and clearly explained, you cannot read this book without realising it is time to change!

Contents

Part 1: Health & Weight-loss in Practice
Let's Get Started; Breakfast: The Most Important Meal of the Day; Eat Real food; Tips for Successful Dieting; The Ideal Diet for Diabetics; Prevention is Better; Dealing With Doctors.

Part Two: The Evidence
Mr Banting's Diet Revolution; It's In Our Genes; The Metabolic Syndrome; Glycaemic Truth; Eat Less, Weigh More? Why Blame Cholesterol? Why Healthy Eating Isn't; Why Your Low-Carb Diet Must be High-Fat, Not High-Protein; Exercise Isn't Necessary; Fat or Fashion?

Appendix
Diseases Helped or Prevented by the Natural Weight-loss and Health Way of Eating; Adult Height/Weight Tables; Glossary; Reliable Sources of Information; Carbohydrate Content and Glycaemic Loads of Foods; Recipes, Menus and advice on Food Preparation.